D1573252

Ecology and Genetics
of Host–Parasite
Interactions

Reports of Linnean Symposia

Speciation in Tropical Environments (Lowe-McConnell)	*Biological Journal of the Linnean Society* Vol. *1* 1969 pp. 1–246
New Research in Plant Anatomy (Robson, Cutler & Gregory)	Supplement to the *Botanical Journal of the Linnean Society* Vol. *63* 1970
Early Mammals (Kermack & Kermack)	Supplement 1 to the *Zoological Journal of the Linnean Society* Vol. *50* 1971
The Biology and Chemistry of the Umbelliferae (Heywood)	Supplement 1 to the *Botanical Journal of the Linnean Society* Vol. *64* 1971
Behavioural Aspects of Parasite Transmission (Canning & Wright)	Supplement 1 to the *Zoological Journal of the Linnean Society* Vol. *51* 1972
The Phylogeny and Classification of the Ferns (Jermy, Crabbe & Thomas)	Supplement 1 to the *Botanical Journal of the Linnean Society* Vol. *67* 1973
Interrelationships of Fishes (Greenwood, Miles & Patterson)	Supplement 1 to the *Zoological Journal of the Linnean Society* Vol. *53* 1973
The Biology of the Male Gamete (Duckett & Racey)	Supplement 1 to the *Biological Journal of the Linnean Society* Vol. *7* 1975

Continued as the Linnean Society Symposium Series

No. 1	**The Evolutionary Significance of the Exine** (Ferguson & Muller) (1976)
No. 2	**Tropical Trees. Variation, Breeding and Conservation** (Burley & Styles) (1976)
No. 3	**Morphology and Biology of Reptiles** (Bellairs & Cox) (1976)
No. 4	**Problems in Vertebrate Evolution** (Andrews, Miles & Walker) (1977)
No. 5	**Ecological Effects of Pesticides** (Perring & Mellanby) (1977)
No. 6	**The Pollination of Flowers by Insects** (Richards) (1978) (*Botanical Society of the British Isles Conference Report, No. 16*)
No. 7	**The Biology and Taxonomy of the Solanaceae** (Hawkes, Lester & Skelding) (1979)
No. 8	**Petaloid Monocotyledons** (Brickell, Cutler & Gregory) (1980)
No. 9	**The Skin of Vertebrates** (Spearman & Riley) (1980)
No. 10	**The Plant Cuticle** (Cutler, Alvin & Price) (1982)

Also published

Botanical Journal of the Linnean Society, Vol. *73*, Nos 1–3 July/Sept./Oct. 1976
Zoological Journal of the Linnean Society, Vol. *63*, Nos 1 & 2 May/June 1978

The Biology of Bracken (Perring & Gardiner)

Sea Spiders (Pycnogonida) (Fry)

Linnean Society Symposium Series   Number 11

Ecology and Genetics of Host–Parasite Interactions

*Papers presented at an International Symposium
organized by the Linnean Society of London
and the British Society for Parasitology,
held at Keele University, 12–13 July 1984*

Editors
D. Rollinson and R. M. Anderson

Published for the Linnean Society of London

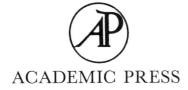

ACADEMIC PRESS

London   Orlando   San Diego   New York
Toronto   Montreal   Sydney   Tokyo

ACADEMIC PRESS INC. (LONDON) LIMITED
24/28 Oval Road
London NW1 7DX
(Registered Office)
(Registered number 598514)

US edition published by
ACADEMIC PRESS INC.
Orlando,
Florida 32887

British Library Cataloguing in Publication Data

Ecology and genetics of Host–parasite interactions.
— (Linnean Society symposium series; no. 11)
1. Host–parasite relationships
I. Rollinson, D.   II. Anderson, R. M.   III. Series
574.5′24   QL757

ISBN 0-12-593690-7

Phototypeset by Dobbie Typesetting Service, Plymouth, Devon
Printed by St Edmundsbury Press, Bury St Edmunds, England

Contributors

ANDERSON, R. M., *Department of Pure and Applied Biology, Imperial College, London University, London SW7 2BB, U.K.*

BARRETT, J., *Department of Genetics, University of Cambridge, Downing Street, Cambridge CB2 3EH, U.K.*

BLACKWELL, JENEFER M., *Department of Tropical Hygiene, London School of Hygiene and Tropical Medicine, Keppel Street, London WC1E 7HT, U.K.*

CROMBIE, J. A., *Department of Pure and Applied Biology, Imperial College, London University, London SW7 2BB, U.K.*

DOBSON, A. P., *Department of Biology, Princeton University, Princeton, New Jersey 08544, U.S.A.*

GILL, D. E., *Department of Zoology, The University of Maryland, College Park, Maryland 20742, U.S.A.*

HUDSON, P. J., *North of England Grouse Research Project, The Game Conservancy, Askrigg, Leyburn, North Yorkshire DL8 3HG, U.K.*

KENNEDY, C. R., *Department of Biological Sciences, The University, Exeter EX4 4PS, U.K.*

KEYMER, ANNE, *Department of Zoology, South Parks Road, Oxford OX1 3PS, U.K.*

LENSKI, R. E., *Department of Zoology, University of Massachusetts, Amherst, Massachusetts 01003, U.S.A.*

LEVIN, B. R., *Department of Zoology, University of Massachusetts, Amherst, Massachusetts 01003, U.S.A.*

LUZZATTO, L., *Department of Haematology, Royal Postgraduate Medical School, Ducane Road, London W12 0HS, U.K.*

MAY, R. M., *Department of Biology, Princeton University, Princeton, New Jersey 08544, U.S.A.*

MOCK, BEVERLY A., *Department of Zoology, The University of Maryland, College Park, Maryland 20742, U.S.A.*

MODIANO, G., *Istituto di Genetica, Citta Universitaria, 00185 Roma, Italy.*

NEWBORN, D., *North of England Grouse Research Project, The Game Conservancy, Askrigg, Leyburn, North Yorkshire DL8 3HG, U.K.*

ROLLINSON, D., *Department of Zoology, British Museum (Natural History), Cromwell Road, London SW7 5BD, U.K.*

SCOTT, MARILYN E., *Institute of Parasitology, Macdonald College of McGill University, 21,111 Lakeshore Road, Ste-Anne de Bellevue, Quebec, Canada H9X 1CO.*

SOUTHGATE, V. R., *Department of Zoology, British Museum (Natural History), Cromwell Road, London SW7 5BD, U.K.*

TAIT, A., *Department of Genetics, University of Edinburgh, West Mains Road, Edinburgh EH9 3JN, U.K.*

USANGA, E. A., *Department of Haematology, Royal Postgraduate Medical School, Ducane Road, London W12 0HS, U.K.*

WAKELIN, D., *M.R.C. Experimental Parasitology Group, Department of Zoology, University of Nottingham, University Park, Nottingham NG7 2RD, U.K.*

Preface

The fourteen papers in this volume draw together information on the ecology, epidemiology and genetics of a wide variety of host–parasite interactions ranging from helminth infections in man to fungal diseases of plants. They reflect a growing interest in research at the interface between population ecology and population genetics, plus excitement with current progress in this field of biological study. It is an area with many implications for other disciplines such as medicine and veterinary science.

Populations of hosts and infectious disease agents are in a state of continuous flux as a result of existing genetic variation, recurrent mutation and recombination. Parasites, by definition, exert a selective pressure on their host population. Conversely, in its battle to survive invasion by the disease agent, the host exerts selective pressures on the parasite via the specific or non-specific responses triggered by infection. Both organisms are therefore evolving as a consequence of their interaction and in response to other features of their environment (both physical and biological). In many cases, additional selective pressures may be imposed by man in the form of drugs, vaccines or chemical pesticides. Any consideration of the ecology or epidemiology of host–parasite interactions must therefore take account of both short-term and long-term changes in the genetic composition of the host and parasite population.

The papers presented here are concerned with various aspects of parasite genetics, host genetics, experimental epidemiology, theoretical ecology, population genetics and observed interactions within natural communities. Some of the central questions addressed are as follows. To what extent do parasites regulate the abundance of their host populations? What determines variation in both the incidence and severity of infection within host communities? How much genetic variation exists in natural populations of host and parasites? To what extent is observed variation and polymorphism a result of selective pressures exerted by either host or parasite? The contributions include both theoretical, experimental and field studies and bring to bear a diverse range of techniques to the study of host–parasite ecology and genetics. Most importantly, however, they illustrate how progress is dependent on a combination of approaches involving techniques at the molecular, cellular, whole organism and population levels of biological study.

The challenge of melding insights gained from ecological and genetical studies of host–parasite interactions is an exciting one. The papers presented in this volume provide a guide to past research and future lines of study. We hope they will stimulate an increased interest in the co-evolution of hosts and parasites and encourage the use of insights gained from ecological and genetical research in the control and management of infectious diseases.

The volume is the result of an international symposium organized by the Linnean Society of London and the British Society for Parasitology on 'Host and Parasite Populations: Genetics and Ecology'. The meeting was held at the University of Keele on 12th and 13th July 1984. We are indebted to the Royal Society and British Council for financial support for overseas speakers and to Professor C. Arme and his colleagues for their hospitality and efficient organization at Keele.

February 1985   *D. Rollinson, British Museum (Natural History), London*
                          R. M. Anderson, Imperial College, University of London

To the memory of Chris Wright

Contents

Interactions of fish and parasite populations: to perpetuate or pioneer?

C. R. KENNEDY

Department of Biological Sciences,
The University,
Exeter, EX4 4PS, U.K.

Mathematical models and laboratory investigations of parasite–fish interactions suggest that parasites can constrain the growth of fish populations and should be of major importance to the fitness of their hosts. Consideration of freshwater habitats predicts extensive spatial variation in fish and parasite population interactions, discrete gene pools with little gene flow between sites and existence of many fish parasite populations in non-equilibrium conditions in which they exert little selection pressure on their hosts. Examples of interactions are reviewed. They confirm the potential of parasites to affect fish fitness, but field data also provide some support for all three predictions. Evidence from a continuous long-term study of several species of parasites and fish in one locality indicates that parasites are existing in non-equilibrium states, and even when interacting with fish are not acting as selection agents. It is argued that this locality is not atypical of contemporary freshwater habitats. The potential of parasites to act as agents of selection upon fish is seldom realized due in part to low natural transmission rates and in part to the speed and extent of human-induced changes taking place in many aquatic habitats, which break down their isolation, perturb them and favour pioneering parasites and non-equilibrium dynamics.

KEY WORDS: — Fish — parasites — ecology — genetics — population dynamics — regulation — equilibrium dynamics.

CONTENTS

Ecology and Genetics of Host–Parasite Interactions
ISBN: 0 12 593 690 7

INTRODUCTION

Although the literature on the ecology of fish parasites is extensive and provides many examples of the ways in which parasites and fish can interact at both the individual and population level, very few of these studies have been concerned in any way with the genetic implications of these interactions and specifically with the selection pressures that parasites may exert upon their fish hosts. This paucity of information is understandable, as it is due in part to the practical difficulties of sampling in the field and of quantifying the effects of parasites and in part to the small number of fish–parasite systems susceptible to experimental laboratory manipulation in view of the complex life cycles of many of the parasites and the long generation times of many parasites and fish. The immediate consequence of this scarcity of data is that this contribution to this symposium will have to adopt a rather different approach to many of the others. It will largely be concerned with field rather than experimental data, and it will have to be theoretical in many places, because of difficulties in relating interpretations of studies undertaken for different reasons to the general body of parasite evolutionary theory.

There is an increasing amount of evidence, derived from models and from experimental investigations of selected host–parasite systems, to suggest that parasites may play a role analogous to predators and resource limitation in constraining the growth of their host populations and that parasite populations often exist in equilibrium states (Anderson & May, 1978, 1979, 1981). Similar evidence also suggests that parasites are of major importance to the fitness of their hosts (Anderson & May, 1982). That much genetic diversity and variability, including that of host immune systems, is due to selection pressure by parasites is now an acceptable view, and indeed forms the theme of several of the papers given here. This view of parasites is not, however, unchallenged. Price (1980) has expressed the view that parasite ecology is concerned with between-patch and within-patch dynamics, and that parasites are adapted to exploit small, discontinuous environments, that evolutionary and speciation rates are high, that adaptive radiation is extensive and that types of speciation other than through geographic isolation are at least as important as allopatric speciation. He thus believes that parasites exist in general in non-equilibrium states. This represents a rather different, though not of necessity contradictory, view of parasites and host–parasite systems. In essence, Anderson & May view parasites as perpetuators, forming stable host-parasite systems, whereas Price views them as pioneers, forming unstable systems. The evolutionary implications of these two views are rather different. If parasites are living in equilibrium states, then it is reasonable to assume that they will persist in a given area for long periods and so exert selection pressures on their host populations and vice versa. On the other hand, if parasite populations are unstable and non-equilibrial, local colonizations and extinctions will be of frequent occurrence and populations are less likely to persist in any given area for a long period. They may be capable of interacting with their host populations, but they are unlikely to exert any strong and persistent selection pressure on their host or to play any major role in maintaining host genetic diversity.

This paper will examine the interactions of fish and parasite populations in the light of these views. Rather than attempt a comprehensive review, which would be difficult in view of the paucity of data and time available, it has been decided instead to divide the approach and the paper into four sections. In the first section, some of the peculiar features of fish and aquatic habitats will be considered, together with their implications for the interactions of fish and parasites: the second part will then review selected examples of interactions: the third part will be concerned with a detailed study of fish and parasite population changes in a single locality over a long period: the fourth part will attempt to reach some general conclusions and relate these to the wider body of parasite evolutionary theory.

AQUATIC HABITATS AND FISH

On the face of it, there seems to be no apparent reason why the parasites of fish should not be similar to those of birds and mammals in their effects on their hosts and in their interactions with the latter. Closer consideration, however, reveals some features of both fish and their habitats that might lead to significant differences. Fish are a very diverse group: they show phylogenetic, structural, immunological and physiological similarities, but a remarkable degree of ecological and habitat diversity. They may be freshwater, euryhaline or marine: anadromous or catadromous or even oceanadromous: they may prefer lentic or lotic conditions: they exhibit a very wide variety of diets. It is deceptive to think in terms of 'fish' as a group and of their living in 'an aquatic habitat': fish are as diverse in their ecological and habitat requirements as are mammals. In fresh water, but to a much lesser extent in the sea, these habitats are separate, discrete and discontinuous. Each lake or river and its catchment is discrete, and separated from its neighbour by a habitat barrier. Each freshwater body is essentially an island or patch, surrounded by an inhospitable environment, within which each host exists as a patch within the matrix of an environment which may be hostile to a parasite. Many of these freshwater bodies are, furthermore, very small and isolated. Many are in addition changeable and changing. In the Northern temperate and arctic regions, most freshwater habitats are of recent, post-glacial origin, and many, if not most, have been influenced by human activities over much if not all of their life (Goudie, 1981). These activities have continued for several thousand years, but both their extent and rate have accelerated in the last century. Changes are also becoming apparent in some areas of the sea, but freshwater habitats are particularly susceptible to change and are thus seldom stable.

In respect of fish and parasite populations and their interactions, it is thus possible to predict that:

(1) Relationships and interactions between different species of fish and parasite will differ and show variation in time and space.

(2) Because of the discrete and isolated nature of each freshwater habitat, there may be little gene flow between them and differences in fish and parasite gene pools between habitats are very likely. The nature of the gene pool may also depend upon the genetic composition of one or a few initial colonizing individuals, and so founder effects may be of enhanced importance. Furthermore, the high reproductive rate of many parasites together with their ability to self-fertilize and/or reproduce asexually can mean that only one parasite individual may be needed to found a colony and that its genotype will be perpetuated, thus further enhancing the genetic differences between populations. Within large freshwater bodies such as lakes, it is also theoretically possible to have discrete populations and gene pools

of both fish and parasites. Relationships and interactions between the same species
of fish and parasite will thus vary from site to site, as will any selection pressure
exerted by parasites on fish and vice versa.

(3) The importance of colonization processes, the stochastic occurrence of
colonizers and the rapidly changing nature of the aquatic habitats themselves,
whether natural or man-induced, suggest that parasites in aquatic systems may
often exist in non-equilibrium conditions. This is most likely in small, isolated and
recent habitats such as small lakes and ponds, and less likely in old, large lakes
and in the sea. Small lakes and rivers may in fact function as islands, in which
colonization, extinction and turnover rates are high.

The implications of these predictions in relation to the selection pressures exerted
by parasites and the genetics of host–parasite interactions in aquatic, especially
freshwater, systems are considerable. Between-habitat differences in interactions
between parasites and fish are as likely to be due to differences in host or parasite
gene pools as to differences in ecology and parasite transmission rates, and within-
habitat differences in infection levels between individual fish are similarly as likely
to be due to differences in host or parasite genotype as to heterogeneity in the
probability of transmission resulting from ecological factors. However, if habitats
are changing rapidly, if parasites are existing in non-equilibrium states and if
parasites do not persist for long periods in a habitat, then they may exert less selection
pressure on their hosts than would otherwise seem likely. One undoubted
consequence of these predictions is the expectation of a great deal of variation in
the interactions of fish and parasite populations, both spatial and temporal.

EXAMPLES OF FISH–PARASITE INTERACTIONS

Differences between species

The first prediction, that interactions between different species of fish and parasite
will differ, is readily verifiable. Fish may serve as intermediate or definitive hosts
for parasites. In the former case, the parasite is often long lived and may alter
the behaviour of the host in such a way as to enhance the probability of predation
upon it and thus directly or indirectly cause the mortality of the host, e.g. *Ligula
intestinalis:* in the latter case, the parasite is generally shorter-lived, and may or
may not have pathogenic effects upon the host. Some species of parasites are
ectoparasites, with a direct life cycle and capable of a rapid build up in
infrapopulation level on fish, whereas others are endoparasites with an indirect
life cycle and a requirement for one or more species of intermediate host. Parasites
of the first group, such as *Ichthyophthirius multifiliis*, may be pathogenic and provoke
a host response that is effective in reducing parasite levels, whereas parasites of
the second group seldom do. In the course of their lives, some species of fish may
change their diet and habitat and thus their parasite community, whereas other
species remain in the same habitat and do not vary their diet significantly. Some
species of parasite, for example monogeneans, are narrowly specific to a single
host species, whereas others may be widely specific. In the case of widely specific
parasites, the host utilized, and hence the nature of the host–parasite relationship,
may vary from site to site: the principle host of *Echinorhynchus salmonis*, for example,
is *Coregonus clupeaformis* in Cold Lake, Alberta (Holmes *et al.*, 1977), *Onchorhynchus
kisutch* and *Osmerus mordax* in Lake Michigan (Amin & Burrows, 1977), *Perca fluviatilis*
in Lake Ontario (Tedla & Fernando, 1970) and *Coregonus nasus* in the Baltic Sea

(Valtonen, 1980). Not only therefore did the flow of the parasite through its host species differ in each habitat, but so also did the interaction between the parasite and each host species, and any effects the parasite might have had on the fitness of its host population will have varied from site to site and from host species to host species between and within sites.

Differences between sites

The second prediction, that variation in interactions between the same species of fish and parasite between sites may have a genetic base, is less easy to verify. There are several examples of differences in the population dynamics of a parasite in different localities, but since the population dynamics of fish parasites are extensively influenced by a variety of biotic and abiotic factors (Kennedy, 1977) and these also vary from site to site, it is difficult to ascertain how much of the variation is due to genetic differences and how much to phenotypic differences.

Differences of sufficient magnitude to permit recognition of different strains of a parasite have been detected in several instances, although the genetic distinction has not been investigated in any of them. For example, *Eubothrium crassum* is believed to comprise two strains at least, one of which is marine and more specific to *Salmo salar* whereas the other is freshwater and more specific to *S. trutta fario* (Kennedy, 1978), and *E. salvelini* is also believed to comprise an American and European strain which differ in their specificity. *Pomphorhynchus laevis* is believed to comprise three strains, an Irish, an English and a Baltic strain, which differ not only in distribution but also in their specificity to their intermediate gammarid and definitive fish hosts (Kennedy, 1984a). *Ligula intestinalis* represents a more complex situation: the relationship between this parasite and *Rutilus rutilus* differs in many respects from that in *Gobio gobio* and Arme (1975) suggested that parasites in *G. gobio* might comprise a different strain, although both strains could co-exist in the same locality. More recent work (Hoole & Arme, 1983) has suggested that parasites in *G. gobio* may be disguising their antigenicity by coating themselves with host protein, but the existence of genetic differences in the parasites in *G. gobio* is still regarded as possible. All the examples of strain differences can be associated with differences in specificity, and, with the exception of *Ligula*, with major habitat differences and/or a substantial degree of geographical isolation. They suggest long periods of co-evolution of hosts and parasites in isolation, and appear to represent a stage in speciation rather than examples of local differences in gene pools.

The best example of genetic variation and local differences in parasite gene pools comes from the studies of Mackiewicz (1981) on caryophyllaeid cestodes. Polyploidy has been detected in several species, and the genetic 'plasticity' of the group appears to be reflected in different genetic forms in different localities, due in turn to the isolation of the localities. For example, examination of three populations of *Glaridacris laruei* revealed two cytologically distinct diploid populations and a third triploid population, and of six populations of *G. catastomi* five were diploid but the sixth triploid (Grey & Mackiewicz, 1980). There had clearly been selection for the triploid form in one locality, but neither its advantages nor the reasons for the selection are yet known. That such genetic differences will be reflected in differences in the population biology of the species in different localities seems likely, but has yet to be demonstrated. *Caryophyllaeus laticeps*, for example, has been shown by Mackiewicz to be genetically heterogeneous and to occur in diploid and triploid populations. There is also evidence of variation in its population biology: in northern latitudes there is a causal relationship between water temperature and parasite mortality (Kennedy, 1971), such that parasites are rejected from fish at summer temperatures. This relationship was confirmed by Anderson (1974), but recent work in heated lakes in Poland has shown that there the parasites can survive in fish at water temperatures well in excess of those at which they are rejected in Britain (Pojmanska, 1984). It would thus seem very likely that such major differences in the temperature tolerance of the parasite are related to differences in the genetic composition of the populations. Similarly, the clinal differences in the stimulus to migration of parenteral plerocercoids of *Proteocephalus ambloplitis* are of such a magnitude (see Kennedy, 1977) as to suggest genetic differences between the populations, although no search for such differences has been undertaken. Many other examples of variation in parasite population biology and parasite–host interactions in different localities can be related to differences in abiotic and biotic conditions in the localities, which in turn influence parasite flow paths and transmission rates. Several examples of these are given by Kennedy (1977), but in no case has the genetic composition of the parasites or hosts been studied and additional genetic differences between the populations may also be present.

Differences in host–parasite interactions between sites may equally reflect differences in the gene pools of the fish, or other hosts, but this possibility appears never to have been investigated. The nearest approach to it is the study by Henricson (1977, 1978) and Henricson & Nyman (1976) on the parasites of two sibling species of *Salvelinus alpinus* in a single locality. He found that there were significant differences in the parasite fauna of the two species, but the differences reflected the food niches of the hosts, which changed if the species were living in sympatric or allopatric situations and in the presence of *Salmo trutta*, and not their genetic differences.

At present, therefore, there is little evidence other than from the caryophyllaeids of genetic differences in parasite populations in different localities, and even less evidence that differences in host–parasite interactions have a genetic basis. On the other hand, even though many of the differences may reflect the phenotypic differences between localities, there is every reason to suppose that genetic differences do also exist.

Differences within sites

The third prediction, that parasites in aquatic systems may often exist in non-equilibrium states, is more controversial, and so therefore are the genetic implications. Theoretical considerations and mathematical models have shown clearly the conditions under which parasite populations may be stable and regulated and equilibrium dynamics are possible (Anderson & May, 1978, 1979, 1981). There is also an increasing body of evidence from laboratory investigations of fish-parasite systems to indicate that regulatory mechanisms may operate on some fish parasite populations: for example on *Transversotrema patialense* (Anderson *et al.*, 1977, 1978), on *Leptorhynchoides thecatus* (Uznanski & Nickol, 1982), on *Gyrodactylus* species (Lester & Adams, 1974; Scott, 1985, this volume), on *Apatemon gracilis* (Gordon & Rau, 1982), on *Ichthyophthirius multifiliis* (Hines & Spira, 1974) and on *Diplostomum spathaceum* (Brassard *et al.*, 1982), amongst others. Field investigations, however, have led to different conclusions. With one or two notable exceptions, such as *Pomphorhynchus laevis* (Kennedy & Rumpus, 1977) and *Eubothrium salvelini* (Smith, 1973), fish-parasite populations appear to be unregulated in natural conditions and Kennedy (1977) was able to conclude that on the present evidence, the majority of fish–parasite populations are unregulated and hence unstable: more recent studies, such as those of Aho *et al.* (1982) and Camp *et al.* (1982), have supported his conclusions.

In the context of any discussion on regulation, differences in infection levels between individual fish, and the reasons for them, assume increased importance. Parasite populations are normally overdispersed throughout their fish host populations, and the proportion of the host population that harbours the heaviest parasite burdens will be the proportion in which the probability of intra-specific competition and/or provoking effective host responses will be the highest. It will, in fact, be the proportion in which regulation will actually occur. It is therefore important to ascertain whether heterogeneity in infection levels in fish is merely a reflection of differences in transmission, or whether it reflects differences in host genotype. Here again there is very little direct evidence to support either view.

Several species of microparasites, particularly protozoans and monogeneans, have been shown to provoke immune responses in their hosts that may be effective against the parasite, and differences in the responses between individual fish are often apparent in such cases. Woo *et al.* (1983) and Woo (1981) were able to demonstrate heterogeneity in fish responses to trypanosomes and Lester & Adams (1974) to *Gyrodactylus*, for example. In virtually all cases where parasites have been shown to provoke immune responses in fish, heterogeneity in the response of fish is evident such that some individuals appear to be capable of mounting an effective response that constrains the parasite, whereas other fish appear to be incapable of such a response and so are susceptible to the parasite. It is not yet clear, however, whether this heterogeneity in immune response has a genetic basis, as in mammals, as this has yet to be investigated. It is clear, though, that in such microparasite–host systems the potential for regulation of the parasite population through its interaction with its fish host does exist.

The situation is less clear in respect of macroparasites, which generally have indirect life cycles. Regulation of such species may take place in hosts other than fish, and there is very little concrete evidence that they provoke effective immune responses in their fish hosts. These species are typically overdispersed throughout their fish hosts, but the causes of the overdispersion are far from clear in most cases. Anderson & Gordon (1982) have shown that the pattern of parasite dispersion is due to conflicting pressures, with parasite induced host mortality tending to result in underdispersion and heterogeneity in probability of exposure to infection resulting in overdispersion. Such heterogeneity may be due to differences in host behaviour, diet or susceptibility, with or without a genetic basis. In very few cases, however, have the mechanisms responsible for the dispersion pattern been investigated: the most detailed study, that of Boxshall (1974), showed that the overdispersion of *Lepeophtheirus pectoralis* on its fish host resulted from aggregation of free-swimming larvae in the sea. In most other cases, the causes of overdispersion are not known, and most authors have suggested heterogeneity in probability of exposure to infection as the most likely cause. Henricson (1977, 1978) specifically suggested individual differences in diet between fish as the most likely cause of overdispersion, thus providing support for the views on the importance of diet advanced by Crompton *et al.* (1984). Parasite-induced host mortality, leading to underdispersion, has been demonstrated in several cases, especially those in which the parasite uses the fish as an intermediate host (Lester, 1977; Henricson, 1977, 1978; Gordon & Rau,

1982; Pennycuick, 1971 amongst others), but there is again no evidence that the most heavily infected hosts are in any way genetically susceptible to infection. There is also no evidence that such mortality is generally regulatory, since in the majority of cases death of heavily infected fish is due to predation and so enhances the probability of transmission of the parasite to its definitive host.

The present situation appears to be one in which a variety of regulatory mechanisms have been demonstrated in the laboratory and it is clear that the potential for regulation exists in many parasite species of fish. A genetic basis for such regulation appears likely in many cases, especially when the regulatory mechanism involves immune responses or other differences in fish susceptibility, but has yet to be demonstrated conclusively. In the field, however, transmission factors appear to be predominant in determining infection levels within a fish population and in individual fish, thus accounting also for much of the variation between sites, and many field investigations suggest that fish parasites exist in non-equilibrium and unregulated states. It would appear that the potential for regulation is seldom realized in practice, in part perhaps because transmission rates in the field are so low that infections seldom if ever reach the levels in individual fish at which regulatory mechanisms have been shown to operate in the laboratory. Physiological and/or immunological factors with, possibly, a genetic basis, may determine whether an individual fish is susceptible to infection and capable of a response that constrains parasite numbers, but unless transmission rates result in infection levels as artificially high as many of those employed in laboratory investigations, the host response will not be manifested in natural populations and the parasites will exist in non-equilibrium states. If this is in fact the generally prevailing situation, then it is unlikely that parasites are actually exerting significant selection pressures on their host populations: they may interact with their hosts and indeed affect their host populations, but such interactions may not influence the genetics of the host populations. In the following section, some of these ideas will be explored further with reference to one specific locality and the long-term parasite population changes that have taken place there.

PARASITE FAUNA OF FISH OF SLAPTON LEY

Background to lake and fisheries

Although Slapton Ley is the largest natural body of fresh water in the south-west of England, it is a small (0.7 km^2), shallow (max. depth 2 m) isolated lake of recent origin ($c.$ 1000 years). The early and recent history of the fishery has been described by Burrough *et al.* (1979). Until recently, the lake was dominated by three species of fish: pike *Esox lucius* L., perch *Perca fluviatilis* L., and rudd *Scardinius erythrophthalmus* (L.), with roach *Rutilus rutilus* (L.) forming a small and insignificant component of the fish fauna. Since the late 1950s, the lake has become increasingly eutrophic (Troake & Walling, 1973) as a result of increased application and run-off of fertilizers from fields in the catchment. This change has benefited the roach population, which expanded considerably after the mid 1960s. Initial growth of roach was good, but the population was so large that the appearance of a strong year class in 1972 resulted in decreased growth rates and stunting (Burrough & Kennedy, 1979). The increase in roach numbers also led to competition with rudd, to the detriment of this species which had virtually disappeared by 1974, and with perch, which had undergone a steady and continuous decline over the same period. A systematic programme of research into the population biology of all four species of fish and their major parasites commenced in 1973 and has continued to the present day.

Population biology of Ligula intestinalis in roach

Ligula appears to have been introduced into the lake in 1973 through the agency of Great Crested Grebes *Podiceps cristatus* L. as a natural chance colonization event, which occurred at a particularly opportune time since the large population of stunted roach was feeding extensively and intensively upon plankton (Kennedy & Burrough, 1981). The *Ligula* population built up rapidly over the next two years (Fig. 1),

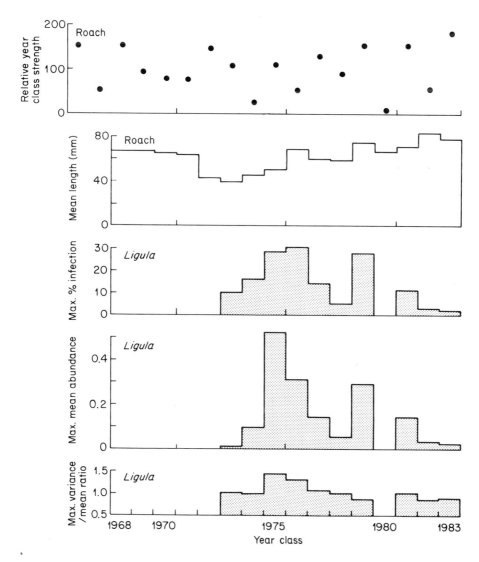

Figure 1. Annual changes in the growth rate and year class strengths of roach and in the infection of *Ligula intestinalis* in roach at the end of their first year of life in Slapton Ley. Data from Burrough & Kennedy (1979), Kennedy & Burrough (1981) and Kennedy (unpublished), with confidence limits omitted for clarity.

causing extensive mortality of roach since *Ligula* renders infected fish more
susceptible to predation as well as sterilizing them (Arme, 1975). This mortality
reduced the roach population, alleviated stunting and so resulted in an immediate
improvement in roach growth, particularly evident by 1976 (Fig. 1). The decline
in the roach population released the rudd from competition, allowing this species
to increase again. Although *Ligula* is capable of infecting rudd (Arme & Owen,
1968), it has never been found to do so in Slapton Ley.

R oach become infected with *Ligula* in their first year of life in autumn, and are
capable of infecting birds if acquired by them over the first winter (Wyatt, pers.
comm.). A few fish may acquire infections in their second year of life, but this
is uncommon as most have ceased to feed on plankton by this time, and the majority
appear to be infected on one occasion only. Infection levels of fish in their first
year can thus be used as an index of infection levels in the population as a whole.
Few infected fish live longer than 18 months (Kennedy & Burrough, 1981): the
major cause of death appears to be selective predation upon parasitized fish by
birds, and mortality rates are greater over the first winter and second summer.
Such parasite-induced host mortality facilitates transmission of *Ligula* to a bird host:
it does not result in death of the parasite and so is unlikely to be regulatory in
its action.

In the years immediately following its appearance, the *Ligula* population built
up rapidly to a peak of prevalence in 1976 and abundance in 1975 (Fig. 1). At
this time, the parasite population was overdispersed, but the degree of overdispersion
was not very pronounced as the maximum number of parasites per fish never
exceeded five. Thereafter, the *Ligula* population declined and, apart from a
temporary reversal in 1979–1981, has continued to decline. Throughout the decline,
parasite dispersion has been close to random (Fig. 1) and infections with more
than one parasite per fish have been exceptionally rare. The growth of roach has
also continued to improve, as the effects of *Ligula* on host reproduction and survival
have prevented any expansion that could lead to resumption of stunting.

It is not easy to interpret the population changes with any degree of certainty.
The pattern observed (Fig. 1) may represent two oscillation cycles, the second one
being of lower amplitude and shorter duration, or the increase in 1979 may just
be a reflection of a temporary improvement in transmission conditions in the lake
and so just 'noise'. This latter explanation is favoured by the fact that 1979 was
a particularly good year for *Ligula* (Kennedy & Burrough, 1981), that there was
no corresponding increase in overdispersion and that there was no significant
improvement in roach growth (Fig. 1). Whatever the explanation, it is clear that
expansion of *Ligula* was checked in 1975–1976 and, thereafter, the trend has been
a fall in transmission rates and parasite levels. The study has failed to provide any
evidence that the *Ligula* population is in any way regulated by its interaction with
roach: on the contrary, it exhibits a number of destabilizing features, including
absence of overdispersion, reduction in host reproductive potential, time lags,
absence of density dependent mortality within fish and parasite-induced host
mortality that facilitates transmission but does not kill the parasite (Kennedy &
Burrough, 1981). This does not preclude the possibility of the *Ligula* population
being regulated in its interaction with its copepod or bird host, in which case, the
population changes could represent oscillation around an equilibrium level, but
the failure to detect regulatory mechanisms and the nature of the population changes
suggest that the population is unregulated and persisting in a non-equilibrium state.

Even the effects of the *Ligula* population upon that of the roach have to be evaluated against the changes in the roach population itself. The roach population in Slapton Ley has been characterized by very considerable variation in year class strengths. These were evident even before the arrival of *Ligula*, when annual variations, e.g. between 1967 and 1968, could exceed 300% (Fig. 1). Following the arrival of *Ligula*, some poor year classes, notably 1974, 1976 and 1980, may be a reflection of heavy parasite levels in the previous years, but the relationship between year class strength and levels of *Ligula* is not always precise. Strong year classes in 1981 and 1983 were not associated with an increase in *Ligula* levels but with a continued decline. Furthermore, the maximum roach mortality in any one year class due to *Ligula* (30% in 1976) should be evaluated in the light of annual changes in year class strength of 300% and greater, and the 3% mortality in the 1982 year class should be seen in the context of a change in year class strength of from 57 in 1982 to 182 in 1983. Thus, although there is no doubt that *Ligula* has interacted with the roach population and has affected both growth and year class strengths of the latter, changes in year class strength are only partly due to *Ligula* and natural variations may have a far greater effect upon roach population size than any mortality due to *Ligula*, which may in any case be compensatory rather than regulatory (Holmes, 1982).

Table 1. Comparison of the infection levels of *Ligula* in Slapton Ley with those in some other British localities

Site	Host	Max. prevalence (%) in young fish	Max. mean abundance per fish	Max. intensity per fish	Authority
Slapton Ley	Roach	30.1	1.75	5	Kennedy & Burrough (1981)
Lake (Northants)	Roach	92.0	1.7	53	Arme & Owen (1968)
Yately Gravel Pit	Roach	92.0	1.5	4	Sweeting (1976)
Chew Reservoir	Roach	96.0	2.6	63	Wilson (1971)
Yeadon Lake	Roach	93.0	4.2	30	Sweeting (1977)
Lake (Swindon)	Roach	62.5	3.4	7	Wyatt (pers. comm.)
R. Thames	Bleak	84.0	3.6	10	Harris & Wheeler (1974)

Many aspects of the *Ligula* infection in Slapton Ley are unusual. Elsewhere, prevalence levels of up to 90% and above are commonly recorded in young fish (Table 1), and may rise in older fish to 100%. Abundance levels are also generally far higher (up to 50 and 60), multiple infections are far commoner and parasites are significantly overdispersed. *Ligula* is generally longer lived in other localities and may also infect rudd. These differences suggested that the *Ligula* in Slapton Ley might constitute a different strain or genotype, but use of isoelectric focusing techniques has so far failed to reveal any significant differences between *Ligula* from Slapton and from other localities (Wyatt, pers. comm.). It is therefore concluded that the peculiarities in the epidemiology of *Ligula* in Slapton Ley reflect the peculiar conditions for, and rates of, transmission there, and so the overall peculiarities in the ecology of the lake.

The effects of *Ligula* on its host population in other localities are similar to, but often more pronounced than, those observed in Slapton Ley. Prevalence levels of 90% and above are followed by dramatic declines in roach numbers, declines in year class strength, and an almost total disappearance of fry in subsequent years (Wilson, 1971; Sweeting, 1976, 1977). The fact that prevalence can reach 100% and that multiple infections may be common or normal suggests that all roach are normally susceptible to infection, and that there are no genetically based differences in individual fish resistance to *Ligula*. Indeed, the normal course of a *Ligula* infection appears to be a rapid rise in population levels leading to a dramatic crash in fish numbers, followed by a similar decline in *Ligula* numbers. No linked oscillation cycles have yet been reported, nor has it even been shown that *Ligula* persists for any length of time in a locality following the population decline or that the population exists in an equilibrium state. This may represent a paucity of long-term studies, or reflect the fact that most reports come from small lakes where the probability of regular or random population fluctuations reducing the population level to extinction point is high. On the other hand, there is evidence that *Ligula* is an opportunistic species (Dubinina, 1964; Kennedy & Burrough, 1981). It is easily dispersed with migratory birds and so can overcome isolation barriers. In small lakes, it may only survive in a non-equilibrium state for short periods but, before such populations become locally extinct, some individuals will have colonized new localities and founded new populations. In larger lakes, *Ligula* may persist for longer periods and even reach equilibrium state, and such sites would provide a permanent reservoir for new colonists. Differences in persistence and epidemiology between lakes would thus largely reflect the differences in conditions and transmission rates there.

Population biology of parasites of perch

The population of perch in Slapton Ley appears to be far more stable than that of roach, perhaps because there appears to be very little variation in year class strengths (Bregazzi & Kennedy, 1982). Recovery of the perch population from the decline caused by competition with roach has been very slow and an adaptive improvement in perch growth has only been apparent from 1976 onwards (Fig. 2). In contrast to roach, growth rates have changed little from year to year, and there is no evidence that the population decline, recovery, growth or year class variations have been influenced in any way by parasitic infections. The changes in parasite populations discussed below have thus taken place against a background of a very stable perch population.

Details of the biology of the species discussed are given by Kennedy & Burrough (1977) and Kennedy (1981a,b) and the following account summarizes these papers and provides additional observations. Prior to 1973, the only species of eyefluke infecting perch was *Diplostomum gasterostei*. Infection levels in the 1973 year class were lower than those in 1972, possibly reflecting the decline in perch density but, thereafter, infection levels in each year class increased in both the first and second years of life until 1977 (Fig. 2), when infection levels declined in the 1977 year class. In 1978, infection levels fell in the 1977 year class, and fell to an unprecedentedly low level in the 1978 year class. Transmission rates have subsequently remained at very low levels, and there is no indication of the population recovering from the crash or rising to its previous levels. There is no indication that the decline was due to regulatory changes within the parasite population itself, or indeed that the population is regulated at all, or to changes in population densities of any of the host species: it is believed to be due instead to interspecific competition

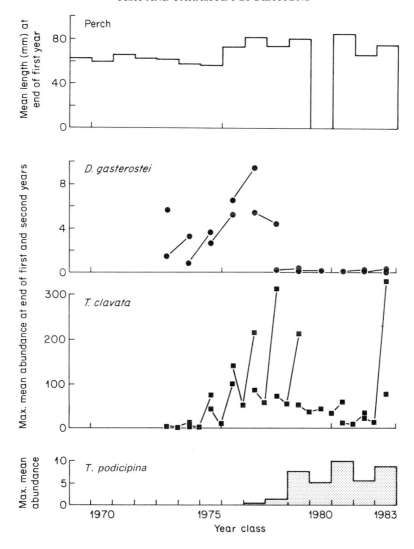

Figure 2. Annual changes in the growth rate of perch and in infection levels of *Diplostomum gasterostei*, *Tylodelphys clavata* and *T. podicipina* in perch in Slapton Ley. Data from Kennedy (1981a,b, unpublished), with confidence limits omitted for clarity.

within perch eyes with *Tylodelphys clavata* and *T. podicipina* (Kennedy, 1981b). Although transmission of the parasite to birds takes place by predation on infected fish, there is no indication that the parasite induces host mortality (Kennedy, 1984b) or indeed has, or has had, any influence at all upon the perch population. Changes in prevalence followed a similar pattern to those in abundance and, prior to 1977, prevalence generally reached 100% and parasites were overdispersed, indicating that all fish were susceptible to single and multiple infections.

In 1973, *T. clavata* was also introduced into the lake, and this again is believed to have been through the agency of *P. cristatus* as a natural chance colonization event. Infection of fish takes place in autumn, but many parasites die over winter and then levels rise again in the following autumn. Following its arrival, the population of *T. clavata* built up rapidly until 1977, showing its cycle of autumn increase and winter decline in each year class (Fig. 2). Infection levels in the first year of life declined for the first time in the 1977 year class, and then in each subsequent year class until that of 1982. The decline in infection levels in the second year of life lagged a year behind. In 1982, infection levels increased slightly and then, in 1983, dramatically in both 1982 and 1983 year classes. The pattern of changes observed is consistent with an oscillation cycle and the start of a new cycle in 1983, but it is possible that 1983 merely represented an exceptionally good year for transmission. There is no evidence of linked oscillation cycles in the populations of snails, fish or birds or in any of the other species of parasites in perch (Fig. 2). Transmission to birds is accomplished by predation on the fish, but there is no evidence that *T. clavata* induces host mortality (Kennedy, 1984b) or indeed that the population is in any way regulated by its interaction with perch (Kennedy, 1981b), or has had any effect on the perch population. Changes in prevalence followed closely those in abundance: by the end of the first year, 100% of the fish were infected, in all cases with multiple infections indicating that there is no resistance of fish to infection.

In 1976, *T. podicipina* was introduced into the lake, again through the agency of *P. cristatus* as a natural chance colonization event. Fish are only susceptible to infection in their first year of life, when levels generally reach 100% and there is no subsequent reinfection. Parasites may survive for up to three years, but there is continuous mortality within the eyes. Following its arrival, the population built up rapidly until 1979 and, thereafter, infection levels in each year class have fluctuated irregularly (Fig. 2). The levels within each year class appear to be determined by the brevity of the infection period, which may last for one to two weeks only when the period of cercarial emission overlaps with the appearance of perch fry in the lake (Kennedy, unpublished). Parasite levels thus appear to reflect transmission events only. There is no evidence that *T. podicipina* causes host mortality (Kennedy, 1984b), or that it is in any way regulated by its interaction with perch (Kennedy, 1981a) or that it has any effect on the perch population. The ability of all young fish to become infected indicates that there is no individual resistance to infection. Parasites are overdispersed, and temporal changes in overdispersion reflect mortality of parasites rather than any effects on the fish.

As far as is known, the population biology of these three species in Slapton Ley is typical of that in other localities. In no localities is there any indication that any of these three species have deleterious, or indeed any, effects upon perch populations, or that individual fish differ in their susceptibility or resistance to infection (other than the resistance of older perch to *T. podicipina*). There have clearly been large changes in transmission rates and population levels of all three species in Slapton Ley over the last 11 years, but there is no evidence that these changes are due to regulatory mechanisms, or that they have affected, or been affected by, the perch population.

Population biology of other parasite species

No other species of parasite in the lake have been studied continuously throughout the period. *Diplostomum spathaceum* was present in roach in all years, and its population levels appear to have undergone large changes. They increased steadily from 1973–1976 (Burrough, 1978), and steeply in 1977, when a mean of 210 parasites per fish was recorded compared with 13 in 1973 and 60 in 1976. Levels have subsequently declined again. Prevalence levels of 100% are common, as are multiple infections, and there is no indication that fish are resistant to infection. Transmission to birds is accomplished by predation on the fish, but the evidence for parasite induced host mortality is not conclusive (Kennedy, 1984b), and the extent of any such mortality would have to be evaluated against the severe mortality due to *Ligula* and the large annual fluctuations in roach year class strength.

The population of *Acanthocephalus clavula* in perch has also undergone pronounced and dramatic changes over the period. Canning *et al.* (1973) reported that prevalence had declined over the previous six years. From 1974–1978, it was present continuously in perch although both prevalence and abundance values were low. In 1979, 35% of the perch were infected, with a mean abundance of 1.25 parasites per fish (max. 15). In 1980, prevalence had fallen to 7.3% and abundance to 0.15 (max. 3). In 1981, however, no parasites were found in perch, nor has *A. clavula* been found in subsequent years up to and including 1984. It can therefore be concluded that the infrapopulation in perch has become extinct or fallen to levels where it is no longer detectable.

The population biology of both these species in Slapton Ley appears to be fairly typical of that in other localities. *Diplostomum spathaceum* is known to be capable of inducing host mortality (Brassard *et al.*, 1982), or of having a deleterious effect upon its hosts (Kennedy, 1984b). By contrast, *A. clavula* has never been shown to have any harmful effects upon its fish hosts, although large declines in population size have been reported from other localities (Kennedy, 1984c).

General comments

The outstanding features of all the parasite populations studied in Slapton Ley over the last 11 years is the extent of the changes that have occurred in their infrapopulation levels in fish. The overwhelming impression of the lake parasite fauna is of its dynamic nature. Three new species have colonized the lake, one of which, *Ligula*, has had a pronounced effect on the dynamics of the fish populations. Of the original inhabitants, levels of *D. spathaceum* have risen and fallen, levels of *D. gasterostei* have fallen sharply to a barely detectable level, and levels of *A. clavula* have fallen to a point at which they are no longer detectable. The whole parasite community has changed dramatically, and the investigation has clearly emphasized the colonizing ability of fish parasites and the importance of chance colonization events in aquatic ecosystems. It has also emphasized the importance of continuous long-term studies in revealing these changes and interpreting them.

Of the six species studied, only *Ligula* has been shown conclusively to interact with a fish population. *Diplostomum spathaceum* may do so, but there is no evidence that any of the other four species do. All fish of both species appeared capable of harbouring multiple infections of all species, and there was no evidence of differences in individual fish, genetically based or otherwise, in their resistance or susceptibility to infection. The effects of *Ligula* on the roach population, and hence on populations of other fish species, have been considerable, but despite these there is no evidence that *Ligula* has actually regulated the roach population or indeed that the *Ligula* population is itself regulated. The *Ligula* population does not appear to be genetically distinct, which is not too surprising since it may not in fact be an isolated population in view of the readiness with which it can be transported to other sites by birds. On the evidence to date, therefore, all the parasite populations in Slapton Ley appear to be existing in non-equilibrium states.

All the species of fish have been influenced, directly or indirectly, by the arrival and persistence of *Ligula*, and indeed the whole aquatic ecosystem was perturbed by this chance colonization. Future changes in the lake will now depend largely upon whether *Ligula* continues to decline to extinction, or whether it persists at present levels or increases again. Clearly, however, the natural rate of change in the fish populations, due to variations in year class strength and interspecific interactions, can be very rapid indeed, and it is very difficult to see how, in the face of such rapid changes and in the absence of any evidence that any species of parasite is regulated by its interaction with its fish host, any species of parasite can be acting as a selection agent. None appears to be able to persist at high enough levels for long enough to be able to affect the host gene pool, even if they have the potential to do so and this is far from certain since most are not pathogenic and all hosts appear to be susceptible to infection. The changes in Slapton Ley illustrate the importance of chance colonizing events and the extent to which one parasite can influence a whole ecosystem: they provide evidence of the colonizing ability of parasites and the importance of pioneers, but they fail to provide any evidence for the importance of perpetuators or for the persistent interaction of parasites and fish in a regulated way, or for the role of parasites as selection agents, or for the existence of parasite populations in equilibrium states.

GENERAL CONCLUSIONS

The investigations at Slapton Ley have verified two of the predictions, namely that interactions between different species of parasite and fish differ and that fish parasites may exist in non-equilibrium states. There was, however, no indication of differences in parasite gene pools, or indeed of any genetic basis to the interactions between parasites and fish. The question therefore arises as to how typical is Slapton Ley and the parasite population changes recorded there?

This question is exceptionally difficult to answer, as there are no comparable studies conducted on several species of parasites and fish simultaneously and continuously for such a long period of time. Long-term data from some localities on single species parasite-fish systems indicate persistence and stability (Peterssen, 1971; Smith, 1973; Kennedy & Rumpus, 1977; Camp *et al.*, 1982), but whilst some of these authors believe that this stability is due to regulation of the parasite population, others do not. By contrast, data from other localities indicate large changes in parasite population levels in at least some species (Hugghins, 1957; Powell & Chubb, 1966; Kennedy, 1984c). Evidence of colonization is equally scarce. *Tylodelphys clavata* and *T. podicipina* have recently colonized a small pool near Slapton Ley (Kennedy, unpublished), and Henricson (1977, 1978) noted that the increase in range and numbers of gulls has often led to an increase in levels of *Diphyllobothrium dendriticum* and to its introduction into some lakes. Realistically, however, there are far too few well-documented studies to permit any generalizations to be made at this stage or to determine whether the parasite population changes in Slapton Ley are typical or not.

It has also been suggested that Slapton Ley is an atypical locality in view of its isolation and small size, and the extent and so impact of the changes in the lake resulting from human activities in recent years. There is certainly no reason to suggest that Slapton Ley is atypical in this respect. It is now clear that lakes have been influenced by human activities for at least 5000 years, and that both the extent and rate of man-made changes have accelerated over the last century and, in some cases, are still accelerating (Pennington, 1978). Cultural eutrophication is a widespread and international problem, affecting lakes as small and isolated as Slapton Ley and as large as the Great Lakes of North America. Many other lakes now serve as regulating reservoirs, or receive thermal effluents, and many of these are localities that have also been the site of parasitological investigations. The full extent of human impact, including alteration in catchments, management, abstraction and addition, upon rivers and lakes and the time over which it has operated is only now becoming apparent (Goudie, 1981) and it is certainly arguable that there is no freshwater body in temperate regions that has not been affected by human activities. In this respect, therefore, Slapton Ley is a typical locality.

It is indeed the extent of human activities that may explain why there is so little evidence of genotypic differences between parasite populations in different localities, and why this prediction is so difficult to verify. The natural isolation of freshwater bodies has been broken down in recent, and distant, years by a whole range of human activities including construction of canals, movement of fish between sites for food and recreation and changes in bird movement patterns as a result of habitat management, whether creative or destructive, stocking and changes in population densities and ranges resulting from human cultural changes. The cumulative effect of all these changes will be mixing of parasite gene pools. A further, and major effect, however, will be to perturb the habitats, often to the extent of breaking down the regulatory mechanisms that produced population and community stability and equilibrium states.

This may be, at least in part, an explanation of the fact that whereas many species of fish parasites clearly have the potential for population regulation and to act as agents of selection on their host populations, this potential seldom seems to be realized in natural populations. Many freshwater habitats are themselves unstable and changing, transmission of parasites to fish is uncertain and probabilities of infection are low and the parasite populations are small and so chance fluctuations can easily lead to extinction. Unstable and changing habitats are likely to contain parasite populations in non-equilibrium states, and they are not the places to seek for evidence of equilibrium dynamics and of parasites exerting selection pressures on their hosts. Such evidence should be sought in stable habitats, such as large and remote lakes where human influence has been minimal, in habitats where natural transmission rates may approach levels employed in laboratory experiments, or in the sea, where conditions are far more stable. Here, probabilities of infection may be low, but may be compensated for by facilitated transmission or behavioural features of free-living parasitic stages. Unfortunately, even less is known about interactions between fish and parasite populations in the sea than in fresh water, but the stability shown by *Gyrocotyle* in chimaerid hosts would seem to provide evidence for the operation of regulatory mechanisms (Halvorsen & Williams, 1968).

It seems highly unlikely that fish parasites do not have the same potential to be of major importance to the fitness of their hosts as do parasites of mammals (Anderson & May, 1982). What seems far more likely is that this potential is either unrealized or is undetectable in many contemporary freshwater habitats and host–parasite systems. The high degree of specificity exhibited by many freshwater parasites, the existence of endemic species in old lakes and the extent of strain formation all suggest long periods of co-evolution and stability in host–parasite relationships. Contemporary conditions, however, generally favour species with high dispersal and colonizing abilities and will tend to result in parasite populations persisting in non-equilibrium states. The discrepancy between predictions from models, laboratory data and results from field investigations is thus not surprising and is readily explicable, as is the inability to verify all the predictions. The extent of the variation in the interaction of fish and parasite populations, of the same and different species and both temporal and spatial, is also readily understandable. Slapton Ley is therefore probably typical of many contemporary freshwater localities, but it would be extraordinarily interesting to see the results of similar investigations conducted in marine localities or in lakes such as Baikal. Until such results are forthcoming, we may never truly understand the relationships between genetics and ecology in fish and parasite populations.

REFERENCES

AHO, J. M., CAMP, J. W. & ESCH, G. W., 1982. Long-term studies on the population biology of *Diplostomum scheuringi* in a thermally altered reservoir. *Journal of Parasitology, 68:* 695–708.

AMIN, O. M. & BURROWS, J. M., 1977. Host and seasonal associations of *Echinorhynchus salmonis* (Acanthocephala: Echinorhynchidae) in Lake Michigan fishes. *Journal of the Fisheries Research Board of Canada, 34:* 325–331.

ANDERSON, R. M., 1974. Population dynamics of the cestode *Caryophyllaeus laticeps* (Pallas, 1781) in the bream (*Abramis brama* L.). *Journal of Animal Ecology, 43:* 305–321.

ANDERSON, R. M. & GORDON, D. M., 1982. Processes influencing the distribution of parasite numbers within host populations with special emphasis on parasite-induced host mortalities. *Parasitology, 85:* 373–398.

ANDERSON, R. M. & MAY, R. M., 1978. Regulation and stability of host–parasite population interactions. I. Regulatory processes. *Journal of Animal Ecology, 47:* 219–247.

ANDERSON, R. M. & MAY, R. M., 1979. Population biology of infectious diseases: I. *Nature, London, 280:* 361–367.

ANDERSON, R. M. & MAY, R. M., 1981. The population dynamics of microparasites and their invertebrate hosts. *Philosophical Transactions of the Royal Society B, 291:* 451–524.

ANDERSON, R. M. & MAY, R. M., 1982. Coevolution of hosts and parasites. *Parasitology, 85:* 411–426.

ANDERSON, R. M., WHITFIELD, P. J. & DOBSON, A. P., 1978. Experimental studies of infection dynamics: infection of the definitive host by the cercariae of *Transversotrema patialense. Parasitology, 77:* 189–200.

ANDERSON, R. M., WHITFIELD, P. J. & MILLS, C. A., 1977. An experimental study of the population dynamics of an ectoparasitic digenean *Transversotrema patialense*: the cercarial and adult stages. *Journal of Animal Ecology, 46:* 555–580.

ARME, C., 1975. Tapeworm–host interactions. *Symposium of the Society of Experimental Biology, 29:* 505–532.

ARME, C. & OWEN, R. W., 1968. Occurrence and pathology of *Ligula intestinalis* infections in British fishes. *Journal of Parasitology, 54:* 272–280.

BOXSHALL, G. A., 1974. The population dynamics of *Lepeoptheirus pectoralis* (Muller): dispersion patterns. *Parasitology, 69:* 373–390.

BRASSARD, P., RAU, M. E. & CURTIS, M. A., 1982. Parasite-induced susceptibility to predation in diplostomiasis. *Parasitology, 85:* 495–501.

BREGAZZI, P. R. & KENNEDY, C. R., 1982. The responses of a perch *Perca fluviatilis* L., population to eutrophication and associated changes in fish fauna in a small lake. *Journal of Fish Biology, 20:* 21–31.

BURROUGH, R. J., 1978. The population biology of two species of eyefluke, *Diplostomum spathaceum* and *Tylodelphys clavata*, in roach and rudd. *Journal of Fish Biology, 13:* 19–32.

BURROUGH, R. J. & KENNEDY, C. R., 1979. The occurrence and natural alleviation of stunting in a population of roach, *Rutilus rutilus* (L.). *Journal of Fish Biology, 15:* 93–109.

BURROUGH, R. J., BREGAZZI, P. R. & KENNEDY, C. R., 1979. Interspecific dominance amongst three species of coarse fish in Slapton Ley, Devon. *Journal of Fish Biology, 15:* 535–544.

CAMP, J. W., AHO, J. M. & ESCH, G. W., 1982. A long-term study on various aspects of the population biology of *Ornithodiplostomum ptychocheilus* in a South Carolina cooling reservoir. *Journal of Parasitology, 68:* 709–718.

CANNING, E. U., COX, F. E. G., CROLL, N. A. & LYONS, K. M., 1973. The natural history of Slapton Ley Nature Reserve. VI. Studies on the parasites. *Field Studies, 3:* 681–718.

CROMPTON, D. W. T., KEYMER, A. E. & ARNOLD, W. E., 1984. Investigating over-dispersion: *Moniliformis* (Acanthocephala) and rats. *Parasitology, 88:* 317–331.

DUBININA, M. N., 1964. Cestodes of the family Ligulidae and their taxonomy. In R. Ergens & B. Rysavy (Eds), *Parasite Worms and Aquatic Conditions*: 168–173. Prague: Czechoslovak Academy of Sciences.

GORDON, D. M. & RAU, M. E., 1982. Possible evidence for mortality induced by the parasite *Apatemon gracilis* in a population of brook sticklebacks (*Culaea inconstans*). *Parasitology, 84:* 41–47.

GOUDIE, A., 1981. *The Human Impact*. Oxford: Blackwell.

GREY, A. J. & MACKIEWICZ, J. S., 1980. Chromosomes of caryophyllidean cestodes: diploidy, triploidy and parthenogenesis in *Glaridacris catastomi*. *International Journal of Parasitology, 10:* 397–407.

HALVORSEN, O. & WILLIAMS, H. H., 1968. Studies on the helminth fauna of Norway. IX. *Gyrocotyle* (Platyhelminths) in *Chimaera monstrosa* from Oslo Fjord, with emphasis on its mode of attachment and regulation in the degree of infection. *Nytt magasin for Zoologi, 15:* 130–142.

HARRIS, M. T. & WHEELER, A., 1974. *Ligula* infection of bleak *Alburnus alburnus* (L.) in the Tidal Thames. *Journal of Fish Biology, 6:* 181–188.

HENRICSON, J., 1977. The abundance and distribution of *Diphyllobothrium dendriticum* (Nitzsch) and *D. ditremum* (Creplin) in the char *Salvelinus alpinus* (L.) in Sweden. *Journal of Fish Biology, 11:* 231–248.

HENRICSON, J., 1978. The dynamics of infection of *Diphyllobothrium dendriticum* (Nitzsch) and *D. ditremum* (Creplin) in the char *Salvelinus alpinus* (L.) in Sweden. *Journal of Fish Biology, 13:* 51–71.

HENRICSON, J. & NYMAN, L., 1976. The ecological and genetical segregation of two sympatric species of dwarfed char (*Salvelinus alpinus* (L.) species complex). *Report of the Institute of Freshwater Research, Drottningholm, 55:* 15–37.

HINES, R. S. & SPIRA, D. T., 1974. *Ichthyophthirius multifiliis* (Foquet) in the mirror carp, *Cyprinus carpio* L. V. Acquired immunity. *Journal of Fish Biology, 6:* 373–378.

HOLMES, J. C., 1982. Impact of infectious disease agents on the population growth and geographical distribution of animals. In R. M. Anderson & R. M. May (Eds), *Population Biology of Infectious Diseases*: 37–51. Dahlem Konferenzen 1982. New York: Springer-Verlag.

HOLMES, J. C., HOBBS, R. P. & LEONG, T. S., 1977. Populations in perspective: community organisation and regulation of parasite populations. In G. W. Esch (Ed.), *Regulation of Parasite Populations*: 209–245. New York: Academic Press.

HOOLE, D. & ARME, C., 1983. Ultrastructural studies on the cellular response of fish hosts following experimental infection with the plerocercoid of *Ligula intestinalis* (Cestoda: Pseudophyllidea). *Parasitology, 87:* 139–149.

HUGGHINS, E. J., 1957. Ecological studies on a strigeid trematode at Oakwood Lakes, South Dakota. *Proceedings of the South Dakota Academy of Science, 35:* 204–206.

KENNEDY, C. R., 1971. The effects of temperature upon the establishment and survival of the cestode *Caryophyllaeus laticeps* in orfe, *Leuciscus idus. Parasitology, 63:* 59–66.

KENNEDY, C. R., 1977. The regulation of fish parasite populations. In G. W. Esch (Ed.), *Regulation of Parasite Populations*: 63–109. New York: Academic Press.

KENNEDY, C. R., 1978. The biology, specificity and habitat of the species of *Eubothrium* (Cestoda: Pseudophyllidea), with a reference to their use as biological tags: a review. *Journal of Fish Biology, 12:* 393–410.

KENNEDY, C. R., 1981a. The establishment and population biology of the eyefluke *Tylodelphys podicipina* (Digenea: Diplostomatidae) in perch. *Parasitology, 82:* 245–255.

KENNEDY, C. R., 1981b. Long term studies on the population biology of two species of eyefluke, *Diplostomum gasterostei* and *Tylodelphys clavata* (Digenea: Diplostomatidae), concurrently infecting the eyes of perch, *Perca fluviatilis. Journal of Fish Biology, 19:* 221–236.

KENNEDY, C. R., 1984a. The status of flounders, *Platichthys flesus* L., as hosts of the Acanthocephalan *Pomphorhynchus laevis* (Muller) and its survival in marine conditions. *Journal of Fish Biology, 24:* 135–149.

KENNEDY, C. R., 1984b. The use of frequency distributions in an attempt to detect host mortality induced by infections of diplostomatid metacercariae. *Parasitology, 89:* 209–220.

KENNEDY, C. R., 1984c. The dynamics of a declining population of the acanthocephalan *Acanthocephalus clavula* in eels *Anguilla anguilla* in a small river. *Journal of Fish Biology, 25:* 665–677.

KENNEDY, C. R. & BURROUGH, R., 1977. The population biology of two species of eyefluke, *Diplostomum gasterostei* and *Tylodelphys clavata*, in perch. *Journal of Fish Biology, 11:* 619–633.

KENNEDY, C. R. & BURROUGH, R. J., 1981. The establishment and subsequent history of a population of *Ligula intestinalis* in roach *Rutilus rutilus* (L.). *Journal of Fish Biology, 19:* 105–126.

KENNEDY, C. R. & RUMPUS, A., 1977. Long term changes in the size of the *Pomphorhynchus laevis* (Acanthocephala) population in the River Avon. *Journal of Fish Biology, 10:* 35–42.

LESTER, R. J. G., 1977. An estimate of the mortality in a population of *Perca flavescens* owing to the trematode *Diplostomum adamsi. Canadian Journal of Zoology, 55:* 288–292.

LESTER, R. J. G. & ADAMS, J. R., 1974. A simple model of a *Gyrodactylus* population. *International Journal of Parasitology, 4:* 497–506.

MACKIEWICZ, J. S., 1981. Caryophyllidea (Cestoidea): Evolution and Classification. *Advances in Parasitology, 19:* 140–206.

PENNINGTON, W., 1978. The impact of man on some English lakes: rates of change. *Polskie Archiwum Hydrobiologii, 25:* 429–437.

PENNYCUICK, L., 1971. Frequency distributions of parasites in a population of three-spined sticklebacks, *Gasterosteus aculeatus* L., with particular reference to the negative binomial distribution. *Parasitology, 63:* 389–406.

PETERSSEN, A., 1971. The effect of lake regulation on populations of cestodan parasites of Swedish whitefish *Coregonus*. *Oikos, 22:* 74–83.

POJMANSKA, T., 1984. The analysis of seasonality of occurrence and maturation of some fish parasites, with regard to thermal factors. II. *Caryophyllaeus laticeps* (Pallas, 1781). *Acta Parasitologica Polonica, 29:* 229–239.

POWELL, A. M. & CHUBB, J. C., 1966. A decline in the occurrence of *Diphyllobothrium* plerocercoids in the trout *Salmo trutta* L. of Llyn Padarn, Caernarvonshire. *Nature, London, 211:* 439.

PRICE, P. W., 1980. *Evolutionary Biology of Parasites*. Princeton, New Jersey: Princeton University Press.

SCOTT, M. E. Experimental epidemiology of *Gyrodactylus bullatarudis* (Monogenea) on guppies (*Poecilia reticulata*): short- and long-term studies. This volume: 21–38.

SMITH, H. D., 1973. Observations on the cestode *Eubothrium salvelini* in juvenile sockeye salmon (*Onchorhynchus nerka*) at Babine Lake, British Columbia. *Journal of the Fisheries Research Board of Canada, 30:* 947–964.

SWEETING, R. A., 1976. Studies on *Ligula intestinalis*. Effects on a roach population in a gravel pit. *Journal of Fish Biology, 9:* 515–522.

SWEETING, R. A., 1977. Studies on *Ligula intestinalis*. Some aspects of the pathology in the second intermediate host. *Journal of Fish Biology, 10:* 43–50.

TEDLA, S. & FERNANDO, C. H., 1970. Some remarks on the ecology of *Echinorhynchus salmonis* Muller, 1784. *Canadian Journal of Zoology, 48:* 317–321.

TROAKE, R. P. & WALLING, D. E., 1973. The Natural History of Slapton Ley Nature Reserve. VII. The hydrology of the Slapton Wood stream. *Field Studies, 3:* 719–740.

UZNANSKI, R. L. & NICKOL, B. B., 1982. Site selection growth and survival of *Leptorhynchoides thecatus* (Acanthocephala) during the prepatent period in *Lepomis cyanellus*. *Journal of Parasitology, 68:* 686–690.

VALTONEN, E. T., 1980. *Metechinorhynchus salmonis* infection and diet in the river-spawning whitefish of the Bothnian Bay. *Journal of Fish Biology, 17:* 1–8.

WILSON, R. S., 1971. The decline of a roach *Rutilus rutilus* (L.) population in Chew Valley Lake. *Journal of Fish Biology, 3:* 129–137.

WOO, P. T. K., 1981. Acquired resistance against *Trypanosoma danilewskyi* in goldfish, *Carassius auratus*. *Parasitology, 83:* 343–346.

WOO, P. T. K., WEHNERT, S. D. & RODGERS, D., 1983. The susceptibility of fishes to haemoflagellates at different ambient temperatures. *Parasitology, 87:* 385–392.

Experimental epidemiology of *Gyrodactylus bullatarudis* (Monogenea) on guppies (*Poecilia reticulata*): short- and long-term studies

MARILYN E. SCOTT

Institute of Parasitology, Macdonald College of McGill University, 21,111 Lakeshore Road, Ste-Anne de Bellevue, Quebec, Canada H9X 1CO

An experimental epidemiological approach was used to study the population dynamics of the viviparous monogenean, *Gyrodactylus bullatarudis*, on the guppy, *Poecilia reticulata*. At 25°C, *G. bullatarudis* has an average fecundity of 1.68 and an average expected life span of 4.2 days. Guppies can be divided into three groups on the basis of the parasite population dynamics on isolated hosts: on some, the parasite never establishes, some fish recover from the infection, and some fish die during the exponential growth of the parasite population. The different patterns observed may reflect genetic differences in the host. Parasite transmission occurs during contact either between live fish or between dead and live fish. The long-term experimental epidemiological study showed that under conditions of continual addition of susceptible fish, *G. bullatarudis* causes recurrent epidemics with cycles of increasing amplitude at medium and high levels of immigration, and cycles of decreasing amplitude at low levels of immigration. In the absence of fish immigration, the parasite population goes extinct after the first epidemic. It is believed that this extinction results either from the low fish densities after the epidemic and/or the unsuitability of the available fish as hosts. The driving force behind the cycles is thought to be associated with a temporary, partial refractory period to reinfection. Parasites are considered to be an important regulatory force as a result of the parasite-induced host mortality. Aggregation is a dominant factor in the association, and is shown to be temporally dynamic.

KEY WORDS: — parasite population dynamics — ecology — colonies — transmission — survival — reproduction — epidemic — parasite-induced host mortality.

CONTENTS

Ecology and Genetics of Host–Parasite Interactions
ISBN: 0 12 593 690 7

INTRODUCTION

Parasite ecologists have historically been considered distinct from epidemiologists primarily because of the differences between the host groups. Recently, the term epidemiology has been extended to include the study of disease spread in non-human populations, and as a consequence, both parasite ecologists and traditional epidemiologists have benefited. One obvious advantage in studying non-human parasites is the ability to manipulate experimentally the host–parasite system in order to test specific hypotheses. When carried out over the long term, this approach can be referred to as experimental epidemiology — that is, the study of the dynamics of disease-spread and persistence under long-term experimental conditions. The pioneers of this approach were Greenwood and Fenner and their co-workers who studied the dynamics of viral and bacterial infections in large laboratory colonies of mice (Greenwood & Topley, 1925; Greenwood *et al.*, 1936; Fenner, 1948, 1949). Park (1948) investigated the consequences of protozoan infections on the long-term competitive interactions of two species of *Tribolium* and Stiven (1964) studied the long-term population dynamics of a protozoan of *Hydra*. During the past 5 years additional experimental epidemiology has been undertaken, including investigations of a fish protozoan (McCallum, 1982), a larval cestode of beetles (Keymer, 1981) and larval and adult stages of *Schistosoma mansoni* in snails and mice (Anderson & Crombie, 1985, this volume). The recent large number of long-term free-running studies attest to the importance modern parasite ecologists place on this technique for aiding in the understanding of the spread and persistence of parasite populations in their host populations.

The experiments reported in this paper have also used a long-term experimental epidemiological approach, in combination with short-term directed experiments and theoretical studies, in order to study the population dynamics of the viviparous monogenean, *Gyrodactylus bullatarudis* Turnbull, 1956, parasitic on the skin and fins of the guppy, *Poecilia reticulata* Peters.

Biology of guppies

Guppies are tropical fish familiar to aquarium hobbyists and researchers. Their natural range includes northern South America and the adjacent eastern Caribbean islands (Rosen & Bailey, 1963), but they have been introduced into a number of other tropical countries, either for culture or as mosquito-control agents. Guppies are benthic feeders, ingesting algae, organic debris and benthic invertebrates predominantly (Dussault & Kramer, 1981). They are live-bearers and have average broods of 20 (Silliman, 1948). A detailed long-term study on guppy population dynamics was undertaken by Silliman & Gutsell (1958) where initial populations of 8–10 guppies in 17 litres of water were monitored over 3 years. They concluded that the equilibrium density was determined by food availability and that regulation occurred through density-dependent cannibalism of young.

Biology of Gyrodactylus species

Gyrodactylus species parasitize many families of teleost fish, both marine and freshwater (Malmberg, 1970). They are recognized pathogens in aquaculture

(Malmberg, 1973) and in the aquarium hobbyist market (Anderson, 1974), where mortality may be direct, or indirect through secondary bacterial or fungal infection.

Gyrodactylids are viviparous and the newborn young contain within the uterus several generations in sequential stages of development. Although the details of this unusual reproductive system have been studied (Kathariner, 1904; Turnbull, 1956; Bychowsky, 1957; Braun, 1966; Khalil, 1970), it is still unclear whether embryos are fertilized. A functional male reproductive system does develop and copulation is frequently observed; however, its biological significance is unknown.

As a consequence of the viviparous reproduction, *Gyrodactylus* do not have the usual dispersal stage of other monogenea, the oncomiracidium. Dispersal therefore relies on the parasite dropping off one host, sinking to the substrate and reattaching to another host, or moving directly from one fish to another during contact. In the case of *G. bullatarudis*, the latter is considered to be the predominant means of transmission (Scott & Anderson, 1984).

Extensive literature is available on the taxonomy and systematics of this genus (e.g. Malmberg, 1970; Ergens, 1981). There is also a large volume of literature describing field surveys, both horizontal and longitudinal, where prevalence and/or mean burden of gyrodactylids are reported (e.g. Parker, 1965; Rawson & Rogers, 1973; Chubb, 1977; Kirby, 1981; Hanzelova & Zitnan, 1982; Heggberget & Johnsen, 1982). Experimental studies of *Gyrodactylus* population dynamics are relatively scarce. Transmission of *Gyrodactylus elegans* Nordmann, 1832 on golden shiners (*Notemigonus crysoleuces*) has been studied by Parker (1965). Lester and Adams (1974a,b) estimated the intrinsic rate of increase of *Gyrodactylus alexanderi* Mizelle and Kritsky, 1967 on sticklebacks (*Gasterosteus aculeatus*) and studied the dynamics of challenge infections on fish which had recovered from a primary infection. They also reported the results of small-scale epidemics involving four fish in a litre of water. More recently, Harris (1982) investigated a number of aspects of the population biology of *Gyrodactylus gasterostei* Glaser, 1974 and *Gyrodactylus pungitii* Malmberg, 1964 on *G. aculeatus*, both in the field and the laboratory.

SHORT-TERM EXPERIMENTS

This paper reviews results from recent work using *Gyrodactylus bullatarudis* on guppies (Scott, 1982; Scott & Anderson, 1984; Scott & Nokes, 1984; Scott & Robinson, 1984; Scott, submitted). This particular host–parasite association is well suited to experimental epidemiological studies. Guppies breed easily under laboratory conditions, thereby providing a source of naïve hosts. The parasites have a short generation time (2.4 days at 25°C) (Scott, 1982), and can be easily and accurately counted on anaesthetized hosts. Thus, the parasite burden can be continually monitored without destructive sampling of the host population.

In understanding the processes occurring under the long-term free-running conditions, it is worthwhile initially to consider the basic life processes of *G. bullatarudis* on isolated guppies.

Parasite reproduction and survival

The birth process in *G. bullatarudis* was first described by Turnbull (1956). She noted that at birth *G. bullatarudis* contain three generations of embryos. Each when born carries with it the future generations and leaves the parent fluke with an empty uterus. At 25°C, newborn young give birth to their first offspring 1 day after they are born and then produce their second and third offspring at intervals of 2.5 and 2 days, respectively (Scott, 1982). The longer time delay for second and third births is a reflection of the extra time required for development of the embryo from the egg as opposed to development from an almost fully formed young. The average fecundity for *G. bullatarudis* is 1.68. As a result of the paedogenesis and the regular release of an egg into the uterus of the innermost embryo, at least nine consecutive generations of *G. bullatarudis* can be produced at daily intervals, in the absence of cross-fertilization, without reducing the average birth rate for each generation (Scott, 1982). Similarly, 12 and 20 consecutive generations have been reported respectively by Braun (1966) for *Gyrodactylus wageneri* Malmberg, 1957 and by Lester and Adams (1974a) for *G. alexanderi*.

Parasites survive on average for 4.20 days (Scott, 1982). As with many other parasites (e.g. Anderson & Lethbridge, 1975; Anderson & Whitfield, 1975; Anderson, Whitfield & Mills, 1977; Evans and Gordon, 1983), the instantaneous death rate increases exponentially with age. Both the birth and death processes were shown to be temperature dependent (Scott & Nokes, 1984). The birth rate and the intrinsic rate of increase peaked at 27.5°C, whereas the maximum average expected life span occurred at 21°C. *G. bullatarudis* was not able to survive at 30°C, but did survive at the lowest temperature tested (17°C).

Population growth and decay characteristics

The consequence of the viviparity and paedogenesis is the ability of the parasite to undergo rapid exponential growth on an isolated fish. Fish infected initially with three *G. bullatarudis* and isolated in 200 ml of water can be divided into three groups based on the resultant parasite population dynamics. On some fish (9% of 284), the parasite population does not establish. Establishment is defined as a) the persistence of the parasite for at least 6 days and b) parasite burden that increases above three at some time during the infection. On a second group of fish (41%), the parasite population becomes established, undergoes exponential growth for a period of time and then plateaus and decreases until the parasite goes extinct. The time scale and peak burden for this group of fish is highly variable. On the third group of fish (50%), the parasite population establishes and continues to grow exponentially until the fish dies. Figure 1 presents a summary of data gathered to date showing the mean patterns for the latter two groups.

Even under the simplified conditions of parasite population growth and decay on isolated guppies, a large degree of variability was noted among the fish. In fact, the parasite population quickly becomes highly overdispersed such that a few fish harbour the majority of the parasites. This high degree of variability can be generated simply by chance in the birth–death process as shown by Scott (1982). This element of chance in generating overdispersion is important in the free-running situation as well.

A theoretical estimate of the probability of extinction due to chance (Bailey, 1964), calculated using the average instantaneous birth and death rates and the initial population size (3), was 0.174. This estimate is almost double the observed initial extinction (group 1) and suggests that chance may have been the dominant factor

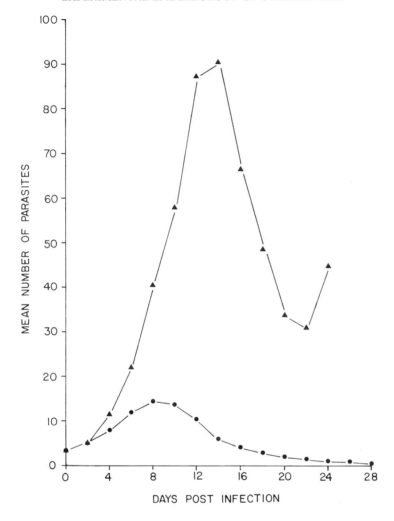

Figure 1. Parasite population dynamics on isolated guppies. The upper curve represents the mean parasite burden on 141 fish that died during infection; the lower curve represents the mean burden on 111 fish that recovered from the infection.

in initial establishment. However, the theoretical estimate is considerably lower than that observed when the recovered fish are included, indicating that processes in addition to chance are important in the extinction of the parasite population on fish that recover.

The fundamental difference between fish that recover and those that die may be genetic. The importance of genetics in host susceptibility/resistance to infectious agents has been demonstrated for a variety of associations (Skamene, Kongshavn & Landy, 1980; Brindley & Dobson, 1981; Blackwell, 1983; Blackwell, 1985, this volume). It is important to note, however, that ability to recover is also likely to be a function of the initial infection dose. Because of the immediate exponential growth in parasite numbers that occurs, it is probable that all fish would succumb if infected with a large enough inoculum.

Transmission

The final process to be considered before addressing the long-term experiments is the ability of *G. bullatarudis* to disperse to other guppies.

Transmission has been investigated in a number of experimental situations. When a single infected fish with a known parasite burden is placed with a single uninfected fish in 200 ml of water for 3 h, the net transmission increases with parasite burden (Fig. 2). Even though this experiment has been replicated 122 times it is still unclear whether the *rate* of transmission is dependent on parasite burden, as more replicates of high donor burdens are required. It would seem reasonable for transmission to be density-dependent, either as a result of an increased tendency of parasites to transfer perhaps due to an unsuitable habitat on the heavily infected fish and/or as a result of an increased tendency for contact between the uninfected and the heavily infected fish. Heavily infected fish become lethargic and the fin rays often stick together resulting in abnormal swimming behaviour. Such differences do attract the attention of other guppies and do increase the number of contacts.

When a single infected guppy is placed with four uninfected guppies in 400 ml of water for 24 h, 20.2% of parasites transfer onto an average of 1.9 naïve guppies. It appears as though there is a considerable risk associated with transmission, however, because in both of these experimental situations, a substantial proportion of the initial parasite population is lost. Scott & Anderson (1984) have estimated that only 35–39% of the parasites, that attempt to transfer, succeed.

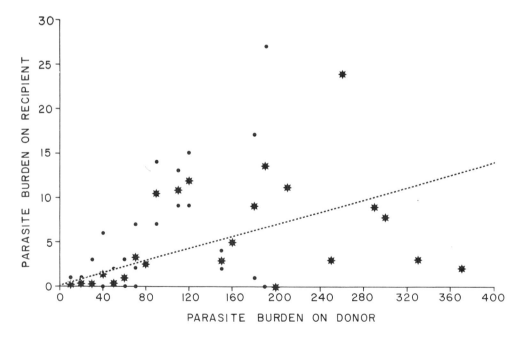

Figure 2. Results of 3-h transmission experiments involving one infected (donor) and one uninfected (recipient) guppy. Stars represent mean numbers of parasites transferring at each donor burden. Dots represent the range of individual values and the dashed line represents the linear regression model, $Y = 0.065 + 0.035X$ ($r = 0.56$, d.f. $= 120$, $P < 0.01$).

An unusual aspect of *G. bullatarudis* transmission is the ability to transfer from dead to live hosts. When a guppy dies, the parasites appear to recognize that the host is dead within approximately 30 min. The behaviour of the parasites then changes. They stop feeding and extend their bodies perpendicular to the fish surface and probe the environment continually. They transfer immediately when another fish passes, and as many as 50–100 parasites will attach in a single sweep of a caudal fin, for instance. The rate of transmission from these dead fish is substantially higher than that from live fish. Once bacterial attack of the fish has begun, the parasites either move off the fish onto the substrate or die. Consequently, although transmission from dead fish is at a higher rate, it occurs over a relatively short time. As was seen for heavily infected fish, dead fish also attract the attention of other guppies and they frequently investigate and eat the dead fish. This also increases the chances of parasite transmission by increasing contacts between hosts.

Parasite transmission also occurs when *G. bullatarudis* drop off one fish and reattach to another. The parasite probably leaves a fish accidentally either on sloughed host tissues, or by attempting an unsuccessful transfer, or by moving onto the substrate or the surface film. The life span of the parasite off the fish is very short (average of 11.6 hours) and the parasite is only able to reattach during a brief portion of this time (pers. obs.). It is considered that this is an infrequent means of transmission.

Data on transmission have thus shown that a) parasites transfer from infected to uninfected hosts during fish contact, b) the number of parasites moving onto the uninfected fish increases with parasite burden, c) there is a risk associated with transferral, and d) parasites are able to transfer from dead fish to live fish at a greater rate than transmission between live fish, presumably due to the tendency of guppies to investigate, and eat dead (or moribund) fish.

EXPERIMENTAL EPIDEMIOLOGY

Protocol

Given this information, it is now appropriate to consider the long-term experiments that were designed to investigate parasite population dynamics and persistence in guppy populations. The details of this study have been reported elsewhere (Scott & Anderson, 1984) and will be summarized here. The protocol for all experiments was based on initially infecting one 10 mm guppy with 10 *G. bullatarudis* and introducing it into 5 litres of water containing 49 uninfected 10 mm guppies. Four different treatments were then applied in which 20, 9, 2 or 0 10 mm guppies were added at intervals every 2 weeks. The four treatments will be referred to as the high, medium, low and zero levels of immigration. All arenas were monitored twice weekly, at which time, all fish were anaesthetized (0.02% tricaine methanesulphonate, MS222), and total parasite counts were recorded. A control uninfected arena was also monitored without fish immigration.

Results

The detailed results of these replicates are shown in Figs 3, 4, 5 and 6, and discussed at length by Scott & Anderson (1984). In all cases, the prevalence of infection increased rapidly. In the absence of fish immigration, however, the parasite population then decreased and became extinct. During this time, fish mortality was extensive. When fish immigration occurred, the parasite population persisted over a 5-month period and showed recurrent epidemic behaviour with cycles of increasing amplitude in the medium and high level immigration arenas and cycles of decreasing amplitude in the low level immigration arenas. The parasite population fluctuated in degree of overdispersion throughout the long-term experiments, with a tendency for highest aggregation (as measured by variance to mean ratios) at high parasite burdens (Fig. 7).

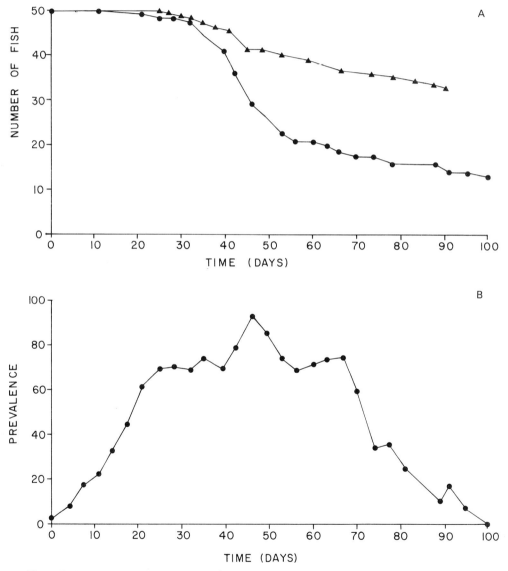

Figure 3. Host and parasite population dynamics in the zero immigration treatment and the control uninfected arena. A, Guppy survival in the control arena (upper curve, triangles) and in the zero immigration arena (lower curve, dots); B, prevalence of infection in the zero immigration arena.

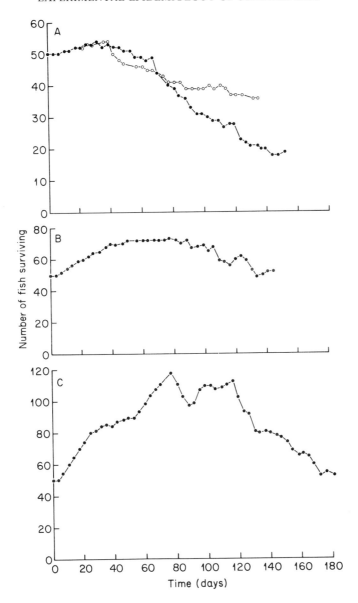

Figure 4. Guppy population dynamics in the low (A), medium (B), and high (C) immigration arenas. The two curves in A represent two replicates (from Scott & Anderson, 1984).

Discussion

These long-term experiments served to highlight several features of the guppy–*Gyrodactylus* association. Firstly, it is clear that under more natural conditions (compared to the isolated guppy situation), *G. bullatarudis* is a pathogen that is capable of substantially reducing host population size. Secondly, in order for parasites to persist over the long term, a continual input of susceptibles seems to

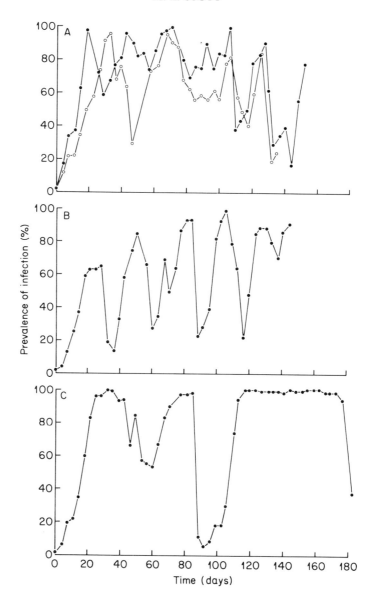

Figure 5. Prevalence of infection in the low (A), medium (B) and high (C) immigration arenas. The two curves in A represent two replicates (from Scott & Anderson, 1984).

be required. Thirdly, parasite aggregation is a dominant feature of the association. Finally, the host–parasite system has a tendency to oscillate.

Parasite-induced host mortality

Host mortality was found to be positively correlated with mean parasite burden (Fig. 8). The substantial mortality caused by *G. bullatarudis* in its natural host serves as an example of parasite-induced host mortality that is capable of regulating the host population. In the arenas with fish immigration, it is probable that fish densities were also acting to regulate the population in a fixed volume of water. Silliman

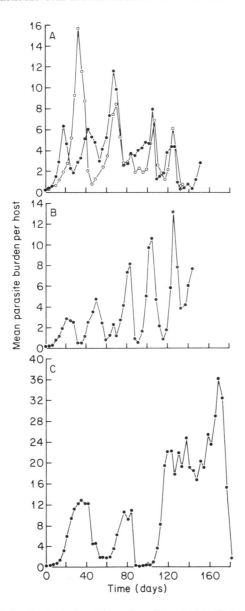

Figure 6. Mean parasite burden in the low (A), medium (B) and high (C) immigration arenas. The two curves in A represent two replicates (from Scott & Anderson, 1984).

& Gutsell (1958) maintained freely breeding colonies of guppies and found that the populations equilibrated at densities of approximately 8/litre. However, in their aquaria, 86% of the population were mature fish. In the present study, only a maximum of 60% of the fish were above 16 mm in length. A comparison of the control uninfected arena with the zero immigration arena indicates that at fish densities of less than 10/litre, the parasite reduced the host population by 50–60%. There is considerable controversy in the literature regarding the compensatory *vs* additive roles of parasite-induced host mortalities in vertebrate populations. This study indicates the additive effect of parasite-induced host mortalities, but as Holmes

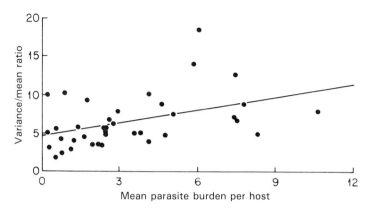

Figure 7. Relationship between variance to mean ratio and mean burden for the medium level immigration arena. The line represents the linear regression model, $Y = 4.51 + 0.57X$ ($r = 0.44$, d.f. $= 37$, $P < 0.01$).

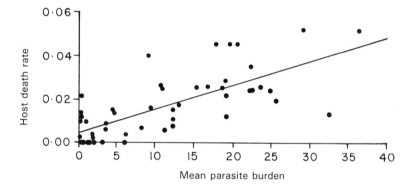

Figure 8. Relationship between instantaneous host death rate and mean parasite burden for the high level immigration arena. The line represents the linear regression model, $Y = 0.0044 + 0.0011X$ ($r = 0.74$, d.f. $= 48$, $P < 0.01$).

(1982) noted, it is still important to obtain field examples where other potential regulating factors act (i.e. predation, competition).

Importance of susceptibles for persistence

It has long been recognized in human epidemiology that disease persistence requires a susceptible population. In fact, a principle goal of many control programs is to increase the level of herd immunity sufficiently so that the parasite is unable to locate a susceptible host. Parasite ecologists are also recognizing the importance of the susceptible portion of the population and theoretical predictions of the threshold susceptible population are available for a range of human and non-human infectious agents (Anderson, 1982a,b,c; Keymer, 1982; Wilson, Smith & Thomas, 1982).

Using a mathematical model to describe the dynamics of G. *bullatarudis* in the long-term experiments, Scott & Anderson (1984) have shown that the critical density of susceptible hosts, X_t, necessary for an epidemic to occur is given by

$$X_t = (b + \hat{\alpha})/\Lambda \qquad (1)$$

and that, for long-term persistence of the parasite, the density of susceptibles, X, must equal or exceed the value

$$X \geqslant (b + \hat{\alpha})/(\Lambda q_1) \tag{2}$$

where

$$q_1 = \exp[-(b + \hat{\alpha})\tau_1] \tag{3}$$

and where b, $\hat{\alpha}$, Λ and τ_1 are the instantaneous natural host mortality rate, the instantaneous infection-induced mortality rate, the instantaneous infection rate and the time period that the hosts remain infected, respectively.

It is probable that the extinction of the parasite in the absence of fish immigration resulted from either the low densities of fish present during the decline of parasite numbers or the potential unsuitability of available fish as hosts.

Temporal dynamics of aggregation

That parasites tend to be overdispersed in their host populations has been well documented for field populations (e.g. Crofton, 1971; Pennycuick, 1971; Anderson, 1974; Gordon & Rau, 1982). Scott (1982) demonstrated the potential for aggregation in *G. bullatarudis* and showed that in a simple birth–death system, as is the case on isolated guppies, stochastic processes are sufficient to generate the overdispersion. Factors tending to generate overdispersion have been summarized by Anderson & Gordon (1982) and include heterogeneity among hosts in behaviour and effective immunity, and direct reproduction of the parasites. Data presented above suggest a distinct heterogeneity among fish in their ability to cope with an initial infection and studies in progress have demonstrated heterogeneity in the responses to challenge infections (Scott, submitted). Direct reproduction is certainly a dominant feature of this host–parasite association and, consequently, it is not surprising to find high levels of parasite aggregation in the long-term arenas.

These experiments have also demonstrated the temporal dynamics of aggregation and it is important that this phenomenon be recognized. Parasite ecologists generally agree with the concept of overdispersion in parasite populations, but often this is seen to be an all or none phenomenon that is static. This view is, in some ways, encouraged by the growing number of theoretical models of host–parasite interactions in which k (a parameter of the negative binomial distribution) is assumed to be a constant (e.g. Anderson, 1978; Scott & Anderson, 1984). The idea of the constancy of aggregation has been most effectively refuted by Anderson & Gordon (1982) where they stressed that, at any point in time, the observed dispersion pattern reflects the current balance between opposing forces, some tending to increase overdispersion and others tending to decrease it, with the result that, through time, a single population may be highly aggregated at some times and randomly dispersed at others.

Data on fish length were collected throughout the long-term experiments and it is worth noting that the degree of aggregation tended to be highest in the smaller fish. The implications of this for the population genetics of the fish population are interesting. It has been demonstrated above that guppies differ in their response to a *G. bullatarudis* infection and it has been suggested that this could have a genetic component. If some guppies are genetically incapable of combatting a *Gyrodactylus* infection, it is probable that they would die as a result of their first exposure to the parasite. Using the high level immigration experiment as an example, the prevalence of infection was maintained at essentially 100% for a period of 45 days, during which time, all introduced guppies became infected within 4 days. During this time, the parasites were extremely aggregated in the younger size classes of fish, and it is probable that substantial mortality occurred in the young size classes as well. If one assumes that mortality will occur predominantly in that component of the population that is unable to combat the infection, one would predict that the genetic heterogeneity of the surviving fish in the arena would be less than that of an uninfected population. Thus, the fish that maintain the infection over the long-term are the ones that are able to control their parasite burdens. The tendency for higher aggregation among the young fish tends to support this, especially in light of the fact that larger guppies are able to harbour much higher parasite burdens than smaller fish.

Tendency to oscillate

Perhaps the most intriguing aspect of the long-term studies is the oscillatory behaviour of parasite prevalence and abundance (in the absence of oscillations in host numbers). Field studies have often shown that species of *Gyrodactylus* cycle in numbers, but these cycles are invariably seasonal, presumably related to temperature fluctuations. In the experimental arenas, temperature was constant, and the cycle had a relatively short period (a month compared to a year in field studies). In an attempt to elucidate the driving force behind these cycles, a number of mathematical models were formulated, with a view to testing specific hypotheses to determine whether oscillatory behaviour could be a potential outcome. A number of features were included in these models, such as time delays, various parasite distribution patterns, density-dependent parasite transmission, density-dependent acquisition of resistance, and partial resistance to reinfection. The results of these attempts were not very satisfactory. It was possible to generate sustained cycles in parasite abundance by incorporating, as a time delay, a temporary refractory period where parasite transmission is reduced, but these cycles did not have the qualitative characteristics of the observed cycles. The mathematical approach did, however, indicate that a temporary refractory period to reinfection could be important and this aspect has since been investigated.

Refractory period to reinfection

Scott & Robinson (1984) demonstrated that fish treated with a weak formalin solution 1 or 2 weeks after an initial infection, and immediately challenged, were less suitable hosts. The percentage establishment of the parasite was lower, the peak burden attained by the challenge infection was lower, and the duration of the challenge infection was shorter (Fig. 9). Research in progress indicates that this reduced suitability persists for at least 2 weeks but appears to be lost after 4–6 weeks. This corresponds well with the pattern observed by Lester & Adams (1974b) for *G. alexanderi* on sticklebacks, where the parasite population dynamics were similar to those on naïve hosts at four weeks after recovery.

The functional basis of the refractory period is not known. Lester (1972) described a strong tissue response by sticklebacks which involved shedding of large sheets of mucoid material. He considered the possibility that this response increased parasite mortality because of dislodgement. In the case of *G. bullatarudis*, gross tissue

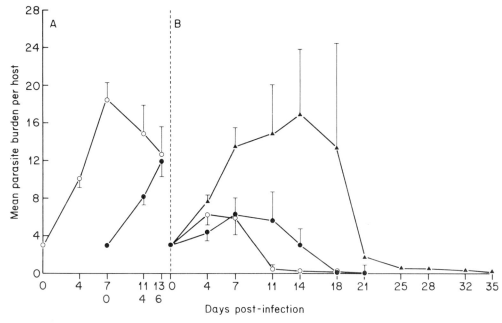

Figure 9. Mean parasite burden per guppy during initial and challenge infections. A, Results of the initial infection of 6 (dots) and 13 (open circles) day duration; B, results of the immediate challenge of the 6 (dots) and 13 (open circles) day initial infections, and a control unchallenged group (triangles). The dashed vertical line represents treatment with formalin and re-infection (from Scott & Robinson, 1984).

changes are frequently observed, and it may be that the surface of recovered fish is not as habitable due to non-specific tissue responses to the initial infection. It is also possible that the guppies mount a specific anti-*Gyrodactylus* immune response, perhaps mediated through mucous-secreted antibodies. Regardless of the mechanism, however, the consequences for the parasite population dynamics are the same.

The inability of the mathematical models to mimic the laboratory experiments highlights the fact that an important process in the biology of *G. bullatarudis* and guppies has not been considered, or is improperly understood, and thus underlines the value of the combined theoretical and experimental approach.

CONCLUSIONS

In conclusion, the observations presented in this paper demonstrate the value of a long-term experimental epidemiological approach combined with short-term experiments and theoretical studies for attempting to understand the population dynamics of host–parasite associations. It is also clear that parasite ecology depends, to a large extent, on interactions between genetics and specific or non-specific immunity. Consequently, it is critical that parasitologists in different disciplines communicate so that host–parasite interactions be considered in the whole.

ACKNOWLEDGEMENTS

Much of this research was undertaken while on a NATO Postdoctoral Fellowship
at Imperial College, London, U.K., in collaboration with Professor Roy M.
Anderson. His assistance and wisdom are gratefully acknowledged. Assistance from
Dr Phil Harris (University of Birmingham), Dr R. Madhavi (Andhra University,
Waltair, India), Dr G. Gibson and Mr R. Bray (British Museum (Natural History))
and from Kathy Keller (McGill University) is greatly appreciated. Funding from
a Winifred Cullis Grant from the International Federation of University Women,
a Natural Sciences and Engineering Research Council Grant (U0204), and the
Faculty of Graduate Studies, McGill University is also acknowledged. Research
at the Institute of Parasitology is supported by NSERC and the Fonds FCAC pour
l'aide et le soutien à la recherche.

REFERENCES

ANDERSON, D. P., 1974. In S. F. Snieszko & H. R. Axelrod (Eds), *Fish Immunology*. Reigate, Surrey: T.F.H.
    Publications Inc. Ltd.
ANDERSON, R. M., 1974. Population dynamics of the cestode *Caryophyllaeus laticeps* (Pallas, 1781) in the bream
    (*Abramis brama* L.). *Journal of Animal Ecology, 43:* 305–321.
ANDERSON, R. M., 1978. The regulation of host population growth by parasitic species. *Parasitology, 76:* 119–158.
ANDERSON, R. M., 1982a. Directly transmitted viral and bacterial infections of man. In R. M. Anderson
    (Ed.), *The Population Dynamics of Infectious Diseases: Theory and Applications:* 1–37. London: Chapman & Hall.
ANDERSON, R. M., 1982b. The population dynamics and control of hookworm and roundworm infections.
    In R. M. Anderson (Ed.), *The Population Dynamics of Infectious Diseases: Theory and Applications:* 67–108. London:
    Chapman & Hall.
ANDERSON, R. M., 1982c. Fox rabies. In R. M. Anderson (Ed.), *The Population Dynamics of Infectious Diseases:
    Theory and Applications:* 242–261. London: Chapman & Hall.
ANDERSON, R. M. & CROMBIE, J., 1984. Experimental studies of age-prevalence curves for *Schistosoma
    mansoni* infections in populations of *Biomphalaria glabrata*. *Parasitology, 89,* 79–105.
ANDERSON, R. M. & CROMBIE, J., 1985. Experimental studies of age-intensity and age-prevalence profiles
    of infection: *Schistosoma mansoni* in snails and mice. This volume: 111–146.
ANDERSON, R. M. & GORDON, D. M., 1982. Processes influencing the distribution of parasite numbers
    within host populations with special emphasis on parasite-induced host mortalities. *Parasitology, 85:* 373–398.
ANDERSON, R. M. & LETHBRIDGE, R. C., 1975. An experimental study of the survival characteristics,
    activity and energy reserves of the hexacanths of *Hymenolepis diminuta*. *Parasitology, 71:* 137–151.
ANDERSON, R. M. & WHITFIELD, P. J., 1975. Survival characteristics of the free-living cercarial population
    of the ectoparasitic digenean *Transversotrema patialense* (Soparker, 1924). *Parasitology, 70:* 295–310.
ANDERSON, R. M., WHITFIELD, P. J. & MILLS, C. A., 1977. An experimental study of the population
    dynamics of an ectoparasitic digenean, *Transversotrema patialense*: the cercarial and adult stages. *Journal of Animal
    Ecology, 46:* 555–580.
BAILEY, N. T. J., 1964. *The elements of stochastic processes*. London: John Wiley.
BLACKWELL, J. M., 1983. Regulation of *Leishmania* populations within the host. V. Resistance to *L. donovani*
    in wild mice. *Journal of Tropical Medicine and Hygiene, 86:* 17–22.
BLACKWELL, J. M., 1985. A murine model of genetically controlled host responses to leishmaniasis. This
    volume: 147–156.
BRAUN, F., 1966. Beiträge zur mikroskopischen anatomie und fortpflanzungsbiologie von *Gyrodactylus wageneri*
    v. Nordmann, 1832. *Zeitschrift für Parasitenkunde, 28:* 142–174.
BRINDLEY, P. J. & DOBSON, C., 1981. Genetic control of liability to infection with *Nematospiroides dubius*
    in mice: selection of refractory and liable populations of mice. *Parasitology, 83:* 51–65.
BYCHOWSKY, B. E., 1957. *Monogenetic trematodes, their systematics and phylogeny*. (translated from Russian by
    P. C. Oustinoff). Washington: American Institute of Biological Sciences.
CHUBB, J. C., 1977. Seasonal occurrence of helminths in freshwater fishes. Part I. Monogenea. *Advances in
    Parasitology, 15:* 133–199.
CROFTON, H. D., 1971. A quantitative approach to parasitism. *Parasitology, 63:* 179–193.
DUSSAULT, G. V. & KRAMER, D. L., 1981. Food and feeding behavior of the guppy, *Poecilia reticulata* (Pisces:
    Poeciliidae). *Canadian Journal of Zoology, 59:* 684–701.

ERGENS, R., 1981. Variability of hard parts of opisthaptor in *Gyrodactylus truttae* Glaser, 1974 (Gyrodactylidae: Monogenea). *Folia Parasitologica (Praha), 28:* 37–42.

EVANS, N. A. & GORDON, D. M., 1983. Experimental studies on the transmission dynamics of the cercariae of *Echinoparyphium recurvatum* (Digenea: Echinostomatidae). *Parasitology, 87:* 167–174.

FENNER, F., 1948. The epizootic behaviour of mousepox (infectious ectromelia of mice). II. The course of events in long-continued epidemics. *Journal of Hygiene, 46:* 383–393.

FENNER, F., 1949. Studies in mousepox (infectious ectromelia of mice). IV. Quantitative investigations on the spread of virus through the host in actively and passively immunized animals. *Australian Journal of Experimental Biology and Medical Sciences, 27:* 1–18.

GORDON, D. M. & RAU, M. E., 1982. Possible evidence for mortality induced by the parasite *Apatemon gracilis* in a population of brook sticklebacks *Culaea inconstans*. *Parasitology, 84:* 41–47.

GREENWOOD, M. & TOPLEY, W. W. C., 1925. A further contribution to the experimental study of epidemiology. *Journal of Hygiene, 24:* 45–110.

GREENWOOD, M., BRADFORD-HILL, A., TOPLEY, W. W. C. & WILSON, J., 1936. Experimental epidemiology. *Medical Research Council Special Report*, No. 209, 204 pp.

HANZELOVA, V. & ZITNAN, R., 1982. The seasonal dynamics of the invasion cycle of *Gyrodactylus katharineri* Malmberg, 1964 (Monogenea). *Helminthologia, 19:* 257–265.

HARRIS, P., 1982. *Studies on the biology of the Gyrodactyloidea (Monogenea)*. Ph.D. Thesis, University of London.

HEGGBERGET, T. G. & JOHNSEN, B. O., 1982. Infestations by *Gyrodactylus* sp. of Atlantic salmon, *Salmo salar* L., in Norwegian rivers. *Journal of Fish Biology, 21:* 15–26.

HOLMES, J. C., 1982. Impact of infectious disease agents on the population growth and geographical distribution of animals. In R. M. Anderson & R. M. May (Eds), *Population Biology of Infectious Disease Agents*, Dahlem Konferenzen. Berlin: Springer-Verlag.

KATHARINER, L., 1904. Uber die Entwicklung von *Gyrodactylus elegans* v. Nordmann. *Zoologische Jahrbücher Suppl., 7:* 519–550.

KEYMER, A., 1981. Population dynamics of *Hymenolepis diminuta* in the intermediate host. *Journal of Animal Ecology, 50:* 941–950.

KEYMER, A., 1982. Tapeworm infections. In R. M. Anderson (Ed.), *The Population Dynamics of Infectious Diseases: Theory and Applications:* 109–138. London: Chapman & Hall.

KHALIL, L. F., 1970. Further studies on *Macrogyrodactylus polypteri*, a monogenean on the African freshwater fish *Polypterus senegalus*. *Journal of Helminthology, 44:* 329–348.

KIRBY, J. M., 1981. Seasonal occurrence of the ectoparasite *Gyrodactylus atratuli* on spotfin shiners. *Transactions of the American Fisheries Society, 110:* 462–464.

LESTER, R. J. G., 1972. Attachment of *Gyrodactylus* to *Gasterosteus* and host response. *Journal of Parasitology, 58:* 717–722.

LESTER, R. J. G. & ADAMS, J. R., 1974a. *Gyrodactylus alexanderi*: reproduction, mortality, and effect on its host *Gasterosteus aculeatus*. *Canadian Journal of Zoology, 52:* 827–833.

LESTER, R. J. G. & ADAMS, J. R., 1974b. A simple model of a *Gyrodactylus* population. *International Journal for Parasitology, 4:* 497–506.

MALMBERG, G., 1970. The excretory systems and the marginal hooks as a basis for the systematics of *Gyrodactylus* (Trematoda, Monogenea). *Arkiv für Zoologi, 23:* 235 pp + 8 plates.

MALMBERG, G., 1973. On a *Gyrodactylus* species from Northern Sweden and the subgeneric position of *G. hrabei* Ergens, 1957 (Trematoda, Monogenea). *Zoologica Scripta, 2:* 39–42.

McCALLUM, H. I., 1982. *Population dynamics of* Ichthyophthirius multifiliis. Ph.D. thesis, University of London.

PARK, T., 1948. Experimental studies of interspecies competition. 1. Competition between populations of the flour beetles, *Tribolium confusum* Duval and *Tribolium castaneum* Herbst. *Ecological Monographs, 18:* 267–307.

PARKER, J. D., 1965. *Seasonal occurrence, transmission and host specificity of the monogenetic trematode* Gyrodactylus elegans *from the golden shiner* (Notemigonus crysoleuces). Ph.D. Thesis, 82 pp. Southern Illinois University.

PENNYCUICK, L., 1971. Frequency distributions of parasites in a population of three-spined sticklebacks, *Gasterosteus aculeatus* L., with particular reference to the negative binomial distribution. *Parasitology, 63:* 389–406.

RAWSON, M. V. & ROGERS, W. A., 1973. Seasonal occurrence of *Gyrodactylus macrochiri* Hoffman and Putz, 1964 on bluegill and largemouth bass. *Journal of Wildlife Diseases, 9:* 174–177.

ROSEN, D. E. & BAILEY, R. M., 1963. The poeciliid fishes (Cyprinodontiformes), their structures, zoogeography, and systematics. *Bulletin of the American Museum of Natural History, 126:* 1–176.

SCOTT, M. E., 1982. Reproductive potential of *Gyrodactylus bullatarudis* (Monogenea) on guppies (*Poecilia reticulata*). *Parasitology, 85:* 217–236.

SCOTT, M. E. (in preparation). Dynamics of challenge infections of *Gyrodactylus bullatarudis* (Monogenea) on guppies (*Poecilia reticulata*). *J. Fish. Dis.*, submitted.

SCOTT, M. E. & ANDERSON, R. M., 1984. The population dynamics of *Gyrodactylus bullatarudis* (Monogenea) within laboratory populations of the fish host *Poecilia reticulata*. *Parasitology, 89:* 159–194.

SCOTT, M. E. & NOKES, D. J., 1984. Temperature-dependent reproduction and survival of *Gyrodactylus bullatarudis* (Monogenea) on guppies (*Poecilia reticulata*). *Parasitology, 89:* 221–227.

SCOTT, M. E. & ROBINSON, M. A., 1984. Challenge infections of *Gyrodactylus bullatarudis* (Monogenea) on guppies, *Poecilia reticulata* (Peters), following treatment. *Journal of Fish Biology, 24:* 581–586.

SILLIMAN, R. P., 1948. Factors affecting population levels in *Lebistes reticulatus*. *Copeia, 1948:* 40–47.

SILLIMAN, R. P. & GUTSELL, J. S., 1958. Experimental exploitation of fish populations. *Fishery Bulletin of the Fish and Wildlife Service, 58, Fishery Bulletin 133:* 215–252.

SKAMENE, E., KONGSHAVN, P. A. L. & LANDY, M., 1980. *Genetic Control of Natural Resistance to Infection and Malignancy*. London: Academic Press.

STIVEN, A. E., 1964. Experimental studies on the epidemiology of the host-parasite system, *Hydra* and *Hydramoeba hydroxena* (Entz). II. The components of a simple epidemic. *Ecological Monographs, 34:* 119–142.

TURNBULL, E. R., 1956. *Gyrodactylus bullatarudis* n.sp. from *Lebistes reticulatus* Peters with a study of its life cycle. *Canadian Journal of Zoology, 34:* 583–594.

WASSOM, D. L., BROOKS, B. O., BABISH, J. G. & DAVID, C. S., 1983. A gene mapping between the S and D regions of the H-2 complex influences resistance to *Trichinella spiralis* infections in mice. *Journal of Immunogenetics, 10:* 371–378.

WILSON, R. A., SMITH, G. & THOMAS, M. R., 1982. Fascioliasis. R. M. Anderson (Ed.), In *The Population Dynamics of Infectious Diseases: Theory and Applications:* 262–319, London: Chapman & Hall.

Genetics, immunity and parasite survival

D. WAKELIN

M.R.C. Experimental Parasitology Group,
Department of Zoology, University of Nottingham,
University Park, Nottingham, NG7 2RD, U.K.

The overdispersion of macroparasites within host populations influences both parasite transmission and survival. It is therefore an important component in theoretical modelling of host–parasite interactions. Many host factors can contribute to the generation of overdispersion, including behaviour, ecology, natural resistance and acquired immunity. In situations where host populations are more or less uniformly exposed to infection with a well-adapted parasite, variations in individual ability to express effective immune responses are likely to play a major role.

Although some progress has been made in analysing the genetic and immunological mechanisms underlying such variation in natural host–parasite populations, there are considerable difficulties associated with the study of genetically and immunologically ill-defined wild hosts. Attention has therefore been focused upon analysis of variation in experimental model systems, using the laboratory mouse as host, and species of parasites which are related, or similar to, species of medical or veterinary interest. The paper discusses the results of work carried out with two species of tapeworms, *Hymenolepis citelli* (*H.c.*) and *Taenia taeniaeformis* (*T.t.*), and four nematodes, *Trichuris muris* (*T.m.*), *Trichinella spiralis* (T.sp.), *Dipetalonema viteae* (*D.v.*) and *Nematospiroides dubius*. For these parasites, the success of transmission between final hosts is influenced by the numbers of larvae accumulating in intermediate hosts (*H.c.*, *T.t.*), by the numbers of eggs released in host faecal material (*H.c.*, *T.t.*, *T.m.*), by the numbers of infective larvae accumulating in host muscle tissue (*T.sp.*) and by the numbers of larvae circulating in the blood (*D.v.*). Consideration is given to the ways in which acquired immunity influences these parameters, to the occurrence of genetically determined variation in the effectiveness of immunity, and to the mechanisms through which this variation is expressed. The ways in which such variation may contribute to overdispersion is then discussed. In the case of *N. dubius*, the emphasis of the discussion is upon variation in the degree of immunodepression associated with infection and on the relationship of such variable immunodepression to overdispersion of third-party species present in the same host.

KEY WORDS: — Genetics — host-parasite relationship — immunity — macroparasites — transmission.

CONTENTS

Ecology and Genetics of Host–Parasite Interactions
ISBN: 0 12 593 690 7

INTRODUCTION

The quantitative analysis of host–parasite population biology is a comparatively recent field of study, but one that is already making significant contributions to our understanding of the epidemiology and control of parasitic disease. It has, in addition, illuminated many aspects of host–parasite relationships hitherto recognized more empirically. One important example that can be cited concerns the distribution of parasites within host populations. It has long been recognized that macroparasites (helminths and arthropods) are not usually randomly or evenly distributed within their hosts, instead their distribution is highly aggregated. Although Milne (1943) characterized one such distribution (tick populations on sheep hosts) as overdispersion, and Fisher (1941), using Milne's results, showed that the data were fully described by the negative binomial distribution, it was not until some 30 years later that the significance of these findings began to be recognized and interpreted in terms of parasite survival and transmission of infection (Crofton, 1971a,b; Bradley, 1972). The last few years have seen an explosion of interest in this aspect of parasite population biology, and the subject has been discussed in several major reviews, notably by Anderson and co-workers (Anderson, 1982a,b; Anderson & Gordon, 1982; Anderson & May, 1978, 1982). It is now accepted that the small number of heavily infected hosts into which parasite populations are aggregated can play a significant role in the maintenance and survival of the parasite species, and can contribute disproportionately to the overall transmission of infection between members of the host species.

Crofton (1971a) identified six situations in which overdispersion of parasites might arise and three of these are particularly relevant to the present paper. Overdispersion may be generated:
(1) As the result of infection increasing the chances of further infection occurring;
(2) As the result of infection decreasing the chances of further infection;
(3) As a result of the variation in host individuals which makes the chances of infection unequal.
No connections were made between any of these situations.

Bradley (1972) considered that the second of these three possibilities would be more likely to reduce, rather than increase, parasite aggregation in the host population, presumably making the reasonable assumption that development of acquired immunity would occur in all members of the host population. Neither author had available to them at that time the very considerable literature on genetically determined variation in immune responsiveness which now exists, and which makes a significant connection between the second and third situations identified by Crofton. In addition, little was then known of the ability of macroparasites to induce specific and non-specific immunosuppression, a phenomenon which extends the limited interpretation given by Crofton for the first situation described above.

The emphasis upon acquired immunity which the present paper places should not be taken to imply that this aspect of the host–parasite relationship is necessarily considered to be the major factor responsible for overdispersion of parasite populations. As Fig. 1 shows, acquired immunity is only one of several influences which determine the outcome of a particular host–parasite association; overdispersion may be generated by any variation which results in the differential

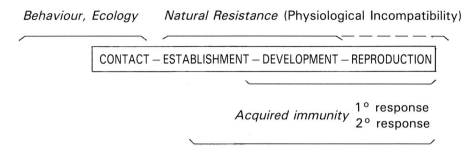

Figure 1. Scheme illustrating the points at which behavioural, ecological and resistance factors may influence the host–parasite relationship.

infection or survival of parasites in individual hosts. Nevertheless, an emphasis upon acquired immunity may be justified when it is considered that the evolution of particular relationships necessarily demands an adaptation of the parasite to the behavioural, ecological and physiological peculiarities of the host. The ability of the host to respond adaptively to the presence of the parasite can, therefore, be seen as the most important way in which it is possible to exert control over infection by those parasites that have become adapted to survive within the conditions specified by the host phenotype. Parasites are, of course, not passive in the face of this host strategy and have evolved many ways of evading the immune response. One such way, that of inducing non-specific immunodepression in the host, not only facilitates survival of the inducing species but reduces the effectiveness of immunity against species present concurrently.

MACROPARASITES AND IMMUNITY

This paper will concentrate exclusively upon helminth parasites, macroparasites which collectively are a major cause of parasitic disease in man and domestic animals. Three groups of helminths are of particular importance in man, the blood flukes or schistosomes, filarial nematodes and gastro-intestinal nematodes. Schistosomes, gastro-intestinal nematodes and larval cestodes are important causes of mortality and economic loss in sheep and cattle. Our knowledge of the operation and basis of acquired immunity against these parasites in man and domestic stock is at present rather limited, but considerable progress has been made using experimental models, i.e. related parasites that can be maintained and studied in laboratory rodents (reviewed in Wakelin, 1978a, 1982; Mitchell, 1979a, 1979b; Cohen & Warren, 1982). It is only in relatively few cases that acquired immunity depends solely upon direct interaction between the parasite and immune effector mechanisms; in the majority, the measurable effects of immunity reflect co-operation between immune effectors (antibodies, T lymphocytes) and a variety of inflammatory cells and inflammatory mediators. The precise details differ between experimental systems but, in general, common mechanisms can be identified as the basis of responses against parasites living in similar locations of the body (e.g. those in tissues as opposed to those in the intestine).

This background of information about immunity to helminths and the ability to study infections in genetically defined laboratory rodents have made it possible to identify the existence of well-defined genetic variations in immune and inflammatory responses, to associate these variations with differential parasite survival, and to analyse the genetic and immunological mechanisms involved. Although much of this research has been pursued at an academic level, it is important to note that it is providing a conceptual framework for related studies in man and domestic animals, and that it provides data relevant to theoretical models of parasite survival and transmission within host populations.

Six experimental models will be discussed here, all of which involve the laboratory mouse as the host species. The parasite species concerned are the tapeworms *Hymenolepis citelli* and *Taenia taeniaeformis*, and the nematodes *Dipetalonema viteae*, *Nematospiroides dubius*, *Trichinella spiralis* and *Trichuris muris* (Table 1). Details of

Table 1. Summary of laboratory models of helminth infections discussed in this paper

Species of helminth	Final host	Infective stage	Useful model for
Hymenolepis citelli	*Peromyscus* (Mouse)	cysticercoid, in beetle	Intestinal tapeworms of man
Taenia taeniaeformis	Cat	cysticercus, in rodent	Larval tapeworms of man and domestic animals
Dipetalonema viteae	Jird (Mouse)	larva 3, in tick	Filarial nematodes of man
Nematospiroides dubius	*Apodemus* (Mouse)	larva 3, free living	Gastro-intestinal nematodes of man and domestic animals
Trichinella spiralis	Any mammal (Mouse)	larva 1, in muscle cyst	*Trichinella* and other gastro-intestinal nematodes of man and domestic animals
Trichuris muris	Mouse	larva 1, in egg	*Trichuris trichiura* of man

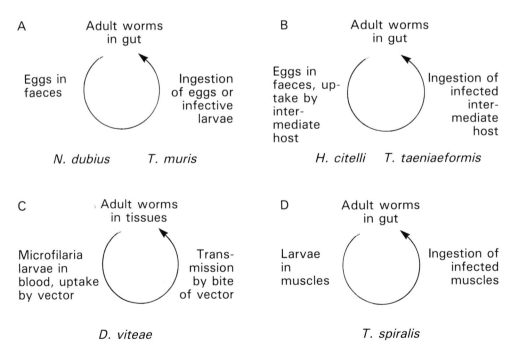

Figure 2. Life cycles of helminth parasites used as laboratory models for genetic studies.

their life cycles are given in Fig. 2, from which it can be seen that the effectiveness of parasite transmission (and thus parasite survival) will be influenced by the numbers of eggs released in host faecal material (A, B), the numbers of larvae circulating in the blood of the host (C) and the numbers of larvae accumulating in the intermediate (B, C) or final host (D). Consideration will be given to the ways in which acquired immunity influences these parameters, to the occurrence of genetically determined variation in the effectiveness of immunity and to the mechanisms through which this variation is expressed. For five of these systems, discussion will centre upon the contribution of variation to overdispersion of the species concerned. In the case of *N. dubius*, the emphasis will be upon the mediation of degrees of non-specific immunodepression leading to overdispersion of third-party species present in the same host.

HYMENOLEPIS CITELLI AND TAENIA TAENIAEFORMIS

Both of these tapeworms are maintained in the field by predator–prey interactions. In both cases, the predator is the final host, i.e. the host in which the adult tapeworm develops and reproduces, and the prey is the intermediate host, i.e. the host in which larval stages develop. Transmission is therefore a function both of the reproductive output of the adult worms, which determines the numbers of eggs released into the environment, and of the success of larval development in the intermediate host, which determines the numbers of infective stages available to the final host.

Hymenolepis citelli, which in nature develops to maturity in the white-footed deermouse *Peromyscus maniculatus*, and utilizes the camel cricket as an intermediate host, was the subject of one of the first detailed studies of host–parasite

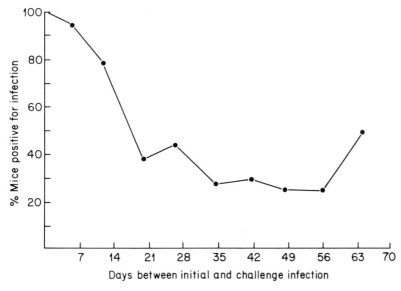

Figure 3. *Hymenolepis citelli* in *Peromyscus maniculatus*. Groups of mice infected with five cysticercoids were challenged with a further five cysticercoids on days 7, 14, 21, 28, 35, 42, 49, 56, or 63. The graph shows the percentage of mice positive for infection with either or both primary and challenge worms when the groups were killed 7 days after challenge. (Redrawn from Wassom *et al.*, 1973.)

immunogenetics (Wassom, Dewitt & Grundmann, 1974). Long-term field collection data had shown that the prevalence of infection in 1094 *P. maniculatus* was only 1.4%, and that the mean number of worms was 3.4. The low prevalence could, in theory, be explained by restricted distribution of intermediate hosts or by the existence of immunity to infection; low levels of infections could reflect the operation of crowding effects, concomitant immunity or thresholds for the operation of protective immunity. Experimental studies showed firstly that there was an effective immunity, which quickly eliminated worms from the intestine, and secondly that not all individual mice were able to express this immunity (Fig. 3; Wassom, Guss & Grundmann, 1973). In the non-responsive mice, worms developed to reproductive maturity, and the hosts remained susceptible to secondary infections. Analysis by selective breeding suggested that the ability to respond protectively to infection was under the control of a single autosomal dominant gene, phenotypically non-responsive mice always breeding true. The theoretical proportion of non-responsive hosts in the population should therefore be higher than the 1.4% recorded in the field. This discrepancy can probably be best explained by the focal distribution of the intermediate host. Transmission of infection would therefore occur only in those foci where there were both adequate numbers of intermediate hosts and of non-responsive individuals. Outside these foci, infections would rapidly die out.

In the life cycle of *T. taeniaeformis*, the final host is a carnivore and the intermediate host a rodent. No field data exist for this system, but there have been intensive studies on the laboratory cycle which is maintained between cats and mice. Early studies (Dow & Jarrett, 1960; Olivier, 1962) showed that infection of mice was unpredictable, some hosts allowing the development of numerous, large larvae within the liver, others failing to produce infective larvae. A more detailed analysis of this variation was carried out by Mitchell, Goding and Rickard (1977), using

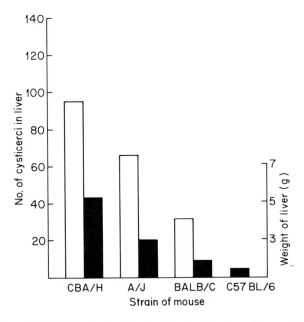

Figure 4. *Taenia taeniaeformis* infections in inbred male mice. Number of larvae in the liver □ and weight of liver ■ 28 days after infection with 200 eggs. (Redrawn from Mitchell *et al.*, 1977.)

a panel of inbred mouse strains. A spectrum of susceptibility to larval development was identified, with particular strains showing markedly different degrees of larval development after infections with a standard number of eggs (Fig. 4). CBA/H mice appeared completely susceptible to infection, whereas C57BL/6 were highly refractory; greater resistance was inherited as a dominant characteristic. The genetic control of this variability was independent of genes linked to the MHC and was expressed primarily through the control of the rate of anti-parasite, IgG antibody production during initial infection (Mitchell, Rajasekariah & Rickard, 1980). Strains which respond before the larval tapeworms develop anti-complementary activity, which interferes with antibody-mediated attack upon the larvae (Hammerberg & Williams, 1978), show resistance to infection; strains with delayed antibody production are susceptible to the initial infection but can effectively resist subsequent challenge.

There is evidence that variation similar to that seen between inbred strains occurs within outbred strains (Olivier, 1962) and it is reasonable to suggest that variation would be expected within wild populations of rodent hosts. Successful transmissions of infection to the final host would therefore depend upon predation by that host upon individual rodents carrying mature infective larvae, and such individuals may be only a small proportion of the total population. Nothing is known of genetically determined variation in susceptibility of the final host to infection by the metacestode larval stages, but, by analogy with *H. citelli* in *P. maniculatus*, it is likely to occur. Thus, there may be a considerable element of chance involved in order for the parasite both to mature as an infective larva and then to mature as an adult tapeworm, despite successful ingestion by rodents of eggs and successful predator–prey interaction.

TRICHURIS MURIS

Trichuris muris is a naturally occurring parasite of house mice, field mice and several other small rodents. There have been few studies of the prevalence of infection in wild populations, but those that have been carried out show relatively low-level and sporadic infections (house mice — Roman, 1951; Behnke & Wakelin, 1973; *Apodemus sylvaticus* — Behnke, pers. comm.). Transmission of infection occurs by ingestion of embryonated eggs. Development of eggs to infectivity under laboratory conditions is relatively slow, taking about 2 months at 20°C (Wakelin, 1969). It can therefore be assumed that by the time eggs released from the host become infective, they would have been freed from faecal pellets and dispersed in the environment.

Explanation of the distribution of *T. muris* may be considered in terms similar to those proposed for *H. citelli* (above). There is good experimental evidence, using laboratory mice, laboratory-bred wild mice and *A. sylvaticus* that protective immunity is expressed during a primary infection and before patency is achieved (Behnke & Wakelin, 1973; Wakelin, 1973). Immunity is elicited above a certain threshold level of infection, approximately equivalent to 10 worms. Superficially, this seems to predict the sort of population regulation (Type III) considered by Bradley (1972), but the difference is that all parasites are expelled when the threshold is exceeded. The threshold therefore appears to place severe restraints upon transmission, but it is important to remember that the threshold level is influenced by factors such as host physiological state and the presence of concurrent infection (Jenkins & Behnke, 1977; Behnke, Ali & Jenkins, 1984). Transmission of infection may therefore depend, in part, upon the maturation of adult worms in individuals with elevated immunological thresholds, for example lactating females, in which immunity is markedly depressed (Selby & Wakelin, 1975). However, there is also evidence for the effects of genetic influences upon immune responsiveness. Threshold levels can vary between inbred strains of mice (Behnke *et al.*, 1984) and it is apparent that there can be wide individual variation in ability to express any degree of protective immunity. Such variation was first described in the outbred Schofield strain, in which some 20% of individuals failed to express immunity (Table 2), thus allowing infections to reach sexual maturity (Wakelin, 1975a). These individuals were also susceptible to challenge infection, despite the presence of circulating anti-worm antibodies capable of transferring protective immunity into competent recipients (Wakelin, 1975b). It can therefore be deduced that the genetic control of this non-responsiveness is expressed through some cell-mediated function, T lymphocyte or myeloid cell in origin.

Table 2. Numbers of *Trichuris muris* recovered from outbred Schofield mice infected with 300 eggs (non-responders underlined)

Days after infection	Individual worm recoveries
13	131, 112, 103, 80, 64
19	126, 86, 76, 8
25	103, 5, 1, 2
35	99, 2, 0, 0, 0

Selective breeding showed that failure to express protective immunity was inherited as a recessive characteristic (Wakelin, 1975a). F_1 progeny from a responder × non-responder cross behaved as responders when infected, and distinct lines of responder and non-responder mice were developed after a few generations of selection, although the latter never bred completely true.

Individual variation in response to infection with *T. muris* is also seen, rather more surprisingly, in the inbred strain DBA/2. A majority of mice expels worms from a primary infection before patency (Worley *et al.*, 1962; Lee & Wakelin, 1982) but the remainder allows worms to mature. The reason for this variation in a genetically homogeneous strain is not fully understood. Worm expulsion in DBA/2 mice is relatively late and it may be that small variations in the time of onset of protective immunity permit worms to reach a stage in development (perhaps size-related) which renders them insusceptible to the immune response.

There is only circumstantial evidence to suggest that these findings in outbred and inbred laboratory mice are paralleled in wild mice, indeed, experimental evidence would be difficult to obtain. However, *T. muris* is not markedly pathogenic in moderate infections and there may not be strong selective pressure against alleles associated with defective responsiveness. If this is correct, then there is no reason to suppose that the situation described by Wassom *et al.* (1974) for *H. citelli* in *P. maniculatus* would not also occur with *T. muris* in wild mice. It may also be reasonable to suggest that similar variation exists in human populations infected with *T. trichiura* or, indeed, with other gastrointestinal nematodes. Overdispersion with these parasites is well documented in man, certain 'wormy persons' (Croll & Ghadirian, 1981) carrying a large proportion of the parasite biomass. Anecdotal evidence suggests that such individuals may reappear regularly at clinics because of the reacquisition of worm burdens after apparently successful anthelmintic treatments.

TRICHINELLA SPIRALIS

The majority of helminths discussed in this paper show restricted host specificities; in contrast, *T. spiralis* has a remarkably wide host range. This ability to develop within many host species implies that natural resistance (insusceptibility) is low and that acquired immunity probably plays an important role in regulating the parasite load carried. If this is so, then genetic variability in immune responsiveness should be a major factor in bringing about overdispersion within the infected population. Surveys of infections in wild populations have been more concerned with identification of infected individuals rather than with assessing the degree of infection present (i.e. the number of larvae/g of muscle). Nevertheless, the data do show irregular and often infrequent infections within host populations, which (at the least) implies a degree of overdispersion. Investigations in laboratory mice have given a detailed picture of the ways in which genetic factors influence the outcome of infection with *T. spiralis*, in particular, the ways in which the burden of muscle larvae (a parameter relevant to transmission) is regulated.

Immunity against *T. spiralis* can operate against the parasite both in the intestinal phase and in the parenteral phase (Wakelin & Denham, 1983). It is probable that the intestinal site of expression is the most important. Enteral responses can interfere with growth, maturation and reproduction of female worms, and bring about their expulsion from the intestine. All of these modes of response serve to reduce the numbers of larvae which eventually establish in the musculature. Variation in the effectiveness of these responses is well documented (Wakelin, 1984) and may influence each parameter separately. As a consequence, there can be marked

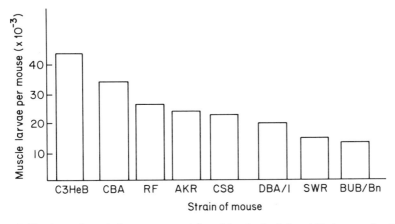

Figure 5. Numbers of muscle larvae recovered from inbred mice infected 30 days previously with a standard inoculum of *Trichinella spiralis*. (Redrawn from Wassom, David & Gleich, 1979.)

differences between individual mice of an outbred strain or between members of different inbred strains in the numbers of muscle larvae present after exposure to a standard infection (Fig. 5).

Resistance to *T. spiralis*, measured in terms of adult worm survival or of total muscle larval burden is inherited in a simple, dominant manner. A number of genes are involved in determining overall responsiveness of mice to *T. spiralis* infection, including both H-2 linked and background genes. Two alleles, designated *Ts-1* and *Ts-2*, have been located within the H-2 complex. One (*Ts-1*) is thought to control lymphocyte responsiveness to parasite antigens, the other may regulate the T lymphocyte interactions necessary for the development of the intestinal inflammatory responses involved in worm expulsion (Wassom *et al.*, 1983, 1984). Background genes clearly regulate intestinal responses at a non-lymphoid level (Wakelin, 1980; Wakelin & Donachie, 1981), possibly controlling the activities of myeloid cell populations (Fig. 6). Genetic control is also evident in terms of resistance to reinfection (Wakelin, 1980; Bell, McGregor & Adams, 1982), though such infections contribute relatively little to the overall number of muscle larvae present and can perhaps be ignored in the context of models of transmission. The ability of the host to regulate parasite reproduction directly, i.e. independently of worm survival in the intestine, has been firmly established (Wassom *et al.*, 1984), but the detailed genetic control of this phenomenon, which perhaps involves anti-worm antibody activity, has yet to be analysed.

T. spiralis antigen presented by worms

Ts-1 (? non-H-2)

T$_H$ response

T$_{AMP}$ response   Ts-2

Myeloid cells   non-H-2

Intestinal inflammation

Expulsion of worms

Figure 6. Hypothesis to explain the operation of H-2 linked (*Ts-1*, *Ts-2*) and non-H-2 alleles in the genetic control of intestinal immunity against *Trichinella spiralis* in mice.

It is difficult to predict what consequences genetic variation of this type would have upon transmission of *T. spiralis* in the wild, if only because little is understood of this process. Accumulation of muscle larvae in the larger carnivores and scavengers has been related to their longevity (Madsen, 1961), but there is, of course, no experimental information about the operation of immunity in such hosts which could validate this suggestion. In rodents, it seems clear that the intensity of infection with muscle larvae is determined by the size of the initial infection experienced, subsequent infections being irrelevant to this parameter. If rodents play an important role in the epidemiology of *T. spiralis* infections (and there is no agreement about this), then variation in ability to regulate parasite reproduction and survival would be expected to have an impact upon transmission. However, as *T. spiralis* can effectively reproduce some 500- or 1000-fold in the host, the effects of variation upon transmission may well be offset and be undetectable.

DIPETALONEMA VITEAE

Transmission of *D. viteae*, as with all filarial nematodes, involves uptake of microfilaria larvae by a blood-feeding arthropod vector, development of the microfilariae into infective stages and the reinjection of the infective larvae into another final host. An important factor in transmission is therefore the availability of microfilaria larvae within the host's body. A relatively small proportion of the microfilariae taken up mature into infective larvae; thus, if microfilarial density is low, infection of the vector will be inefficient. If microfilarial density is too high, then the vector may become overinfected and die before infective larvae develop. Regulation of microfilaraemia (the number of microfilaria per unit volume of blood) is imperfectly understood, although it is clearly under immunological control. Control can be exerted through responses directed against the survival or reproduction of adult female worms (the source of microfilariae) or against the microfilariae themselves.

Dipetalonema viteae is a parasite of the jird which can be passaged in hamsters. Jirds appear to have little immunity to infection whereas hamsters express immunity against adult reproduction and microfilarial survival. Marked strain-dependent variation in immune responsiveness has been described in hamsters (Neilson, 1978) but this model is not amenable to detailed analysis. Although mice cannot be infected by exposure to infective larval stages, it is possible to implant adult worms subcutaneously, and these worms will survive, reproduce and establish a patent infection. Under these conditions, strain-dependent variation in microfilaraemia is readily apparent (Haque *et al.*, 1980; Storey, Wakelin & Behnke, 1985), being reflected in the duration and level of microfilaraemia. As with all the other cases discussed in this paper, resistance (i.e. short-lived, low microfilaraemia) is inherited as a dominant trait, F_1 hybrids from crosses of resistant and susceptible parents behaving as resistant individuals. No influence of genes linked to the mouse MHC has been identified, H-2 congenic lines of mice on resistant or susceptible backgrounds (B10 and BALB respectively) maintaining the response patterns characteristic of the background strains.

It is clear that the striking difference seen between B10- and BALB-line mice is independent of adult worm survival, as implanted females die at approximately the same time in mice of each line. It is also independent of non-immunological, structural and physiological characteristics of the host, as response phenotype is reversed in radiation chimaeras given bone marrow cells from donors of the opposite phenotype. Thus, BALB/b mice reconstituted with B10.D2 bone marrow behave indistinguishably from B10.D2 mice. The immunological basis of resistance is not yet fully analysed but appears to involve IgM antibodies with specificity for the microfilarial cuticle. Inability to produce such antibody, as in BALB/c mice (Storey,

Wakelin & Behnke, unpublished) or in CBA/N mice (Thompson *et al.*, 1979) results in prolonged microfilaraemia.

In hamsters, once microfilariae have been cleared from the circulation, the blood remains negative even after reinfection. Mice, on the other hand, do develop a microfilaraemia after reinfection, but this is low level and of short duration (Storey *et al.*, 1984). Both findings imply that host animals could act as significant sources of infection to vectors only during an initial infection — and that their value as sources of infection would be related to their genetically determined response status. In the absence of adequate data, it is difficult to extrapolate from these experimental conclusions to transmission in the field. Nevertheless, several aspects of filarial infections in man suggest that such extrapolation may be justified. Even in endemic areas, where uniform vector transmission can be assumed, microfilaraemia status is very variable. It is also known that development of immunity is associated with disappearance of microfilariae from the bloodstream and appearance of anti-microfilarial antibodies (Piessens & Mackenzie, 1982). Some correlation has already been established in both the lymphatic filariases and in onchocerciasis, between individual clinical status, microfilarial burden and immunological responsiveness. All of these factors point to an important role for genetic influences upon the degree to which individuals can control infection and thus act as sources of microfilariae for the arthropod vectors.

NEMATOSPIROIDES DUBIUS

Nematospiroides dubius has been recorded from a wide variety of small rodents (Forrester, 1971) and it is a common parasite of the field mouse *Apodemus sylvaticus* in the U.K. (Lewis, 1968). Unlike the other gastro-intestinal parasites discussed earlier, infections in laboratory mice are characterized by their chronicity. In many strains of mice, the duration of primary infections, which can exceed 8 months, is little affected by host immunity, although some strains do expel adult worms after a period of time (Wakelin, 1978b). Under normal conditions, therefore, it may be assumed that genetic variability within the host population does not seriously interfere with the survival of the parasite and its ability to reproduce. Such an assumption appears justified when one considers the data on prevalence and intensity of infection provided by Lewis (1968). Of greater relevance to the theme of this paper are the mechanisms by which *N. dubius* survives in rodent hosts and the consequences of these mechanisms for the survival and transmission of other helminth parasites. In the laboratory mouse, infections with *N. dubius* are associated with a pronounced immunodepression, and it is becoming apparent that this depression operates against both homologous and heterologous antigens (see Behnke, Hannah & Pritchard, 1983; Pritchard, Ali & Behnke, 1984). *Nematospiroides dubius* may therefore promote its own survival at the expense of other immune responses. In this context, it is of particular interest that infections with *N. dubius* markedly diminish the responses mice can make against unrelated helminths such as *Trichinella spiralis* (Behnke, Wakelin and Wilson, 1978), *Trichuris muris* (Jenkins & Behnke, 1977; Behnke *et al.*, 1984), *Nippostrongylus brasiliensis* (Colwell & Westcott, 1973; Jenkins, 1975) and *Hymenolepis diminuta* (Hopkins, 1980). This is reflected in delayed expulsion, raised immunological thresholds, higher reproductive output and interference with resistance to reinfection. Each of these could contribute to greater transmission of the species concerned. The mechanisms underlying homologous and heterologous suppression have been the subject of several recent papers and there is evidence for selective induction of suppressor cell activity by immuno-modulatory factors released from *N. dubius* (see Pritchard *et al.*, 1984). Hagan & Wakelin (1982) found that *N. dubius* infection prevented the normal expression of anti-*T. spiralis* immunity by adoptively transferred immune lymphocytes, and interfered with the induction of inflammatory changes in the intestinal mucosa. The effects of *N. dubius* upon heterologous responses are dose-dependent, but the data of Lewis (1968) show that the levels of infection which occur in wild-populations are such that immunodepressive consequences would be predicted.

A recent finding is that there is strain variability in the effects exerted by *N. dubius* upon the immunological competence of the host, some strains being immunodepressed to a greater degree than others (Ali, 1983; Jacobson, pers. comm.). This observation may reflect the fact that there is mouse strain variation in the ease with which suppressor cells are induced. For the present purposes, the significance of the finding is that, in an outbred population, there may well be variation between individuals in the degree of suppression accompanying infection with *N. dubius*. This variation may lead, as a secondary consequence, to variation in intensity or duration of infection with parasites that are normally well controlled by immune responses. Thus, the transmission of certain species of helminth may be influenced by genetic variation in parameters relevant, not to itself, but to a third-party species.

CONCLUSIONS

Identification and analysis of genetic variation in immune responsiveness to macroparasites is most readily achieved in controlled laboratory systems, where it is possible to hold many variables constant. The heterogeneity of wild populations, and the problems of experimentation with these hosts, makes it difficult to extend similar studies into natural host–parasite relationships. Nevertheless, as Wassom *et al.* (1974) have shown, the difficulties are not insuperable and it is possible to draw clear-cut conclusions from such work. The system studied by these workers, *H. citelli* in *P. maniculatus*, was one in which the genetic differences within the host population were expressed in a qualitative fashion, the mice being apparently either responders, capable of eliminating both primary and subsequent infections, or non-responders, in which the infections survived unhindered. It may be felt that differences of this nature would be exceptional, because complex macroparasites are likely to elicit complex immunological and inflammatory responses in their hosts, and defective responsiveness in one component may well be cancelled out by enhanced responsiveness in another. The limited number of examples that have been discussed here show, however, that qualitative differences in responsiveness are not uncommon, being recorded in *T. taeniaeformis*, *T. muris* and *D. viteae*. This reflects the fact that, although the total host response to a macroparasite may indeed be complex, relatively few elements of that total response will contribute to a protective immunity, i.e. one that allows the host to control the parasite. Of course, other experimental systems show more quantitative genetically based differences in response to infection. One such system, which well illustrates the complexities which genetic control can display, is *N. dubius* in the mouse, not considered from the point of view of immunodepression, as here, but considered from the point of view of immunity, as in the work of Dobson and his colleagues (see Brindley & Dobson, 1983).

It is beyond the scope of this paper to discuss whether selection pressures operating upon wild populations exposed to infection by macroparasites are more likely to lead to qualitative or quantitative differences in protective immune responses. Each host–parasite system may well have to be considered separately, because each parasite will exert a particular pressure upon the overall fitness of the host. The purpose of the paper has been to show that genetically determined differences in protective immunity do exist, that it is posisble to analyse and explain the ways in which these differences are generated, and that awareness of such differences is of importance not only at the level of theoretical modelling of parasite transmission, but also in terms of practical application to the proiblems of human and veterinary parasitology.

REFERENCES

ALI, N. M. H., 1983. *The effect of infection with* Nematospiroides dubius *on the immune responsiveness of mice.* Ph.D. Thesis, University of Nottingham.

ANDERSON, R. M., 1982a. Epidemiology of infectious disease agents. In F. E. G. Cox (Ed.), *Modern Parasitology*: 204–251. Oxford: Blackwell Scientific Publishers.

ANDERSON, R. M., 1982b (Ed.). *The Population Dynamics of Infectious Diseases: Theory and Applications.* London, New York: Chapman & Hall.

ANDERSON, R. M. & GORDON, D. M., 1982. Processes influencing the distribution of parasite numbers within host populations with special emphasis on parasite-induced host mortalities. *Parasitology, 85:* 373–398.

ANDERSON, R. M. & MAY, R. M., 1978. Regulation and stability of host–parasite population interactions. I. Regulatory processes. *Journal of Animal Ecology, 47:* 219–247.

ANDERSON, R. M. & MAY, R. M., 1982. The population dynamics and control of human helminth infections: control by chemotherapy. *Nature (London), 297:* 557–563.

BEHNKE, J. M. & WAKELIN, D., 1973. The survival of *Trichuris muris* in wild populations of its natural hosts. *Parasitology, 67:* 157–164.

BEHNKE, J. M., ALI, N. M. H. & JENKINS, S. N., 1984. Survival to patency of low-level infections with *Trichuris muris* in mice concurrently infected with *Nematospiroides dubius. Annals of Tropical Medicine and Hygiene, 78:* 509–517.

BEHNKE, J. M., HANNAH, J. & PRITCHARD, D. I., 1983. *Nematospiroides dubius* in the mouse: evidence that adult worms depress the expression of homologous immunity. *Parasite Immunology, 5:* 397–408.

BEHNKE, J. M., WAKELIN, D. & WILSON, M. M., 1978. *Trichinella spiralis*: delayed rejection in mice concurrently infected with *Nematospiroides dubius. Experimental Parasitology, 46:* 121–130.

BELL, R. G., McGREGOR, D. D. & ADAMS, L. S., 1982. *Trichinella spiralis*: characterization and strain distribution of rapid expulsion in inbred mice. *Experimental Parasitology, 53:* 301–314.

BRADLEY, D. J., 1972. Regulation of parasite populations. A general theory of the epidemiology and control of parasitic infections. *Transactions of the Royal Society of Tropical Medicine and Hygiene, 66:* 696–708.

BRINDLEY, P. J. & DOBSON, C., 1983. Genetic control of liability to infection with *Nematospiroides dubius* in mice: direct and correlated responses to selection of mice for faecal parasite egg counts. *Parasitology, 87:* 113–127.

COHEN, S. & WARREN, K. S., 1982 (Eds). *Immunology of Parasitic Infections.* Oxford: Blackwell Scientific Publishers.

COLWELL, D. A. & WESTCOTT, R. B., 1973. Prolongation of egg production of *Nippostrongylus brasiliensis* in mice concurrently infected with *Nematospiroides dubius. Journal of Parasitology, 59:* 216.

CROFTON, H. D., 1971a. A quantitative approach to parasitism. *Parasitology, 62:* 179–193.

CROFTON, H. D., 1971b. A model of host parasite relationships. *Parasitology, 63:* 343–364.

CROLL, N. A. & GHADIRIAN, E., 1981. Wormy persons: contributions to the nature and patterns of overdispersion with *Ascaris lumbricoides, Ancylostoma duodenale, Necator americanus* and *Trichuris trichiura. Tropical and Geographical Medicine, 33:* 241–248.

DOW, C. & JARRETT, W. F. H., 1960. Age, strain and sex differences in susceptibility to *Cysticercus fasciolaris* in the mouse. *Experimental Parasitology, 10:* 72–74.

FISHER, R. A., 1941. The negative binomial distribution. *Annals of Eugenics, 11:* 182–187.

FORRESTER, D. J., 1971. *Heligmosomoides polygyrus* (= *Nematospiroides dubius*) from wild rodents of Northern California: natural infections host specificity and strain characteristics. *Journal of Parasitology, 57:* 498–503.

HAQUE, A., WORMS, M. J., OGILVIE, B. M. & CAPRON, A., 1980. *Dipetalonema viteae*: microfilariae production in various mouse strains and in nude mice. *Experimental Parasitology, 49:* 398–401.

HAMMERBERG, B. & WILLIAMS, J. F., 1978. Interaction between *Taenia taeniaeformis* and the complement system. *Journal of Immunology, 120:* 1033–1038.

HAGAN, P. & WAKELIN, D., 1982. *Nematospiroides dubius*: effect of infection on lymphocyte responses to *Trichinella spiralis* in mice. *Experimental Parasitology, 54:* 157–165.

HOPKINS, C. A., 1980. Immunity and *Hymenolepis diminuta*. In H. Arai (Ed.), *Biology of the Tapeworm Hymenolepis diminuta*: 551–614. New York: Academic Press.

JENKINS, D. C., 1975. The influence of *Nematospiroides dubius* on subsequent *Nippostrongylus brasiliensis* infections in mice. *Parasitology, 71:* 349–355.

JENKINS, S. N. & BEHNKE, J. M., 1977. Impairment of primary expulsion of *Trichuris muris* in mice concurrently infected with *Nematospiroides dubius*. *Parasitology, 75:* 71–78.

LEE, T. D. G. & WAKELIN, D., 1982. The use of host strain variation to assess the significance of mucosal mast cells in the spontaneous cure response of mice to the nematode *Trichuris muris*. *International Archives of Allergy and Applied Immunology, 67:* 302–305.

LEWIS, J. W., 1968. Studies on the helminth parasites of the long-tailed field mouse, *Apodemus sylvaticus sylvaticus* from Wales. *Journal of Zoology, 154:* 287–312.

MADSEN, H., 1961. The distribution of *Trichinella spiralis* in sledge dogs and wild mammals in Greenland under a global aspect. *Meddelelser orn Grønland, 159:* 1–124.

MILNE, A., 1943. The comparison of sheep-tick populations (*Ixodes ricinus* L.). *Annals of Applied Biology, 30:* 240–253.

MITCHELL, G. F., 1979a. Responses to infection with metazoan and protozoan parasites in mice. *Advances in Immunology, 28:* 451–511.

MITCHELL, G. F., 1979b. Effector cells, molecules and mechanisms in host-protective immunity to parasites. *Immunology, 38:* 209–223.

MITCHELL, G. F., GODING, J. W. & RICKARD, M. D., 1977. Studies on immune responses to larval cestodes in mice: increased susceptibility of certain mouse strains and hypothymic mice to *Taenia taeniaeformis* and analysis of passive transfer with serum. *Australian Journal of Experimental Biology and Medical Science, 55:* 165–186.

MITCHELL, G. F., RAJASEKARIAH, G. R. & RICKARD, M. D., 1980. A mechanism to account for mouse strain variation in resistance to the larval cestode, *Taenia taeniaeformis*. *Immunology, 39:* 481–489.

NEILSON, J. T. M., 1978. Primary infections of *Dipetalonema viteae* in an outbred and five inbred strains of golden hamsters. *Journal of Parasitology, 64:* 378–380.

OLIVIER, L., 1962. Studies on natural resistance to *Taenia taeniaeformis*. I. Strain differences in susceptibility of rodents. *Journal of Parasitology, 48:* 373–378.

PIESSENS, W. F. & MACKENZIE, C. D., 1982. Immunology of lymphatic filariasis. In S. Cohen & K. S. Warren (Eds), *Immunology of Parasitic Infections*: 622–653. Oxford: Blackwell Scientific Publishers.

PRITCHARD, D. I., ALI, N. M. H. & BEHNKE, J. M., 1984. Analysis of the mechanism of immunodepression following heterologous antigenic stimulation during concurrent infection with *Nematospiroides dubius*. *Immunology, 51:* 633–642.

ROMAN, E., 1951. Étude écologique et morphologique sur les acanthocéphales et les nématodes parasites des rats de la région Lyonnaise. *Mémoires du Muséum National d'Histoire Naturelle. Série A. Zoologie, II:* 49–270.

SELBY, G. R. & WAKELIN, D., 1975. Suppression of the immune response to *Trichuris muris* in lactating mice. *Parasitology, 71:* 77–85.

STOREY, N., WAKELIN, D. & BEHNKE, J. M., 1985. The genetic control of host responses to *Dipetalonema viteae* (Filarioidea) infections in mice. *Parasite Immunology* (in press).

THOMPSON, J. P., CRANDALL, R. B., CRANDALL, C. A. & NEILSON, J. T., 1979. Clearance of microfilariae of *Dipetalonema viteae* in CBA/N and CBA/H mice. *Journal of Parasitology, 65:* 966–969.

WAKELIN, D., 1969. The development of the early larval stages of *Trichuris muris* in the albino laboratory mouse. *Journal of Helminthology, 43:* 427–436.

WAKELIN, D., 1973. The stimulation of immunity to *Trichuris muris* in mice exposed to low-level infections. *Parasitology, 66:* 181–189.

WAKELIN, D., 1975a. Genetic control of immune responses to parasites: selection for responsiveness and non-responsiveness to *Trichuris muris* in random-bred mice. *Parasitology, 71:* 377–384.

WAKELIN, D., 1975b. Genetic control of immunity to parasites. *Parasitology, 71:* xxv.

WAKELIN, D., 1978a. Immunity to intestinal parasites. *Nature (London), 273:* 617–620.

WAKELIN, D., 1978b. Genetic control of susceptibility and resistance to parasitic infection. *Advances in Parasitology, 16:* 219–308.

WAKELIN, D., 1980. Genetic control of immunity to parasites. Infection with *Trichinella spiralis* in inbred and congenic mice showing rapid and slow responses to infection. *Parasite Immunology, 2:* 85–98.

WAKELIN, D., 1982. Mouse models of genetic variation in resistance to helminth parasites. In D. G. Owen (Ed.), *Animal Models in Parasitology*: 53–68. London: MacMillan.

WAKELIN, D., 1984. Genetic variation in immunity to *Trichinella spiralis* in the mouse — a review. *Proceedings of the International Commission for Trichinellosis, Wiadomosci Parazytologiczne, 29:* 375–385.

WAKELIN, D. & DONACHIE, A. M., 1981. Genetic control of immunity to *Trichinella spiralis*. Donor bone marrow cells determine responses to infection in mouse radiation chimaeras. *Immunology, 43:* 787–792.

WAKELIN, D. & DENHAM, D. A., 1983. The Immune Response. In W. C. Campbell (Ed.), *Trichinella and Trichinosis*: 265–308. New York: Plenum Press.

WASSOM, D. L., DAVID, C. S. & GLEICH, G. J., 1979. Genes within the major histocompatibility complex influence susceptibility to *Trichinella spiralis* in the mouse. *Immunogenetics, 9:* 491–496.

WASSOM, D. L., DEWITT, C. W. & GRUNDMANN, A. W., 1974. Immunity to *Hymenolepis citelli* by *Peromyscus maniculatus*: genetic control and ecological implications. *Journal of Parasitology, 60:* 47–52.

WASSOM, D. L., GUSS, V. M. & GRUNDMANN, A. W., 1973. Host resistance in a natural host–parasite system. Resistance to *Hymenolepis citelli* by *Peromyscus maniculatus. Journal of Parasitology, 59:* 117–121.

WASSOM, D. L., BROOKS, B. O., BABISCH, J. G. & DAVID, C. S., 1983. A gene mapping between the S and D regions of the H-2 complex influences resistance to *Trichinella spiralis* infections of mice. *Journal of Immunogenetics, 10:* 371–378.

WASSOM, D. L., WAKELIN, D., BROOKS, B. O., KRCO, C. J. & DAVID, C. S., 1984. Genetic control of immunity to *Trichinella spiralis* infections of mice. Hypothesis to explain the role of H-2 genes in primary and challenge infections. *Immunology, 51:* 625–631.

WORLEY, D. E., MEISENHELDER, J. E., SHEFFIELD, H. G. & THOMPSON, P. E., 1962. Experimental studies on *Trichuris muris* in mice with an appraisal of its use for evaluating anthelmintics. *Journal of Parasitology, 48(3):* 433–437.

Experimental epidemiology:
Nematospiroides dubius and the laboratory mouse

ANNE KEYMER

Department of Zoology,
South Parks Road,
Oxford OX1 3PS, U.K.

Nematospiroides dubius is a common trichostrongylid infection of microtine and murine rodents. Although the genetics and immunology of its interaction with the laboratory mouse have been intensively studied, its epidemiology has received relatively little attention. The aim of this paper is to review some of the laboratory based data which may be of relevance in this regard, and to evaluate the suitability of *N. dubius* as an experimental model for the epidemiology of endemic human hookworm infection. Aspects of the population biology of the parasite in hosts subject to primary, repeated and trickle infection are considered.

KEY WORDS: — *Nematospiroides dubius* — nematoda — epidemiology — population biology — trickle infection.

CONTENTS

INTRODUCTION

Nematospiroides dubius, or synonymously *Heligmosomoides polygyrus*, is a common trichostrongylid infection of microtine and, to a lesser extent, murine rodents. It was introduced as an experimental model in laboratory mice by Spurlock (1943) and, over the last 20 years, it has become one of the most intensively studied nematode parasites from both immunological and genetic points of view. Its epidemiology, on the other hand, has received relatively little attention. Its

Ecology and Genetics of Host–Parasite Interactions
ISBN: 0 12 593 690 7

life-history exhibits a combination of the features of the directly transmitted
nematodes of public health concern: it lives in the small intestine and the eggs
released by the females into the faeces hatch after a period of between 24 and 36 h
and then develop through two complete bacterial feeding larval stages in the external
environment (Bryant, 1973; Fig. 1). Moulting to the non-feeding L_3 larva occurs
after between 2 and 6 days, and this stage takes up a vertical stance at the highest
point in its microhabitat to await ingestion by a passing host. There is no extensive
larval migration inside the animal, instead development through the L_4 stage to
adulthood occurs within a mucosal cyst in the small intestine (Liu, 1965). As an
experimental system, *Nematospiroides* combines the advantages of large size and short
generation time, with an ease of manipulation in inexpensive and easily maintained
hosts.

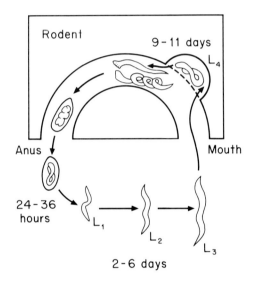

Figure 1. The life-cycle of *N. dubius*.

The use of a mouse-*Nematospiroides* system as an epidemiological model for
endemic human hookworm infection was specifically suggested by Bartlett & Ball
(1972), but the suggestion does not appear to have been followed up. The
methodological requirements for such a system to be of value with respect to
helminth epidemiology perhaps suggest the collection of two quite distinct kinds
of data. The first represents an overview of the complete epidemiological behaviour
of the parasite in its host population. The second requires some experimental
dissection of the life-history, in order to gain numerical measurements of each of
the population parameters, together with estimates of their dependence on, and
interaction with, other biological processes and also with physical variables. The
sum of the component parts can then be compared with the observed population
patterns of infection in order to gain insight into what may be the complex interaction
of many parameters, and perhaps to be of additional use in a more predictive mode.

The first question in a consideration of *N. dubius* as an epidemiological model might then perhaps be to ask what is known of its dynamic behaviour in naturally occurring rodent populations. The work of Elton *et al.* (1931) shows a degree of temporal constancy in a prevalence of infection of about 85% over a period of 31 months, combined with a seasonal fluctuation of infection intensity, which seems to vary in both this and other studies around mean values ranging from 10 to 25 parasites per host (Fig. 2). (Rather disconcertingly, a clearly seasonal oscillation has also been detected in the worm burden of laboratory mice infected experimentally with a standard number of *N. dubius* larvae at different times of year (Sitepu & Dobson, 1982); perhaps the repeatability and cause of this phenomenon should be one of the primary aims of an experimental study of the epidemiology of this species.) The basic characteristics of the population biology of *N. dubius* are thus not unlike those relating to endemic human hookworm infection but, unfortunately, any further similarity is obscured by the seasonal and longer term periodicity which characterizes both the abundance and age-structure of microtine rodent populations (e.g. Krebs & Myers, 1974). Leaving aside the question of whether helminth parasites may have any direct or indirectly causal role in the generation of 'wildlife's 4-year cycle' (see, e.g. Potts, Tapper & Hudson, 1984), one might at very least expect the population behaviour of the parasite to track the fluctuations of its host. Unfortunately, there appear to be no data relating to the way in which host and parasite dynamics are coupled for *N. dubius* and it

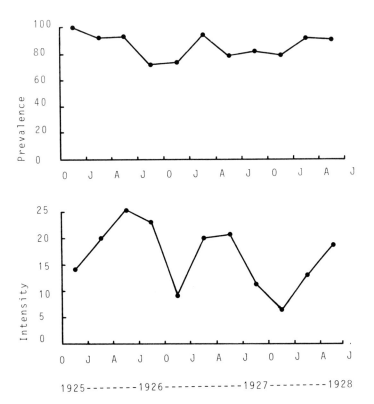

Figure 2. The prevalence and intensity of *N. dubius* infection in adult members of a wild population of *Apodemus sylvaticus* (Elton *et al.*, 1931).

is perhaps unrealistic to expect that any detailed epidemiological information could be easily extracted from such a complex and difficult to monitor system. The conclusion to be drawn, perhaps, is that if *N. dubius* is to be successfully utilized as an epidemiological model, the complete investigation must be brought into the laboratory, or at least into an experimentally controlled field situation.

The aim of this paper is to review some of the laboratory based data which may be of relevance in this regard and to give a personal opinion of the direction which experimental helminth epidemiology may take over the next few years.

LARVAL BIOLOGY

The development of *N. dubius* has been studied by several authors including Bryant (1973), and the survival characteristics of the third-stage larvae have been intensively investigated (Kerboeuf, 1978a,b; Mallet & Kerboeuf, 1984). Given appropriate environmental conditions, larval survival in this species is very high, with no loss of infectivity over the first 17 weeks of maintenance at 4°C (Kerboeuf, 1978a; Liu, 1966; Keymer, in prep.), followed by gradual decline in infectivity to zero at about 73 weeks of age (Kerboeuf, 1978a). This age-dependence in larval mortality is essentially lost at higher temperatures, such that the expected infectivity span of larvae maintained under equivalent conditions at 22°C is only approximately 7 weeks (Kerboeuf, 1978a; Fig. 3). Practical experience indicates that no larval development occurs in the absence of adequate moisture or in the presence of intense illumination (Keymer, in prep.).

PRIMARY INFECTION

Survival

It seems that no studies have yet been carried out to investigate the dynamics of the transmission process itself, but much is known about the establishment and survival of adult worms in primary infections. Mouse strain was first demonstrated to be of importance in this regard by Spurlock (1943); worm persistence and pathogenicity have now been documented in at least 20 different defined mouse strains (Liu, 1966; Scofield, 1975; Cypess *et al.*, 1977; Jenkins & Carrington, 1981). Parasite longevity varies from a few days in some strains to many months in others, and it is perhaps not surprising therefore that the manifestation of density-dependence in parasite survival also appears to be strain-related (Fig. 4). The percentage recovery of worms 28 days after the experimental infection of male and female Quakenbush mice with between 100 and 150 larvae was found to be significantly related to density (Dobson & Owen, 1977); similar results have been presented for the recovery of worms from male white mice (strain unknown) after 58 days (Liu & Ivey, 1961). In contrast, there appears to be no density-dependence in the number of parasites present in male CD1 mice 40 days after infection with between 50 and 700 *N. dubius* larvae (Kerboeuf, 1982).

Data from experiments using S-W (Van Zandt, Cypess & Zidian, 1973) and Swiss strains (Dobson, 1961), indicate that mature male mice have a greater innate susceptibility to primary infection than females. Evidence for the development of innate age-resistance appears equivocal, although some results clearly suggest that whereas immature male and female Swiss mice are equally susceptible to infection,

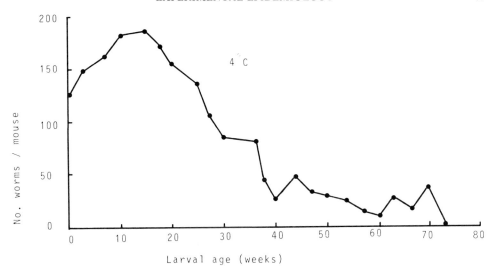

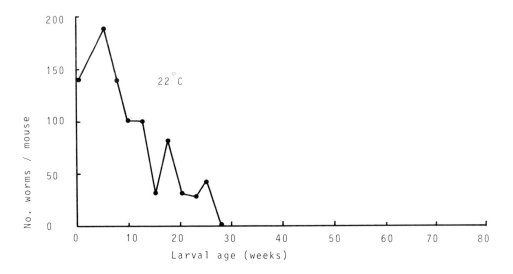

Figure 3. Age-dependent changes in the infectivity of living *N. dubius* larvae, as measured by the number of worms recovered from male Swiss mice 3 weeks after infection with 200 larvae of known age (Kerboeuf, 1978a). Upper, larvae stored at 4°C; Lower, larvae stored at 22°C.

only males become increasingly resistant with age (Dobson, 1961). The generality of sex-related differences in innate susceptibility is supported by field data from microtine rodent populations, which in general indicate higher levels of infection in male compared with female hosts (Lewis, 1968; Lewis & Twigg, 1972); other explanations for these differences are of course possible.

Experimental results relating to the survival of primary infections of 52 ± 3 and 110 ± 6 *N. dubius* larvae in adult male MF1 mice are shown in Figs 5 and 6 (Keymer, in prep.). No significant loss of worms was detected over a 16-week period in mice infected with 52 ± 3 larvae; the low values of the variance to mean ratio of worm numbers per host throughout this period indicated no significant heterogeneity between members of the mouse population in their innate susceptibility to this

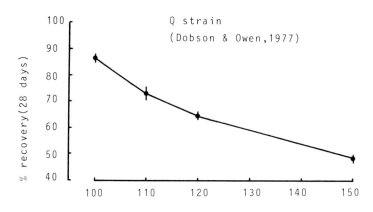

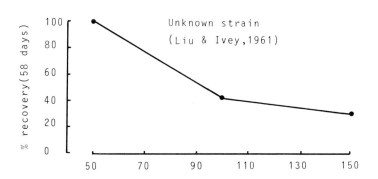

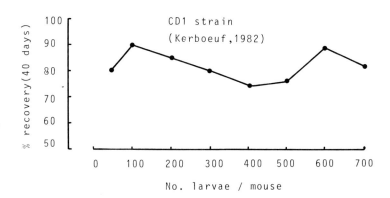

No. larvae / mouse

Figure 4. Density-dependent changes in the survival of *N. dubius* in primary infection. No. of worms recovered from the small intestine expressed as a percentage of the number of larvae administered. Upper, 28 days after infection of male and female Quakenbush mice (Dobson & Owen, 1977); Middle, 58 days after infection of male white mice of unknown strain (Liu & Ivey, 1961); Lower, 40 days after infection of male CD1 mice (Kerboeuf, 1982).

level of primary infection (Fig. 5a). This was supported by the results of the infection of each of 50 8-week-old male MF1 mice with 18 ± 1 *N. dubius* larvae. The number of worms recovered from the small intestine of each mouse on day 14 post-infection (12.5 ± 0.7; $S^2\sqrt{x} = 2.0$; k (negative binomial) = 12.7) indicated very little

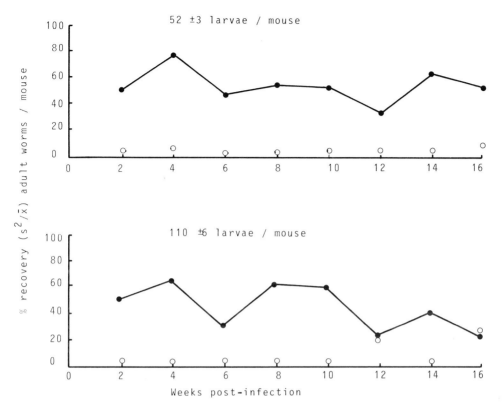

Figure 5. The survival of *N. dubius* in primary infection in adult male MF1 mice (Keymer, in prep.). Closed circles represent the number of worms recovered from the small intestine expressed as a percentage of the number of larvae administered. Open circles represent the variance to mean ratio of the number of worms recovered per mouse. Upper, Mice infected with 52 ± 3 larvae; Lower, mice infected with 110 ± 6 larvae.

difference between hosts in ability to support a primary infection of this size.

There was no significant difference in the percentage recovery of worms from the small intestine of mice from 2 to 10 weeks post-infection with either 52 or 110 larvae per mouse (Fig. 5). In contrast to the lower level of infection, however, a significant loss of worms may be detected from mice infected with 110 larvae between weeks 10 and 16 post-infection. Increases in the variance to mean ratio of worm numbers per host during this time (Fig. 5b), indicated that worm loss occurred faster in some mice than in others, perhaps suggesting some degree of heterogeneity between individuals in their ability to respond immunologically to the prolonged presence of higher antigen levels. It would obviously be improper to attach much significance to the results of experiments at just two levels of infection. Nevertheless, the experimental worm burden range did overlap that observed in naturally occurring infection, and the results may perhaps be taken to indicate that horizontal laboratory investigations undertaken at a single point in time may not always be reliable indicators of the presence or absence of density-dependence in parasite population parameters.

These results also indicate that there may be a density-dependent shift in the sex-ratio of surviving worms. Whereas there appeared to be little overall deviation from unity at a dose of 52 larvae per mouse (Fig. 6a), significant female bias may

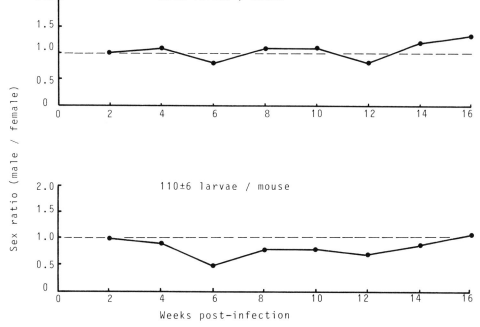

Figure 6. Sex-ratio (male/female) of the worms recovered from a primary infection of *N. dubius* in adult male MF1 mice (Keymer, in prep.). Upper, Mice infected with 52 ± 3 larvae; Lower, Mice infected with 110 ± 6 larvae.

be detected in the worms recovered from mice infected with 110 larvae (Fig. 6b). The implication that female worms may be better able to establish and survive in the host than male worms at high parasite density, is supported by various published reports in which a female-biased sex ratio has been detected (Lewis, 1968; Bawden, 1969; Cypess *et al.*, 1977; Kerboeuf and Jolivet, 1980). Further experimental investigation of this possibility is required.

Fecundity

The published results of several experimental studies may be used to investigate aspects of the fecundity of *N. dubius* in primary infection. It has been suggested that faecal egg counts may be used as a reliable indicator of worm burden (Sitepu & Dobson, 1982); results obtained on day 21 after the infection of a strain derived by crossing Quakenbush and wild mice, indicated no density-dependence in the number of eggs per gram (epg) of faeces produced by each female worm (Fig. 7a). The results of similar experiments carried out by Brindley and Dobson (1983a) indicated a positive correlation between epg and worm burden, perhaps related to reduced mating success at low worm density (Fig. 7b) but, in both cases, epg and worm burden exhibited clear evidence of direct proportionality.

The need for caution in the interpretation of faecal egg counts is highlighted by the results of Brindley & Dobson (1982) and Kerboeuf & Jacob (1983), both showing that the egg output of *Nematospiroides* females may be subject to diurnal fluctuation (Fig. 8). The existence of independent rhythms of egg and faecal output (Kerboeuf and Jacob, 1983) suggest that the phenomenon does not result simply

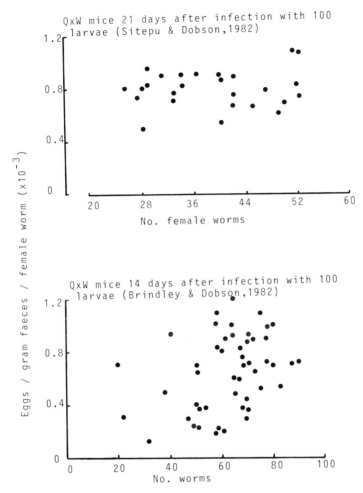

Figure 7. The fecundity of *N. dubius* in primary infection. Relationship between epg and number of worms present in the small intestine. Upper, 21 days after infection with 100 larvae, Q × W mice (Sitepu & Dobson, 1982); Lower, 14 days after infection with 100 larvae, Q × W mice (Brindley & Dobson, 1982).

from periodicity in host feeding behaviour. As a consequence of these results, it seems likely that the accuracy of measurements of worm fecundity will be improved by the collection of 24 h faecal samples and the expression of data in terms of eggs per female worm per day (epd). Results obtained by this method indicate a clear density-dependent constraint on worm fecundity in CD1 mice given primary infections of between 50 and 700 *N. dubius* larvae (Kerboeuf, 1982; Fig. 9). Results from the same experimental system (Fig. 10) indicated that worm fecundity was clearly age-related, the decline in the egg output of older female worms not being coincident with any changes in the number of worms present in the small intestine.

The age-dependent nature of worm fecundity was also illustrated by data relating to primary infections of 52 ± 3 or 110 ± 6 *N. dubius* larvae in adult male MF1 mice (Keymer, in prep.; Fig. 11). The pattern of egg production was very similar to that observed by Kerboeuf, although in this case no significant differences were detected in the pattern of egg production at the two levels of infection, indicating

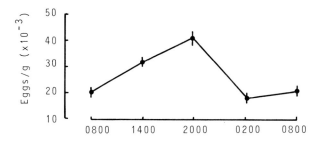

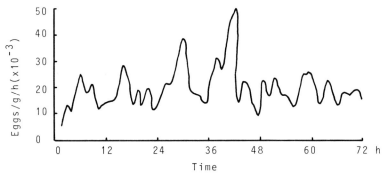

Figure 8. Diurnal fluctuation in egg release by *N. dubius*. Upper, Q × W mice infected with 100 larvae (Brindley & Dobson, 1982); Lower, CD1 mice harbouring approximately 340 worms (Kerboeuf & Jacob, 1983).

no density-dependent constraint on fecundity in this system over the experimental range and duration of primary infection. One possible explanation for the observed decline in fecundity with age would be to postulate some change in the copulatory behaviour of the worms. Mating is known to begin in this species as soon as the adults enter the small intestine and to continue periodically for several months thereafter (Somerville & Weinstein, 1964). Unlike most other nematode species, *N. dubius* is often seen *in copulatione* at *post mortem* examination, indicating that mating is not a transitory phenomenon. In the present experiments (Keymer, in prep.), no age or density-related changes could be detected in the mating behaviour of the worms (Fig. 12); on average, 37 % of all female worms were found to be mated at any time between 2 and 16 weeks post-infection. It is likely, therefore, that decline in fecundity is related to some physiological rather than behavioural change. All *post mortem* examination in these experiments was carried out between the hours of 0800 and 1200, but further experiments should be undertaken to investigate whether any diurnal rhythm is apparent which might explain the already detected periodicity in egg release.

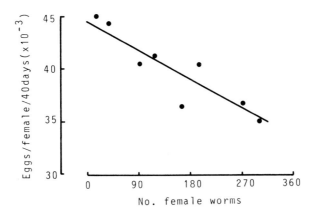

Figure 9. The fecundity of *N. dubius* in primary infection. Relationship between number of eggs/female worm/40 days and the number of female worms present in the small intestine of male CD1 mice 40 days after infection with between 50 and 700 larvae (Kerboeuf, 1982).

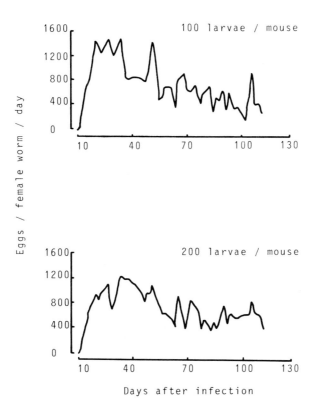

Figure 10. The fecundity of *N. dubius* in primary infection. Changes in the egg production of female worms through time in male NMR1 mice (Kerboeuf, 1982). Upper, 100 larvae/mouse; Lower, 200 larvae/mouse.

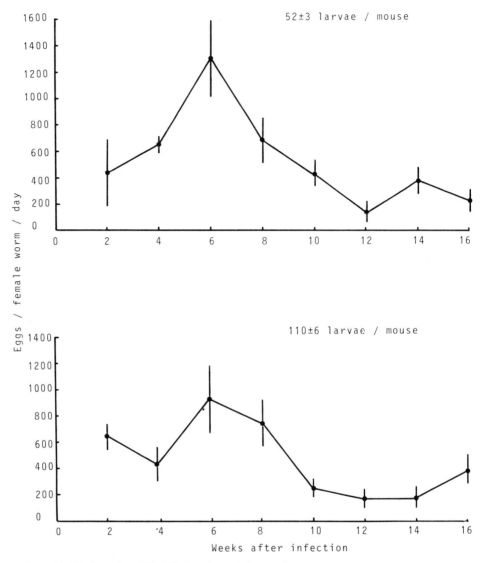

Figure 11. The fecundity of *N. dubius* in primary infection. Changes in the egg production of female worms through time in male MF1 mice (Keymer, in prep.). Upper, 52 ± 3 larvae/mouse; Lower, 110 ± 6 larvae/mouse.

Because of the ease with which copulation may be observed, *N. dubius* would appear to be a very good experimental model for the study of the influence of parasite density on mating success and the impact of mating behaviour on the dynamics of egg production; experiments to this end are underway at present.

REPEATED INFECTION

What has become known in the immunological literature as 'primary infection' involves the exposure of immunologically naive hosts to relatively large numbers of parasitic larvae at a single point in time: such conditions would never occur

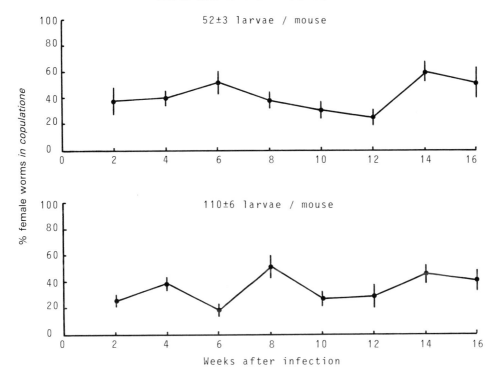

Figure 12. The reproductive behaviour of *N. dubius* in primary infection. Changes through time in the percentage of female worms observed *in copulatione* at *post mortem* examination of male MF1 mice (Keymer, in prep.). Upper, 52 ± 3 larvae/mouse; Lower, 110 ± 6 larvae/mouse.

in the real world. In studies of experimental epidemiology, particularly those involving mammals, it is thus of considerable interest to determine whether the dynamics of infection is modified by repeated exposure, and to investigate the influence of acquired immunity on the population biology of the parasite–host interaction.

In addition to interstrain variability in the persistence of a primary infection of *N. dubius* in the laboratory mouse, there appears also to be heterogeneity between mouse strains in the ability to mount a protective immunity to reinfection (Scofield, 1975; Cypess & Zidian, 1975; Cypess *et al.*, 1977; Behnke & Wakelin, 1977; Jenkins & Carrington, 1981). Although variation exists both in the level of immunity acquired and also in the ease with which it may be induced, published results indicate that for most strains of mice, the induction of complete protection against reinfection necessitates a very complex procedure involving several immunizing infections, each separately terminated by anthelmintic treatment. This has led to the suggestion that the larval stages may be highly immunogenic, with the degree of immunity therefore related to the duration of the immunogenic larval phase as well as to the intensity of infection (Panter, 1969; Behnke & Wakelin, 1977). As pointed out by Cypess & Zidian (1975), the effects of an acquired immune response may be sixfold: (1) 'self-cure' (2) a reduction in the proportion of infecting larvae which develop to adulthood (3) retarded larval development (4) mortality of encysted larvae (5) reduction in the size and fecundity of adult worms and (6) expulsion of adult parasites following emergence. The extent and combination of these effects in natural infections will undoubtedly be of primary importance in the epidemiology of host–parasite interactions and it is therefore of some importance that experiments are undertaken to investigate the dynamics of the parasite in hosts subject to repeated exposure to infection.

Although Behnke & Parish (1979) have both suggested and demonstrated that the reduction of the adult worm burden in immunized mice may be due in some degree to the arrested development of larvae in inflammatory nodules in the intestinal wall, most of the recent literature on the subject has compared the reactions to challenge infection at a single point in time, of naïve hosts and those subject to an immunization regime involving multiple infection followed by anthelmintic termination. The dynamics and immunology of the parasite–host relationship in repeatedly infected, untreated hosts, still remains to be investigated. The potential importance of arrested development in this respect is illustrated by a comparison of challenge infection in immunized NIII mice, naïve mice and immunized mice treated with cortisone (Behnke & Parish, 1979). Cortisone treatment in these experiments was found to allow the development to maturity of previously arrested larvae in immunized mice, possibly as a direct result of its anti-inflammatory properties. The results indicated that whereas the percentage of the challenge infection present in the intestine on days 23 and 24 post-infection is independent of larval dose in both naïve and immunized mice, the recovery of worms from immunized animals treated with cortisone was inversely related to the size of the challenge infection administered (Fig. 13). The absence of density-dependence in primary infection is therefore no guarantee that some regulatory constraint on worm numbers will not be manifest under certain other conditions relating to the much more complex dynamics of repeated exposure. This work also draws attention to the importance of host condition on worm dynamics, particularly the potential significance of immunocompromise induced by factors such as malnutrition, lactation, or the presence of other infections.

The influence of host genetics on *N. dubius* has been recently defined (Brindley & Dobson, 1981; 1983a,b; Sitepu & Dobson, 1982), and distinction made between the traits of innate liability to infection and immune responsiveness. Beginning with a cross of Quakenbush and wild mice, selective breeding over a series of 10 generations has allowed the isolation of two separate strains which diverge in terms

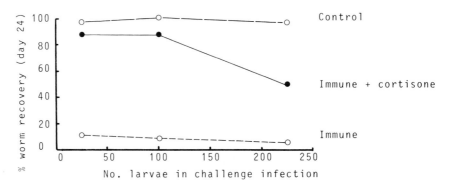

Figure 13. The survival of *N. dubius* in immunized NIH mice (Behnke & Parish, 1979). The relationship between the number of larvae in challenge infection and the percentage of the challenge infection recovered from the small intestine 24 days after infection in control mice (○—— ——○), immunized mice (○————○) and immunized mice treated with cortisone (●————●).

of their liability and refractoriness to initial infection, and two further strains differing in immune responsiveness to repeated exposure. The authors suggest that the two traits are linked, with each under the control of a few genes, heritability being estimated as 0.45 for liability and 0.49 for immune responsiveness. Furthermore, it has been deduced that innate susceptibility is controlled by two genetic units, one influencing larval establishment and the other interfering with the reproduction and growth of established worms.

Selection of host strains with respect to liability to infection has been found to influence parasite biology (Brindley & Dobson, 1982); worms inhabiting liable mice are both larger and more fecund than those in refractory hosts. As well as the influence of genetically mediated changes in host environment on parasite biology, experimental evidence exists to suggest that genetic changes in the parasite may also be induced experimentally. Passage through different strains of mice for only 10 generations results in parasites which have increasingly enhanced immunogenicity for the chosen mouse strain (Dobson & Owen, 1977). The ease of rejection of selected parasites by their hosts possibly relates to an increased concentration of structurally uniform immunogens and indicates that parasites may, under experimental conditions, be selected for increased infectivity for a given host, in spite of the trade-off between this and the risk of enhanced immunoresponsiveness and, therefore, rejection. This kind of investigation illustrates the overriding importance of both host and parasite genetics for epidemiology, and also draws attention, first to the complete absence of experimental data in this area and, secondly, to the suitability of *N. dubius* in the laboratory mouse as an experimental model for future studies.

TRICKLE INFECTION

Figure 14 shows the results of a preliminary experiment in which adult male MF1 mice were subject to repeated infection with *N. dubius*, by the oral administration of 52 ± 3 larvae at 2-weekly intervals (Keymer, in prep.). The mean worm burden per mouse rises after just 4 weeks to a plateau at a level of about 67 worms per host (Fig. 14a) although, by the end of the experiment, each mouse had received an average of 416 parasite larvae. These results alone give no indication of the dynamics of the parasite in each individual host: there could be a continual turnover of the worm population in the small intestine (in which case it would be necessary to postulate an expected life span for each worm of only 2.6 weeks) or, at the other extreme, there could be some kind of 'concomitant' immunity, whereby the survival of the originally established adult worms was accompanied by destruction of all newly invading larvae. Some indication of the real situation is given by the temporal change in the variance to mean ratio of worm numbers per host (Fig. 14b). In direct contrast to primary infection (Fig. 5), the variance to mean ratio increased dramatically through time, to reach a plateau after about 10 weeks. This is indicative of the development of great heterogeneity in the worm burdens harboured by the mice; what seemed to happen as the experiment proceeded was that some mice developed a protective acquired immunity and were successful in eliminating all the parasites they harboured, whereas others accumulated greater and greater numbers of adult worms. The maximum burden observed during this experiment was 211 adult worms per mouse, indicating the accumulation of parasites in this particular host at a rate of 50% of the administered larvae at every infection. As

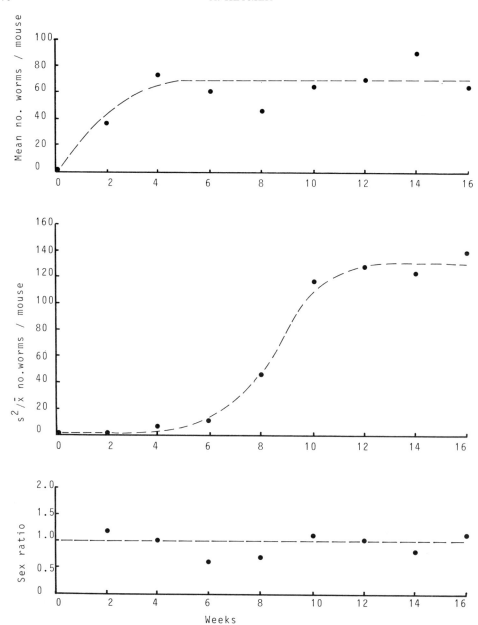

Figure 14. The dynamics of *N. dubius* in adult male MF1 mice subject to a trickle infection of 52 ± 3 larvae every 2 weeks (Keymer, in prep.). Upper, Changes in the mean worm burden of the mice through time; Middle, changes in the variance to mean ratio of the number of worms per mouse; Lower, changes in the sex-ratio of the surviving adult worms.

with the primary infection (Fig. 6), there was some evidence to suggest female bias in the sex ratio of surviving worms (Fig. 14c).

Parasite fecundity (Fig. 15a) is indistinguishable from the primary infection at week two, but the age-dependent nature of the egg production of each worm (Fig. 11) is obscured by the accumulation of parasites of different ages within a single host. These results emphasize the difficulties associated with the interpretation

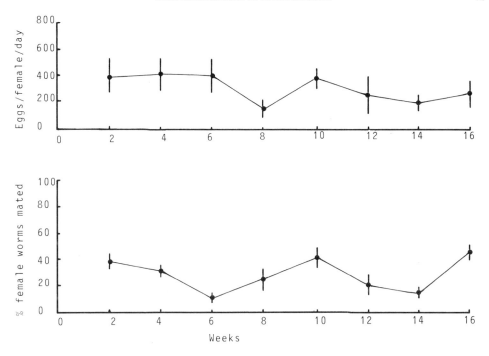

Figure 15. The fecundity of *N. dubius* in adult male MF1 mice subject to a trickle infection of 52 ± 3 larvae every 2 weeks (Keymer, in prep.). Upper, Temporal changes in egg production; Lower, temporal changes in reproductive behaviour.

of faecal egg counts for the diagnosis of the level of human geohelminth infection, where the observed egg output is the complex result of variable factors such as worm age, worm density, diurnal egg release, periodic faecal output and, perhaps most importantly, host response (both innate and acquired) to infection. Again, the percentage of female worms found to be *in copulatione* at *post-mortem* examination was fairly stable throughout the experimental period (Fig. 15b) and was very similar to that observed in primary infection (Fig. 12).

The form of the results observed in this experiment seems to be a direct function of host genetic variability. MF1 is an outbred strain, obviously with much heterogeneity in immune responsiveness to this particular parasite. It would seem likely that the use of an inbred strain could produce a very similar temporal pattern of infection intensity, but that the component dynamics of infection within individual hosts would be very different. This seems to be an area which could support a great deal of further experimental research.

The dynamics of infection within individual hosts could be followed by labelling procedures, as originally suggested by Bartlett & Ball (1974), but a much simpler method such as length measurement would probably provide a great deal of worthwhile information: size heterogeneity in the parasite burden is very apparent after repeated exposure to infection.

The consequences of these experimental results with respect to the epidemiology of *Nematospiroides* infection are clear. If this is a reflection of the way in which host genetic heterogeneity operates in the natural host–parasite interaction, it might be predicted that the degree of overdispersion in parasite numbers per host would rise with host age. Unfortunately, this cannot be tested for *Nematospiroides dubius* at present, although there is evidence that high levels of overdispersion do occur in wild rodent populations (Lewis, 1968; Fig. 16). On the other hand, the effect of host genetic variability may be obscured under natural conditions by other causes of overdispersion in parasite numbers per host, for example, heterogeneity in host behaviour or condition, or aggregation in the spatial distribution of parasite-infective stages. That this may in fact be the case is indicated by the apparent absence of age-dependence in the level of overdispersion of parasite numbers per host in human hookworm infection (Anderson, in press).

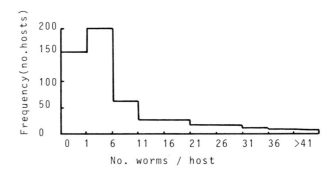

Figure 16. The frequency distribution of *N. dubius* in a wild population of *Apodemus sylvaticus* (Lewis, 1968).

A further implication to be drawn from these results concerns the form of epidemiological data presented as age-prevalence curves (Fig. 17). The experimental data suggested that, in cases where this degree of host heterogeneity is operative, an age-related decline in the prevalence of infection would be expected as a result of the development of protective immunity on continual exposure (Fig. 17a). Again, it seems likely that this effect might be obscured by other variables under natural conditions, but it is interesting to note that this is a feature of the epidemiology of human hookworm infection (Anderson, in press). Data relating to *Nematospiroides* in wild rodent communities are perhaps inevitably related to host size rather than host age, and are therefore more difficult to interpret, but two distinct patterns of age-prevalence have been demonstrated (Elton *et al.*, 1931; Kupwehbnat, 1938; Fig. 17b and c).

CONCLUSIONS

As suggested in the introduction to this paper, data of two kinds may be required in order for a host–parasite system to be successfully developed as an experimental model in epidemiology. The results described here seem to indicate that *N. dubius* in the laboratory mouse provides an extremely suitable system for the experimental study of component population processes. An appropriate method for the study of its overall epidemiological behaviour, however, remains to be developed. Field populations are subject to so many complex variables, often both uncontrollable and unmeasurable, that assessment of the influence of each individual factor on the overall dynamics in many cases is impossible to achieve. What seems to be required is a system whereby the behaviour of infected populations can be studied

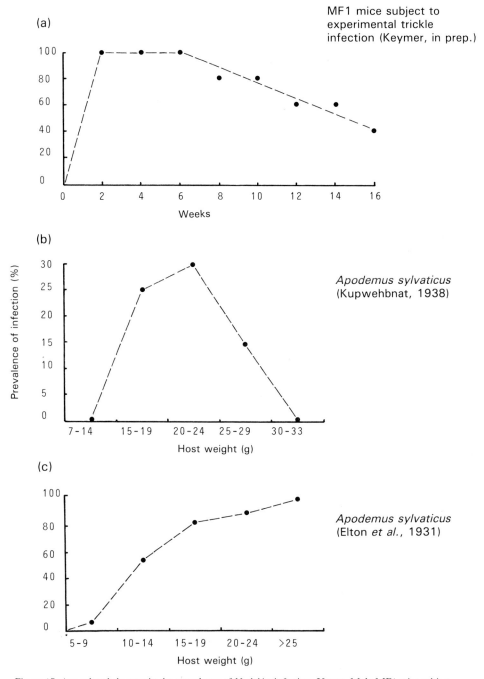

Figure 17. Age-related changes in the prevalence of *N. dubius* infection. Upper, Male MF1 mice subject to experimental trickle infection of 52 ± 3 larvae/2 weeks (Keymer, in prep.); Middle, naturally infected *Apodemus sylvaticus* (Kupwehbnat, 1938); Lower, naturally infected *Apodemus sylvaticus* (Elton *et al.* 1931).

under controlled conditions. There exists a range of possibilities for this type of study of varying degrees of complexity, from experimental populations in large laboratory cages to breeding populations in an enclosed field situation subject to the normal range of environmental fluctuation. (The latter system would allow further investigation of the potentially important phenomenon of parasite-mediated change in host behaviour (Freeland, 1981).) Under these conditions, the interaction of the various parameters in the generation of observed epidemiological patterns should be relatively transparent; again *Nematospiroides dubius* would seem to be eminently suitable for this kind of investigation.

Epidemiological studies of viral and bacterial infections completed a similar progression from experimentation on the individual to population studies of the experimentally infected herd, almost 50 years ago (Greenwood *et al.*, 1936). The major advantage for helminth epidemiology undergoing this change at the present time is that there now exist established theoretical frameworks to guide the design of experiments and to allow a formal, quantitative interpretation of their results (Anderson & May, 1979; May & Anderson, 1979).

The powerful influence of genetic heterogeneity on epidemiology has long been apparent, as illustrated by the statement: "standardized animals, like pure reagents in chemistry, should provide a means of elucidating many of the quantitative problems in infectious disease" (Webster, 1946). Although genetically defined mouse strains have now been available for some time, they have not perhaps yet been used to full advantage in population studies. With both the methods and the tools at hand, experimental helminth epidemiology now seems set for considerable expansion, with a collaborative approach involving genetics, immunology and population biology perhaps providing the most fruitful way ahead.

ACKNOWLEDGEMENTS

I am grateful to the Royal Society for the provision of a Research Fellowship and to the Wellcome and Nuffield Foundations for financial support.

REFERENCES

ANDERSON, R. M. Helminth infections of humans: mathematical models, population dynamics and control. *Advances in Parasitology* (in press).
ANDERSON, R. M. & MAY, R. M., 1979. Population biology of infectious diseases. Part I, *Nature, 280:* 361–7.
BARTLETT, A. & BALL, P. A. J., 1972. *Nematospiroides dubius* in the mouse as a possible model of endemic human hookworm infection. *Annals of Tropical Medicine and Parasitology, 66:* 129–34.
BAWDEN, R. J., 1969. Some effects of the diet of mice on *Nematospiroides dubius. Parasitology, 59:* 203–13.
BEHNKE, J. M. & PARISH, H. A., 1979. *Nematospiroides dubius*: arrested development of larvae in immune mice. *Experimental Parasitology, 47:* 116–27.
BEHNKE, J. M. & WAKELIN, D., 1977. *Nematospiroides dubius*: stimulation of acquired immunity in inbred strains of mice. *Journal of Helminthology, 51:* 167–76.
BRINDLEY, P. J. & DOBSON, C., 1981. Genetic control of liability to infection with *Nematospiroides dubius* in mice: selection of refractory and liable populations of mice. *Parasitology, 83:* 51–65.
BRINDLEY, P. J. & DOBSON, C., 1982. *Nematospiroides dubius* in mice selected for liability to infection: modification of parasite biology through host selection. *International Journal for Parasitology, 12:* 573–8.
BRINDLEY, P. J. & DOBSON, C., 1983a. Genetic control of liability to infection with *Nematospiroides dubius* in mice: direct and correlated responses to selection of mice for faecal parasite egg count. *Parasitology, 87:* 113–27.
BRINDLEY, P. J. & DOBSON, C., 1983b. Partitioning innate and acquired immunity in mice after infection with *Nematospiroides dubius. International Journal for Parasitology, 13:* 503–7.
BRYANT, V., 1973. The life-cycle of *Nematospiroides dubius*, Baylis, 1926 (Nematoda Heligmosomidae). *Journal of Helminthology, XLVII:* 263–8.
CYPESS, R. H., LUCIA, H. L., ZIDIAN, J. L. & RIVERA-ORTIZ, C. I., 1977. *Heligmosomoides polygyrus*: temporal, spatial and morphological population characteristics in LAF, IJ mice. *Experimental Parasitology, 42:* 34–43.

CYPESS, R. H. & ZIDIAN, J. L., 1975. *Heligmosomoides polygyrus*: the development of self-cure and/or protection in several strains of mice. *Journal of Parasitology, 61:* 819–24.

DOBSON, C., 1961. Certain aspects of the host–parasite relationship of *Nematospiroides dubius* (Baylis). *Parasitology, 51:* 173–9.

DOBSON, C. & OWEN, M. E., 1977. Influence of serial passage on the infectivity and immunogenicity of *Nematospiroides dubius* in mice. *International Journal of Parasitology, 7:* 463–6.

ELTON, C., FORD, E. B., BAKER, J. R. & GARDNER, A. D., 1931. The health and parasites of a wild mouse population. *Proceedings of the Zoological Society of London,* 657–721.

FREELAND, W. J., 1981. Parasitism and behavioural dominance among male mice. *Science, 213:* 461–2.

GREENWOOD, M., BRADFORD-HILL, A., TOPLEY, W. W. C. & WILSON, J., 1936. Experimental epidemiology. *Medical Research Council Special Report Series, 209.*

JENKINS, D. C. & CARRINGTON, T. S., 1981. *Nematospiroides dubius*: the course of primary, secondary and tertiary infections in high and low responder Biozzi mice. *Parasitology, 82:* 311–8.

KERBOEUF, D., 1978a. The effects of time and temperature of storage on the infectivity of L_3 of *Heligmosomoides polygyrus*. I. Effects on the development to the adult stage in mice. *Ann. Rech. Vet. 9:* 153–9.

KERBOEUF, D., 1978b. The effects of time and temperature of storage on the infectivity of third-stage larvae of *Heligmosomoides polygyrus*. II. Studies on the fecundity of female worms as a function of the infectivity of the third stage larvae. *Ann. Rech. Vet. 9:* 161–8.

KERBOEUF, D., 1982. Egg output of *Heligmosomoides polygyrus* in mice infected once only. *Ann. Rech. Vet. 13:* 69–78.

KERBOEUF, D. & JACOB, C., 1983. Rhythmic egg release by *Heligmosomoides polygyrus*, parasitic trichostrongylid of the murine rat. *Chronobiologia, 10:* 255–67.

KERBOEUF, D. & JOLIVET, G., 1980. Repeated anthelmintic treatments and receptivity of mice to experimental infections with *Nematospiroides dubius. Ann. Rech. Vet. 11:* 185–93.

KREBS, C. J. & MYERS, J. H., 1974. Population cycles in small mammals. *Advances in Ecological Research, 8:* 267–399.

KUPWEHBNAT, R. A., 1938. Regularities in the dynamics of the parasitofauna of mouse-type rodents., *Publications of Leningrad State University.*

LEWIS, J. W., 1968. Studies of the helminth parasites of the long-tailed field mouse *Apodemus sylvaticus sylvaticus* from Wales. *Journal of the Zoological Society of London, 154:* 287–312.

LEWIS, J. W. & TWIGG, G. I., 1972. A study of the internal parasites of small rodents from woodland areas in Surrey. *Journal of the Zoological Society of London, 166:* 61–77.

LIU, G. Y. H. & IVEY, M. H., 1961. Effect of several nematodes on an initial infection of *Nematospiroides* in mice. *Journal of Parasitology, 47:* 433–6.

LIU, S. K., 1965. Pathology of *Nematospiroides dubius*. I. Primary infections in C_3H and Webster mice. *Experimental Parasitology, 16:* 123–35.

LIU, S. K., 1966. Genetic influence on resistance of mice to *Nematospiroides dubius. Experimental Parasitology, 18,* 311–9.

MALLET, S. & KERBOEUF, D., 1984. Relation between enzyme activity and infectivity during ageing of *Heligmosomoides polygyrus* infective larvae. *C.R. Acad. Sci. Paris, 298:* 39–44.

MAY, R. M. & ANDERSON, R. M., 1979. Population biology of infectious diseases. Part II. *Nature, 280:* 455–61.

PANTER, H. C., 1969. Host–parasite relationships of *Nematospiroides dubius* in the mouse. *Journal of Parasitology, 55:* 33–7.

POTTS, G. R., TAPPER, S. C. & HUDSON, P. J., 1984. Population fluctuations in red grouse: analysis of bag records and a simulation model. *Journal of Animal Ecology, 53:* 21–36.

SCOFIELD, A. M., 1975. Differences in immunity to *Nematospiroides dubius* in inbred and outbred mice. *Journal of Parasitology, 61:* 158–9.

SITEPU, P. & DOBSON, C., 1982. Genetic control of resistance to infection with *Nematospiroides dubius* in mice: selection of high and low immune responder populations of mice. *Parasitology, 85:* 73–84.

SOMERVILLE, R. I. & WEINSTEIN, P. P., 1964. Reproductive behaviour of *Nematospiroides dubius in vivo* and *in vitro. Journal of Parasitology, 50:* 401–9.

SPURLOCK, G. M., 1943. Observations on host–parasite relations between laboratory mice and *Nematospiroides dubius. Journal of Parasitology, 29:* 303–11.

VAN ZANDT, P. D., CYPESS, R. H. & ZIDIAN, J. L., 1973. Development of age and sex resistance to *Nematospiroides dubius* in the mouse following single and multiple infections. *Journal of Parasitology, 59:* 977–9.

WEBSTER, L. T., 1946. Experimental epidemiology. *Medicine, 25:* 77–110.

Cyclic and non-cyclic populations of red grouse: a role for parasitism?

P. J. HUDSON, A. P. DOBSON* & D. NEWBORN

*North of England Grouse Research Project,
The Game Conservancy, Askrigg, Leyburn,
North Yorkshire DL8 3HG, UK., and
*Biology Department, Princeton University,
Princeton, New Jersey 08544 U.S.A.*

The hypothesis that parasitism is a key element influencing the pattern of fluctuations in red grouse numbers was investigated. Data were collected from estates in the north of England which exhibited either cyclic, intermediate or non-cyclic bag records. Cyclic populations were associated with greater worm burdens of *Trichostrongylus tenuis* and more rainfall than non-cyclic but there was no difference in the nitrogen content of food or mean bag size. It is proposed that low humidity reduces the survival of free-living stages resulting in lower levels of infection and reduced effects on host fecundity in non-cyclic populations. By modelling, it was shown that the interaction of a long-lived free-living stage and parasite induced reduction in fecundity could be of prime importance in producing the cycles in grouse density. These findings are discussed in relation to previous hypotheses and studies on grouse population cycles.

KEY WORDS: — Red grouse — cyclic and non-cyclic populations — *Trichostrongylus tenuis* — parasitism — population fluctuations.

CONTENTS

Ecology and Genetics of Host–Parasite Interactions
ISBN: 0 12 593 690 7

INTRODUCTION

The cause of the cyclic fluctuations in numbers of red grouse *Lagopus l. scoticus* (Lath.) has interested population biologists since Lack (1954) and Chitty (1954) independently analysed data from an early study of red grouse (Lovat, 1911) and arrived at conflicting conclusions. Lack suggested that regulation was due to parasitism and starvation whereas Chitty thought it was due to inherent changes within the birds' population. In later years, Chitty developed these and other ideas into a general hypothesis for cycles (Chitty, 1967) and proposed that the genetic composition of a population changes during a cycle; selection at high densities favours aggressive animals with low reproductive rates and, at low densities, less aggressive (subordinate) animals with high reproductive rates. This hypothesis, often referred to as the genetic hypothesis, was later tested for the red grouse. Inherent changes in dominance were found during a population fluctuation (Moss, Watson & Rothery, 1984) but the proportion of subordinate birds increased before the population started to decline, suggesting that changes in dominance were a result of, rather than a cause of population change. Modelling of the population (Watson *et al.*, 1984) found that direct losses due to extrinsic factors such as food, predation and parasitism provided only a poor fit to observed changes in numbers; a better fit was obtained when intrinsic factors causing dispersal were incorporated. It was proposed by Moss *et al.* (1984) that intrinsic changes in tolerance may be the cause of population cycles.

The importance of parasitism as a factor that may regulate a host's population density has gained stature in recent years through the development of theoretical models (Anderson, 1978; 1979; 1980; Anderson & May, 1978, 1979; May & Anderson, 1978, 1979). These models illustrate the potential importance of disease in a variety of parasite–host systems, many of which exhibit a tendency to oscillate. Potts, Tapper & Hudson (1984) have produced a simulation model of a grouse population based on data from the north of England which proposes that the effect of the nematode parasite *Trichostrongylus tenuis* (Eberth) on breeding production is a key element causing cycles in grouse numbers. To test a prediction from this model, Hudson (in press) has experimentally reduced parasite burdens in wild grouse and shown that parasites reduce breeding production. These manipulative experiments provide an insight into how the system operates but need not exclude intrinsic factors even in a system where parasites have the potential to operate as an important selective force.

One question which may help to throw further light on the problem is why some populations of red grouse exhibit cyclic fluctuations whilst others do not. To explore this question we looked at empirical differences in parasite burdens from cyclic and non-cyclic populations of grouse and then investigated the dynamical consequences of *T. tenuis* for grouse populations using a model of a parasite–host system originally developed by May & Anderson (1978). This analysis suggests that the interaction between the grouse and the nematode may be of prime importance in determining the cycling of the grouse populations. We conclude by discussing other studies of grouse populations in areas where parasitism has been suggested to be unimportant.

METHODS

Analysis of population fluctuations

The number of red grouse shot each year from 63 estates in the north of England were obtained from landowners in 1979 and 1980. Each estate manages and harvests the grouse independently from their neighbours and, although some estates were contiguous, each series of bag data were considered a separate 'population'. The series were analysed using time series analysis (Poole, 1974) which simply correlates numbers shot in one year with those shot in each succeeding year at increasing time intervals. In a series exhibiting cycles, high correlations occur when intervals correspond to phases of the cycle. A detailed account of the analysis of this data has been presented elsewhere by Potts *et al.* (1984). Populations were considered cyclic if coefficients were found greater than two large-lag errors (Box & Jenkins, 1970), equivalent to 95% confidence limits. Populations were considered non-cyclic if coefficients were less than one large-lag error and intermediate if greater than 1 but less than two large-lag errors. Mean density was estimated for each population as the mean number of birds shot per km^2 in the 30-year span from 1949 to 1979.

Environmental data

Altitude of each grouse moor was estimated from 1:50 000 Ordnance Survey maps and taken as the altitude in the centre of the heather moorland. Mean rainfall figures from 1916 to 1950 were obtained from H.M.S.O. (1973) and taken from the rainfall stations closest to each grouse moor.

Samples of building heather *Calluna vulgaris*, the main food plant of grouse were taken from the centre of 36 estates during April 1981. At each moor, several handfulls of heather were taken, combined as a sample and dried to constant weight in an oven set at 27°C. Samples were ground and nitrogen content estimated using a Technicon Autoanalyser II. Results are expressed as percentage nitrogen of dry matter.

Prevalence and intensity of infection with T. tenuis

Samples of grouse guts were collected from 46 estates on shooting days (August to November) in all years from 1979 to 1983. Birds were picked at random from the days bag and aged as either old (> 1 year old) or young (production of that season) from plumage characteristics, claw scars and relative skull strength (Watson & Miller, 1976). From each gut sample, a caecum was removed and the contents washed with water over a 210 μm gauze, the residue collected and mixed with 300 ml of water and then subsampled to estimate the number of worms per bird (after Wilson, 1983).

RESULTS

Pattern of fluctuations in grouse bags

Of the 63 sets of bag records, 51 provided sufficient data for analysis. Of these, 30 (58%) showed negative coefficients greater than two large-lag errors, 12 less than two but greater than one, and nine had coefficients less than one large lag-error.

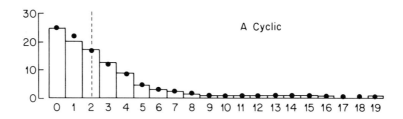

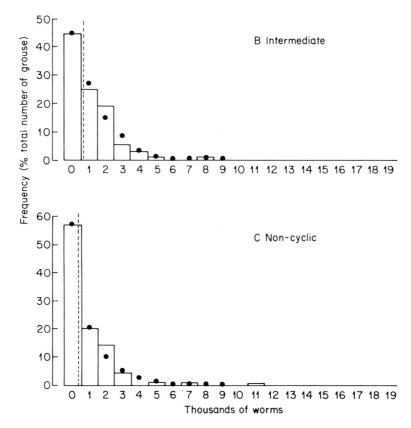

Figure 1. Frequency distribution of *T. tenuis* numbers in old grouse. Bars show observed frequency, circles the frequency predictions of the negative binomial probability distribution and broken lines the means. Note each category represents number of birds within a span of worm burdens so 0 is 0 – 1000 worms. A, Cyclic grouse populations, $s^2/x = 2.67$, $k = 1.41$; B, intermediate grouse populations, $s^2/x = 2.1$, $k = 1.4$; C, non-cyclic populations $s^2/x = 3.0$, $k = 0.60$.

Mean bag records along with mean altitude, rainfall and nitrogen content of heather for each respective type of grouse population are shown in Table 1. There were no significant differences in altitude and mean number shot between the three population types. Rainfall from stations near to 'cyclic moors' was significantly greater than 'non-cyclic moors' (*t* test, $t = 3.3$, d.f. = 35, $P<0.01$) and 'intermediate moors' had significantly greater rainfall than 'non-cyclic moors' (*t* test, $t = 2.25$, d.f. = 18, $P<0.05$). The levels of nitrogen in the heather taken from intermediate 'moors' was greater than both cyclic and non-cyclic but the differences were not significant (Table 1, cyclic versus non-cyclic, $t = 1.72$, d.f. = 29, $P > 0.1$).

Table 1. Bag records and environmental data from different types of red grouse populations. Figures show mean ± standard deviation

| | Type of grouse population | | | |
	Cyclic	Intermediate	Non-cyclic	Significance
Number of estates	30	12	9	
Mean bag/km^2	76.4 ± 6.0	58.4 ± 4.9	57.2 ± 12.3	N.S.
Mean rainfall (mm)	1409 ± 57	1357 ± 109	1030 ± 77	$P < 0.001$
Mean altitude (m)	439 ± 18	388 ± 20	377 ± 31	N.S.
Nitrogen content (%)	1.39 ± 0.02	1.42 ± .03	1.31 ± .04	N.S.

Prevalence and intensity of infection with T. tenuis

A total of 1858 old grouse were examined and all contained *T. tenuis* worms. Of 1512 young grouse examined, only in 18 were no *T. tenuis* worms found.

The frequency distribution of *T. tenuis* numbers in old grouse, for each type of population, is shown in Fig. 1. Each distribution has a variance to mean ratio ($s^2/\bar{x}$) greater than 1 and conforms to the negative binomial; the degree of aggregation (k) for cyclic populations = 1.41, intermediate = 1.40 and non-cyclic = 0.60. The distribution of worm numbers from cyclic populations was significantly different from non-cyclic (Goodness of fit, $\chi^2 = 48.3$, d.f. = 6, $P < 0.001$) and intermediate was significantly different from non-cyclic ($\chi^2 = 37.2$, d.f. = 6, $P < 0.001$) but no difference was found between cyclic and intermediate populations ($\chi^2 = 3.37$, d.f. = 3, $P > 0.1$). On cyclic moors, 24% of the old grouse inspected had parasite burdens greater than 4000 worms per bird, at a level likely to have a significant effect on the bird (Hudson, unpublished), while from non-cyclic populations only 3.6% of grouse inspected had such high worm burdens.

Young grouse from cyclic populations carried less worms per bird than old grouse ($\chi^2 = 781.1$, d.f. = 10, $P < 0.001$) and, although the $s^2/\bar{x} = 1.15$, the distribution (Fig. 2) does not conform to the Poisson ($\chi^2 = 214$, d.f. = 3, $P < 0.001$) as there were a few birds with very high worm burdens. It is possible that a few old birds were aged incorrectly as young birds, and conceivable that high levels of infection may alter plumage characteristics (see Hamilton & Zuk 1982) and make some old birds appear young.

Few young grouse ($N = 165$) were taken from the intermediate and non-cyclic populations although the frequency distribution of both was slightly different from the young collected from cyclic populations (cyclic versus non-cyclic, $\chi^2 = 9.21$, d.f. = 2, $P < 0.01$; cyclic versus intermediate, $\chi^2 = 6.64$, d.f. = 2, $P < 0.05$) but were not different from each other ($\chi^2 = 0.95$, d.f. = 1, $P < 0.01$).

MODEL

Trichostrongylus tenuis is a directly transmitted nematode, the life cycle of which is described in Lovat (1911), by Wilson (1979) and is summarized in Fig. 3. As with all directly transmitted nematodes, there are two basic populations of the

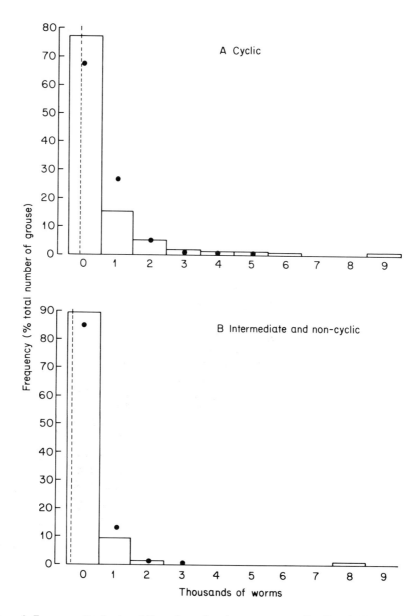

Figure 2. Frequency distribution of *T. tenuis* numbers in young grouse. Details as in Fig. 1 but here circles represent predictions of the Poisson distribution. A, Cyclic grouse populations, $s^2/x = 1.15$; B, non-cyclic and intermediate grouse populations combined, $s^2/x = 1.13$.

parasite; the sexually mature worms living in the birds' caecae and the free-living stages. Parasite burdens cannot increase within the host and infection is by ingestion of the infective larvae with food.

The population dynamics of the host and parasite populations may be readily described using one of the models developed by May & Anderson (1978). This consists of two coupled differential equations which describe changes in the populations of grouse, *H*, and adult parasites, *P*:

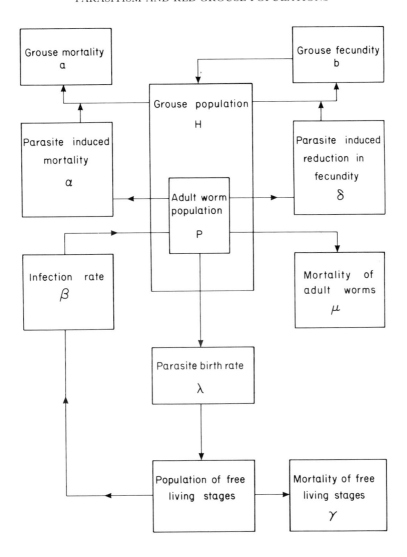

Figure 3. Flow chart summarizing the life cycle of *T. tenuis* in grouse and the principle features of the model.

$$dH/dt = (a - b)H - (\alpha + \delta)P \qquad (1)$$

$$dP/dt = \lambda PH/(H_0 + H) - (\mu + b)P - \alpha P^2/(k + 1/k) \qquad (2)$$

This is essentially the same as May & Anderson's (1978) Model D. The parameters are defined in Table 2, where estimates are made from the data presented in this and other studies. A formal local stability analysis of this model is presented in the Appendix, which follows that presented in Anderson & May (1978). As with their Model D, there are two conditions which have to be met if a stable joint equilibrium is to be established. The first requires

$$\lambda > \mu + b + \alpha + (a - b)\alpha(k + 1)/(\alpha + \delta)k \qquad (3)$$

Table 2. Population parameter estimates for *T. tenuis* and red grouse

Parameter	Symbol	Value
Grouse Fecundity	*a*	0.6–2.5/grouse/year
Grouse Mortality	*b*	0.55/grouse/year
Infection rate	λ	10^4–10^6/worm/year
Adult worm mortality	μ	0.556/worm/year
Parasite pathogenicity	α	0.0001–0.001/grouse/year
Parasite reduction in host fecundity	δ	0.0004/grouse/year
Aggregation of parasites in hosts	k	0.5–1.5

This will be met if the parasites have a very high rate of egg production, as found in this system (Table 2). The second condition determines the stability of any joint equilibrium and requires

$$\alpha > k\delta \qquad (4)$$

When k is around unity, this condition will be met if the pathogenicity of the parasite α, is greater than the parasite-induced reduction in fecundity. As the degree of aggregation increases and k gets smaller, the stability of the system increases. However, if k is around unity and δ is larger than α, then the system will show a propensity to oscillate when perturbed from equilibrium (Fig. 4). This tendency will become increasingly marked as the life expectancy of the free-living larval stages increases. When these are of similar order to that of the host species, the system will cycle with a period determined by the expression given in the Appendix. For the parameters given in Table 2, this suggests cycles in the order of 4–5 years for

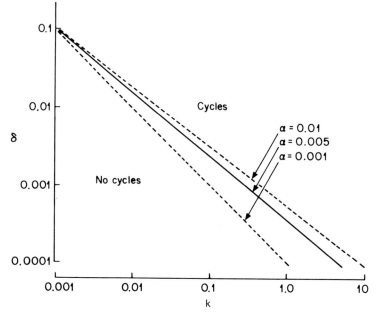

Figure 4. The relationship between the effects of parasites on grouse fecundity (δ) and k, the degree of aggregation of parasites in grouse. See text for details.

the grouse — *T. tenuis* system. This compares with a mean value of 4.8 years described by Potts *et al.* (1984).

The tendency for the system to oscillate is highly dependent on the mortality rate of the free-living stages. When these are short lived, *Ho* is large and the effective infection rate remains low, parasite burdens decline and cycles do not occur. However, when these free-living stages are long lived *Ho* is small and large parasite burdens can build up. Although these may ultimately lead to crashes in the hosts' population, and consequently the parasite population, there will still be viable stages around to reinfect the surviving grouse when the hosts' population starts to increase. The differences observed in rainfall between cyclic and non-cyclic moors are likely to be of prime importance in determining the survival of the free-living stages.

The effects of varying the survival of the free-living stages may be more accurately modelled using a three-equation model which incorporates a term for the dynamics of the free-living stages (May & Anderson 1978). Initial numerical simulations support the observations made above for the simple two equation model which essentially captures the interaction between parasite-induced reduction in fecundity, pathogenicity and degree of parasite aggregation.

Similar predictions can be derived from the simulation model of grouse and *T. tenuis* developed by Potts *et al.* (1984). In this model, a change in the stochastic elements influencing breeding production (i.e. plane of nutrition) or infection rate can alter the outputs from cyclic to non-cyclic fluctuations.

DISCUSSION

The data and analysis presented in this paper suggest that infections with the nematode parasite *T. tenuis* may be an important factor influencing the cyclic patterns observed in grouse populations in the north of England. This final discussion briefly outlines some of the biological features which determine the magnitude and relative importance of the parameters used in the model and this is then discussed in the context of previous hypotheses and work on grouse population cycles.

The model indicated that there were three important features which could determine the pattern of population fluctuations in a simple one host, direct-life cycle parasite system. Firstly, cycles are likely to be found in systems where the mortality of the free-living stages is low. Although this was not studied directly, the higher levels of infection found in cyclic as opposed to non-cyclic grouse populations and associated differences in rainfall between moors provided some evidence to support this prediction. Survival of *Trichostrongylus* species is known to be dependent on humidity (Prasad, 1959); low humidity increases the chances of larval desiccation and would reduce infection rate. Thus, the lower rainfall on the non-cyclic moors indicates that there is a difference in humidity between cyclic and non-cyclic populations and this could affect the survival of the free-living larvae.

Secondly, cycles will not exist if the pathogenicity of the parasite is high relative to its effects on host fecundity. Both of these parameters will be influenced by the host's plane of nutrition, so when food quality is low the relative impact of the parasite is increased. The plane of nutrition measured as the nitrogen and phosphorous content of heather has been found to be an important factor influencing the breeding production of red grouse (Moss, Watson & Parr, 1975). In this study, no significant difference was found between the nitrogen content of heather taken from cyclic and non-cyclic populations. However, in years when severe weather conditions reduce food quality, the effects of parasitism on fecundity will be particularly intense and these effects will increase the tendency of populations with high parasite burdens to oscillate.

Thirdly, the propensity of populations to oscillate will be dependent on the statistical distribution of the parasites within the host population. Cyclic fluctuations will be expected if the degree of aggregation of the parasites is low. Although the data illustrated the expected differences in the degree of parasite aggregation between cyclic and non-cyclic populations, both estimates of k (of the negative binomial) were close to unity and it seems likely that variations in the previously discussed parameters were more important in determining differences between the two types of population.

In summary, evidence for two of the three conditions predicted by the model were found when parameters from cyclic and non-cyclic populations were compared. Differences in the aggregation of parasites will influence the stability of host numbers but, even in non-cyclic populations, the model predicts that parasitism will regulate host numbers. Since parasite burdens are low in non-cyclic populations, a more likely explanation is that some grouse populations are not cyclic because they have low parasite burdens and this comes about through low infection rate and survival of free-living stages. Although it was not tested in this study, the low rainfall figures do suggest that humidity is lower on moors supporting non-cyclic populations and this can be expected to reduce infection and survival of larvae. This study does not provide conclusive proof that parasitism causes cycles but when considered with findings from other studies (Potts *et al.*, 1984; Hudson, in press) it does imply that parasitism has a role to play in the population fluctuations of grouse numbers in the north of England.

Since this study was designed to refute the parasitism hypothesis, we can make little comment on hypotheses invoking inherent factors unless the two are considered mutually exclusive. The long-term and detailed studies in Scotland (Moss *et al.*, 1984; Watson *et al.*, 1984) have suggested that parasitism does not play a significant role in the population fluctuations they have studied. This difference probably reflects differences between areas and to some extent differences in definition. The following five points note some of these differences:

(1) What some workers classify as cyclic populations others may consider non-cyclic. In this respect, Potts *et al.* (1984) conducted a time series analysis of bag records from Kerloch, the principle study area of Watson, Moss and co-workers and found no significant cycles. This is not to say that the population did not cycle since harvesting techniques may vary (Hudson, 1984) and an analysis of combined bag records from an area of north-east Scotland (Williams, unpublished BSc dissertation quoted by Moss *et al.*, 1984) found significant cycles, albeit of a longer period than those observed in the north of England. As this study would have classified Kerloch 'non-cyclic' it would predict low levels of infection with *T. tenuis* and hence reduced effects. As such it is perhaps not surprising that the Scottish workers have considered parasitism an unimportant factor.

(2) The hypotheses invoking intrinsic factors include genetic and non-genetic effects on birds before hatching (Moss *et al.*, 1984), some are correlated to density in previous years (Watson *et al.*, 1984) and could include some direct and indirect

effects of parasitism. As an example of direct effects, it is known that parasitism can influence the aggressiveness of mammals (Freeland, 1981; Rau, 1983, 1984) so it is conceivable that infections of *T. tenuis* could influence the spacing behaviour of red grouse. The effects of parasitism on breeding success may also have an indirect effect on spacing behaviour. Levels of aggression can be expected to vary as a function of the coefficient of relatedness between neighbours, which is a function of breeding success and dispersal (Charnov & Finnerty, 1980). Low levels of aggression between cocks from the same covey (i.e. probably siblings) have been demonstrated in red-legged partridges *Alectoris rufa* (Green, 1983) and there is some evidence for this in red grouse (Lance, 1978; Hudson unpublished). If such a system operates then changes in aggression during a population cycle could be a result of breeding success and not necessarily the cause of population change.

(3) Analysis of long-term population cycles is based on the number of grouse harvested each autumn. A major contribution to these numbers is the production of young in the preceding summer. Studies, such as this, which concentrate on bag records may tend to emphasize the factors influencing breeding production. On the other hand, studies following changes in spring breeding density may tend to emphasize the factors causing winter losses.

(4) Population studies usually monitor changes in density within an area which is much smaller than the actual boundaries of the population. This study has taken data from managed estates which average $17\,km^2$ while the intensive study of Watson *et al.* (1984) was from an area of $1.77\,km^2$. The variation in habitat quality, density and the factors regulating density can be expected to change with respect to the size of a study area. Small study areas will tend to emphasize dispersal whilst also concentrating on factors regulating density within a small and somewhat restricted area of habitat.

(5) The relative importance of intrinsic and extrinsic factors can be expected to vary both temporally and spatially. Spacing behaviour can be expected to regulate density in some situations, particularly in prime habitats (*sensu* Fretwell & Lucas, 1969) and after particularly high production. As such, intrinsic factors may only limit density when the effects of extrinsic factors such as predation, food quality and parasitism are low. This is similar to the general hypothesis of Watson & Moss (1979) and is demonstrated in the demographic study of Watson *et al.* (1984).

In conclusion, studies on red grouse have indicated a range of factors which influences population dynamics. The relative importance of these factors can be expected to vary in time and space and it may be naïve to invoke a simple explanation for all populations.

ACKNOWLEDGEMENTS

The Earl Peel and landowners in the north of England kindly provided access to their estates and bag records. Willie Wint kindly helped with estimates of nitrogen content at Oxford University. Stephen Tapper conducted the time-series analysis and Richard Barnes the negative binomial. Dick Potts and Roy Anderson provided constructive discussion and comments on the manuscript.

REFERENCES

ANDERSON, R. M., 1978. The regulation of host population growth by parasite species. *Parasitology, 76:* 119–157.
ANDERSON, R. M., 1979. The influence of parasitic infection on the dynamics of host population growth. In R. M. Anderson, B. D. Turner & L. R. Taylor (Eds), *Population dynamics:* 245–282. Oxford: Blackwell.
ANDERSON, R. M., 1980. Depression of host population abundance by direct life cycle macroparasites. *Journal of Theoretical Biology, 82:* 283–311.
ANDERSON, R. M. & MAY, R. M., 1978. Regulation and stability of host–parasite population interactions: I Regulatory processes. *Journal of Animal Ecology, 47:* 219–249.
ANDERSON, R. M. & MAY, R. M., 1979. Population biology of infectious diseases: I. *Nature (London), 280:* 361–367.
BOX, G. E. & JENKINS, G. H., 1970. *Time Series Analysis: Forecasting and Control.* San Francisco: Holden-Day.
CHARNOV, E. L. & FINNERTY, J. P., 1980. Vole population cycles: a case for kin selection. *Oecologia, 45:* 1–2.
CHITTY, D., 1954. Tuberculosis among wild voles: with a discussion of other pathological conditions among certain mammals and birds. *Ecology, 35:* 227–237.
CHITTY, D., 1967. The natural selection of self-regulatory behaviour in animal populations. *Proceedings of the Ecological Society of Australia, 2:* 51–78.
FREELAND, W. J., 1981. Parasitism and behavioural dominance among male mice. *Science, 213:* 461–462.
FRETWELL, S. D. & LUCAS, H. L., 1969. On territorial behaviour and other factors influencing habitat distribution in birds. I Theoretical development. *Acta Biotheoretica, 19:* 16–36.
GREEN, R. E., 1983. Spring dispersal and agonistic behaviour of the Red-legged Partridge *(Alectoris rufa). Journal of Zoology, London, 201:* 541–555.
H.M.S.O., 1973. *British Rainfall 1967.* Meteorological Office, London.
HUDSON, P. J., 1984. Harvesting red grouse in the north of England. *Game Harvest Management*, Texas: Caesar Kleberg Research Institute (in press).
HUDSON, P. J. The effect of a parasite nematode on the breeding production of red grouse. *Journal of Animal Ecology*, in press.
LACK, D., 1954. *The Natural Regulation of Animal Numbers.* Oxford: Clarendon Press.
LANCE, A. N., 1978. Survival and recruitment success of individual young cock Red Grouse *Lagopus l. scoticus* tracked by radio-telemetry. *Ibis, 120:* 369–378.
LOVAT, Lord, 1911. *The Grouse in Health and Disease.* 2 vols; London: Smith & Elder & Co.
MAY, R. M., 1975. *Stability and complexity in model ecosystems.* (2nd edition). Princeton: Princeton University Press.
MAY, R. M. & ANDERSON, R. M., 1978. Regulation and stability of host–parasite population interactions. Part II Destabilising processes. *Journal of Animal Ecology, 47:* 249–268.
MAY, R. M. & ANDERSON, R. M., 1979. Population biology of infectious diseases: II. *Nature (London), 280:* 455–461.
MAYNARD SMITH, J., 1974. *Models in Ecology.* Cambridge: Cambridge University Press.
MOSS, R., WATSON, A. & PARR, R., 1975. Maternal nutrition and breeding success in red grouse *(Lagopus lagopus scoticus). Journal of Animal Ecology,* 44: 171–190.
MOSS, R., WATSON, A. & ROTHERY, P., 1984. Inherent changes in the body size, viability and behaviour of a fluctuating red grouse *(Lagopus l. scoticus)* population. *Journal of Animal Ecology, 53:* 171–189.
POOLE, R. W., 1974. *An Introduction to Quantitative Ecology.* Kogaskuha, Tokyo: MacGraw-Hill.
POTTS, G. R., TAPPER, S. C. & HUDSON, P. J., 1984. Population fluctuations in red grouse: analysis of bag records and a simulation model. *Journal of Animal Ecology, 53:* 21–36.
PRASAD, D, 1959. The effects of temperature and humidity on the free-living stages of *Trichostrongylus retortaeformis. Canadian Journal of Zoology, 37:* 305–316.
RAU, M. E., 1983. Establishment and maintenance of behavioural dominance in male mice infected with *Trichenella spiralis. Parasitology, 86:* 319–322.
RAU, M. E., 1984. Loss of behavioural dominance in male mice infected with *Trichinella spiralis. Parasitology, 88:* 319–373.
WATSON, A. & MILLER, G. R., 1976. *Grouse management.* Fordingbridge: The Game Conservancy.
WATSON, A. & MOSS, R., 1979. Population cycles in the Tetraonidae. *Ornis Fennica, 56:* 87–109.
WATSON, A., MOSS, R., ROTHERY, P. & PARR, R., 1984. Demographic causes and predictive models of population fluctuations in red grouse. *Journal of Animal Ecology, 53:* 639–662.
WILSON, G. R., 1983. The prevalence of caecal threadworms *(Trichostrongylus tenuis)* in red grouse *(Lagopus lagopus scoticus). Oecologia, 58:* 265–268.
WILSON, G. R. 1979. Effects of the caecal threadworm *Trichostrongylus tenuis* on red grouse. Unpublished PhD thesis, University of Aberdeen.

APPENDIX

This appendix outlines the analysis of the stability properties of the model presented in the main text. It is essentially that presented in Anderson & May 1978).

The equation (1) aND (2) can be rewritten to have the general form:

$$dH/dt = c1\ H - c2\ P \tag{A1}$$

$$dP/dt = P\{\lambda H/H + Ho - c3 - c4\ P/H\} \tag{A2}$$

where $c1 = a - b$; $c2 = \alpha + \delta$; $c3 = \mu + b + \alpha$ and $c4 = \alpha(k + 1/k)$

The two populations are at equilibrium when $dH^*/dt < dP^*/dt = 0$. This occurs when the mean number of parasites per host,

$$P^*/H^* = c1/c2 \tag{A3}$$

$$\text{and } H^* = Ho\ (c3 + c1\ c4/c2)/(\lambda - c3 - c1\ c4/c2) \tag{A4}$$

Thus, we will only achieve a positive equilibrium when

$$\lambda > c3 + c1\ c4/c2 \tag{A5}$$

A linearized stability analysis is carried out along standard lines (see May, 1975). Writing $H(t) = H^* + x(t)$ and $P(t) = P^* + y(t)$, and linearizing by neglecting higher order terms, we get from equations A1 and A2

$$dx/dt = c1\ x - c2\ y \tag{A6}$$

$$dy/dt = c5\ x - (c1\ c4/c2)y \tag{A7}$$

As with Anderson & May (1978), $c5$ is defined as

$$c5 = (\lambda Ho + H^*)/(Ho + H^*) + c1\ c4/c2)c1/c2 \tag{A8}$$

The temporal behaviour of $x(t)$ and $y(t)$ then goes as $\exp(\Lambda t)$, where the stability determining eigen values Λ are obtained from (A6) and (A7) by the quadratic equation:

$$\Lambda^2 + A\Lambda + B = 0 \tag{A9}$$

Here

$$A \equiv (c1/c2)\ (c4 - c2) \tag{A10}$$

$$B \equiv c2\ c5 - c1^2\ c4/c2 \equiv c1\lambda HoH^*/(Ho + H^*) \tag{A11}$$

The requirement for neighbourhood stability is that the real part of both eigen values be negative; the necessary and sufficient criterion for this to be so is given by the Routh–Hurwitz criterion $A > 0$ and $B > 0$. We can see from (A11) that B is always positive, therefore the equilibrium point will be locally stable if $A > 0$, that is if $c4 > c2$ or

$$\alpha(k + 1)/k > \alpha + \delta \tag{A12}$$

When this important constraint is not met, providing that Ho is small (i.e. the free-living stages have a low mortality rate), the system will show a propensity to oscillate and may enter a stable limit cycle. The period of the cycles may be roughly estimated using the following formula (Maynard Smith, 1974):

$$\text{Cycle length} = 4\pi/\sqrt{(4B - A^2)} \tag{A13}$$

Here, A and B are as defined in (A10) and (A11). Substitution of the parameters given in Table 2 into this formula gives an estimated cycle length in the order of 4–5 years.

Schistosome and snail populations: genetic variability and parasite transmission

DAVID ROLLINSON AND VAUGHAN R. SOUTHGATE

Department of Zoology,
British Museum (Natural History),
Cromwell Road, London SW7 5BD, U.K.

This paper aims to bring together a variety of studies pertaining to the genetic interaction of schistosomes and their snail hosts, particular emphasis being given to the application of electrophoretic techniques. Information concerning the genetic mechanisms of schistosome–host interactions is reviewed. Enzyme variation relating to schistosome isolates is discussed and an example of variation in the worms of an individual host is provided by studies on *Schistosoma leiperi* infections of *Kobus leche kafuensis*. The contribution of enzyme analyses and the significance of hybridization is explored with reference to *S. mattheei* and *S. haematobium* in S. Africa; data concerning hybridization of *S. haematobium* and *S. intercalatum* in Loum, Cameroun, are presented which indicate that in children urinary schistosomiasis is replacing the intestinal form. The possibility of finding linkage between enzyme markers and susceptibility or infectivity genes is considered. Attention is drawn to the use of enzymes for detecting multiple infections in snails. Enzyme studies are considered to be useful for examining the population structure of both *Biomphalaria* and *Bulinus* but may not necessarily reflect observed susceptibility patterns. Reproductive strategies of snails, including sperm storage, sperm sharing, cross- and self-fertilization and multiple insemination, are discussed. The continued integration of ecology and genetics to the study of microevolutionary processes involved in schistosome–snail interactions is encouraged.

KEY WORDS: — schistosomes — snails — population genetics — transmission — enzymes — polymorphism — hybridization — breeding biology

CONTENTS

Ecology and Genetics of Host–Parasite Interactions
ISBN: 0 12 593 690 7

INTRODUCTION

In recent years, knowledge of genetic differentiation and diversity in a variety of organisms has been greatly enhanced by the study of protein variation. By providing a means to characterize, unambiguously, genetic variation among individuals, enzyme electrophoresis has become an invaluable method for the study of population genetics. Such studies have revealed, somewhat unexpectedly, a large amount of protein polymorphism in natural populations and considerable debate has ensued concerning the forces responsible for generating and maintaining such variation; indeed, it has been argued that genetic interactions between parasites and their hosts might play some role in maintaining protein polymorphisms (Clarke, 1976). The application of electrophoretic techniques to the study of parasites and their hosts has had a considerable impact in four main areas of research. First and foremost in providing a method for differentiating genetically distinct, but often morphologically similar, forms; secondly, in allowing a quantitative assessment to be made of the relationship between closely related organisms; thirdly, in providing markers for inheritance and linkage studies and, fourthly, by allowing an insight into the genetic structure of populations and the breeding biology of both parasites and their hosts. In this paper, electrophoretic data pertaining to genetic variation in schistosomes and their snail hosts are considered and particular emphasis is given to the ways in which a knowledge of protein variation can enhance investigations concerned with the interaction of natural populations.

The majority of the 19 or so recognized species of *Schistosoma* utilize relatively large mammalian species for their definitive hosts and are long-lived as mature adults (Loker, 1983). Unlike most other parasitic flatworms, which are hermaphrodite, schistosomes are dioecious. The adult worms reside in the blood vessels where, it is assumed, they are monogamous.

As the eggs produced must leave the body to continue the life cycle, the worm population of a definitive host can only increase in number by the successful invasion of new parasites. The sexual phase alternates with an asexual phase in intermediate snail hosts. Like many other digenea, schistosomes show a marked specificity for their molluscan hosts. It is customary to recognize three species groups within the genus, typified by *S. mansoni*, *S. haematobium* and *S. japonicum*, and each group is associated with particular genera of snails. Of the five species which are important parasites of man, *S. mansoni* is transmitted by *Biomphalaria* spp. in Arabia, Africa, South America and some of the Caribbean islands; *S. haematobium* and *S. intercalatum* by *Bulinus* spp. in Africa and adjacent regions; *S. japonicum* by *Oncomelania hupensis* in Japan, China, Formosa and the Philippines, and *S. mekongi* by *Tricula aperta* in Cambodia. Both *Biomphalaria* and *Bulinus* are hermaphrodite freshwater snails belonging to the Planorbidae, whereas *Oncomelania* and *Tricula* are dioecious prosobranchs belonging to the Pomatiopsidae (Davis, 1979). Despite the seemingly narrow host range of the parasites, schistosomiasis is one of the most widespread parasitic diseases of man, being endemic in 73 countries (Iarotski & Davis, 1981). The wide distribution reflects the geographical range of the intermediate hosts which, in spite of their parasite burden, have successfully colonized large areas of the world.

GENETIC MECHANISMS OF SCHISTOSOME-SNAIL INTERACTIONS

The close association of schistosomes and snails is shown by the often specific and indeed local nature of the host–parasite relationship. This can be considered in terms of overall compatibility, comprising both infectivity of the parasite and susceptibility of the snail. In compatible interactions, the sporocyst develops without a host tissue reaction, while in incompatible interactions, the larval schistosome is rapidly surrounded by amoebocytes and eventually destroyed. Following on from the earlier work of Newton (1952, 1953, 1955), Richards has demonstrated that there are a number of genetic factors in *Biomphalaria glabrata* governing susceptibility of this species to infection with defined strains of *S. mansoni* (Richards, 1973, 1975a,b, 1976a,b, 1984). By selection and self-fertilization, he succeeded in establishing strains with different susceptibility characteristics including: non-susceptible at any age, susceptible at any stage, juvenile susceptible and adult non-susceptible; a fourth susceptibility type showed juvenile susceptibility but modification of adult susceptibility with unpredictable infection frequencies and delayed parasite development. It seems that although host and parasite compatibility might be under simple genetic control, susceptibility might vary during a snail's life and the nature of the control might vary for each parasite–snail combination considered. The complexity of the interaction is well illustrated by a recent study of Richards (1984) in which six Puerto Rican *B. glabrata* stocks were exposed to 13 genetically different Puerto Rican *S. mansoni* isolates, giving a total of 78 snail stock/parasite strain combinations. Each snail stock gave a different susceptibility pattern to the parasite strains, with only one stock being susceptible at any age to any strain. Juvenile susceptibility was common to all but three of the combinations, whereas adult non-susceptibility or variability was shown by 51 combinations. That similar kinds of control mechanisms might operate in *Oncomelania hupensis* and *S. japonicum* interactions has been suggested by the early work of Davis & Ruff (1973) and, more recently, Chiu *et al.* (1981).

Detailed studies concerning the infectivity of schistosomes are logistically more difficult to carry out but much has been learnt by the study of hybridization (Le Roux, 1954; Taylor, 1970; Wright & Southgate, 1976) and from experiments using different species of *Schistosoma* and a single species of host snail. The latter kind of experiment has shown that certain closely related parasites (species or strains) can produce quite different reactions by the snail; thus, certain parasites elicit the snail's immunological response, whereas others develop undetected. Whether the failure of the snail to recognize a parasite as foreign is due to the blocking of the host recognition system by the parasite or by the parasite's adoption of some form of molecular camouflage or a combination of the two is a question of some debate (Wright & Southgate, 1981; Lie, 1982).

Experimental crosses of schistosomes in the laboratory require the infection of the laboratory host with the appropriate male and female genotypes. This is normally achieved by exposing snails to single miracidia and then exposing the definitive host to cercariae emanating from two snails; asexual reproduction of the parasite within the snail ensures tne production of identical cercariae. Due to difficulties in determining the sex of cercariae, each cross is conducted blind, the sex and charac-teristics of the selected parasites being determined by the use of control infections.

Most hybrid miracidia that have been studied combine, to a greater or lesser degree, the infectivities of their parental species. For example, in the experiments reported by Wright (1974), the progeny of a cross between *S. mattheei* male × *S. intercalatum* female were equally infective to *B. globosus* and *B. scalaris*, whereas the parental forms were restricted in the case of *S. mattheei* to *B. globosus* and in the case of *S. intercalatum* to *B. scalaris*. This duel infectivity persisted through to the F_3 generation, even though the parasite was passaged solely through *B. globosus*; it was not until F_4 that infectivity to *B. scalaris* was apparently lost.

GENETIC MECHANISMS OF
SCHISTOSOME-DEFINITIVE HOST INTERACTIONS

Many schistosome species show less specificity to their mammalian host than to their molluscan host. *S. japonicum*, for example, is reputed to occur naturally in 31 species representing five orders of mammals (Mao & Shao, 1982) and yet utilizes the snail host *Oncomelania hupensis* throughout its range. Whereas infection by schistosomes is known to reduce the fitness of infected snails, and there may well be selective pressures towards increasing resistance in snail populations, little is known concerning the influence of schistosomes on the reproductive fitness of their mammalian hosts. Schistosomiasis can be a severely debilitating disease but probably plays a minor role as a selective agent in terms of pre-reproductive mortality. Nevertheless, a number of studies have now shown the importance of the host genotype in susceptibility to infection and evidence also suggests that the pathological manifestations of schistosomiasis may be modified by the genetic background of the host (Abdel Salem *et al.*, 1979; Claas & Deelder, 1978; Dean, Bukowski & Cheever, 1981; Fanning *et al.*, 1981). Marked differences in the proportion of *S. mansoni* cercariae which ultimately develops into adult worms have been noted among different mouse strains (Bickle *et al.*, 1980; Colley & Freeman, 1980; Dean *et al.*, 1981; Deelder *et al.*, 1978). This variability could be due to parasite factors such as heterogeneity in the capacity of cercariae to mature (Smith & Clegg, 1979), host factors which limit development of the helminth, or to a combination of the two. Fanning & Kazura (1984) adopted a strictly quantitative approach and measured the number of adult worms recovered from eight inbred and two congenic strains of mice infected with 30 cercariae of *S. mansoni*. The number of adult worms recovered showed a segregation pattern among strains. The mode of inheritance of susceptibility to infection was assessed in F_1 offspring and backcrosses of two strains with relatively high or low susceptibility to *S. mansoni* infection. The results were consistent with homozygosity for a polygenic phenomenon controlling susceptibility to primary *S. mansoni* infection. Studies in congenic mice further suggested that genes within the major histocompatibility complex do not have a great influence in determining the ability of schistosomes to develop into mature adult worms.

In summary, therefore, the limited evidence available suggests that susceptibility and infectivity are probably under the control of a small number of genes and that, as far as snail–schistosome interactions are concerned, different gene combinations may be involved with each local host–parasite interaction. Unfortunately, there are problems in gathering data relating to genetic variation in compatibility within local populations of schistosomes and their hosts. Even though it is apparent that a clear understanding of parasite transmission must take into account genetic as well as environmental factors, there remains an unbridged gap between observations on the inheritance of characters in the laboratory and our understanding of how populations interact in nature. The following sections seek to illustrate how electrophoretic studies are contributing to our knowledge of genetic diversity and interactions between schistosome and snail populations.

SCHISTOSOMA: ENZYME VARIATION AND POPULATION STRUCTURE

Cercariae from snails, and eggs in excretions from the definitive host, are the schistosome life-cycle stages normally encountered in the natural situation. Isolation of the parasite depends on hatching eggs and infecting snails with miracidia or on exposing animals to cercariae from naturally infected snails. Isolates, therefore, may not necessarily provide an adequate assessment of genetic variation in the original parental populations. Little is yet known concerning the amount of variability within the schistosome population of a single host or whether differences in gene frequencies exist between schistosomes from different hosts. Analysis of laboratory isolates has revealed a certain amount of enzyme variation. In a study of 14 enzymes in individual adult worms representing 22 isolates of *S. mansoni*, Fletcher, LoVerde & Woodruff (1981b) recorded a range of genetic variation. Estimates of the proportion of enzyme loci that were polymorphic in a population (P) ranged from 0–0.33, although P averaged over all *S. mansoni* strains was low in comparison with other invertebrate groups at 0.13 ± 0.02. Perhaps, not surprisingly, the proportion of polymorphic loci was higher for six recent isolates than for 15 mouse-adapted strains. The highest P values, 0.28–0.33, were for two samples from a *S. mansoni* strain from Kenya that had been maintained in baboons; a much lower P value (0.06) was obtained for the same isolate passaged in mice. The results undoubtedly reflect the population bottlenecks inherent in laboratory passage, since the baboon adapted line had been through three generations as opposed to 30–40 for the mouse adapted line. Long periods of laboratory maintenance might also explain the lack of polymorphism in strains of *S. japonicum* and *S. mekongi* reported by Fletcher, Woodruff & LoVerde (1980). It is also possible that passage of the parasite through particular definitive hosts may select against particular alleles. Changes in the malate dehydrogenase patterns of schistosomes during passage have been noted by Coles (1971a,b) and Ross, Southgate & Knowles (1978). The possibility of host induced selection was examined by LoVerde, Dewald & Minchella (1982). A line of *S. mansoni* which had originally been passaged through baboons was enzyme typed and was subsequently passaged through murine hosts for three generations. Allele frequencies were found to drift away from frequencies for populations maintained in baboons towards values found for parasites passaged through mice.

That genetic differences might exist between the worm populations of different hosts was suggested by the results of a study utilizing six separate isolates of *S. haematobium* from individual patients living in the SE of Mauritius (Rollinson, Ross & Knowles, 1982). Each isolate was typed for glucose-6-phosphate dehydrogenase (G6PDH) and marked differences in the frequencies of the four recognized alleles in each of the six isolates were observed. However, the differences could also be accounted for by the selection procedures in the isolation of the parasites. A better way of looking at the genetic variation within the schistosome population of an individual host would be to examine adult worms recovered from naturally infected animals.

Schistosome infections of lechwe

Lechwe (*Kobus leche kafuensis*) are antelope closely associated with permanent waters in southern Zambia. They are known to harbour two species of schistosome, *S. margrebowiei* and *S. leiperi*. The former are large worms and many small eggs are found in the female uterus, whereas *S. leiperi* are smaller worms with fewer, larger uterine eggs; hence, the worms can usually be readily identified in mixed infections. An interesting relationship, depicted in Fig. 1, exists between the age of the animal and the species of schistosome by which it is infected (Wright, Southgate & Howard, 1979; Howard, Wright & Southgate, 1982). Examination of 27 animals has shown that lechwe under 1 year old had pure *S. margrebowiei* infections and those over 4 years old had *S. leiperi* only; a changeover from one species to the other occurred during the second, third and fourth years of life of the host. Wright *et al.* (1979) suggested that the early infection with *S. margrebowiei* was related to the distribution of the snail hosts of the two parasites and the annual migration of the lechwe across the Kafue flats as dictated by the flood cycle. It is, as yet, unclear as to why *S. leiperi* sometimes takes so long to become established and why *S. margrebowiei* is not found in older animals. The finding of multiple infections of *S. leiperi*, *S. margrebowiei* and *S. mattheei* in adults of the closely related defassa waterbuck (*Kobus kobus defassa*) suggests that the same kind of interaction is not operating in this definitive host. *S. leiperi* and *S. margrebowiei* from lechwe can be clearly distinguished by alleles at the phosphoglucomutase and glucose-6-phosphate dehydrogenase loci. In adult *S. leiperi* worms, collected directly from culled lechwe, two out of seven enzymes, G6PDH and malate dehydrogenase (MDH), were found to be polymorphic. Two alleles were recognized for G6PDH and three alleles at the MDH-1 locus. The results of an analysis of individual worms

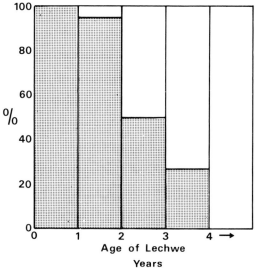

Figure 1. Proportion of *S. margrebowiei* and *S. leiperi* in lechwe antelope of different ages. (Based on Howard *et al.*, 1982.) ▨ *S. margrebowiei*; ▢ *S. leiperi*.

from two 4-year-old male lechwe are shown in Table 1. Theoretically, disregarding sex, there are 18 possible combinations of alleles for G6PDH and MDH. In one animal, five schistosome genotypes were identified and in the other 10, indicating that these animals had been infected by cercariae emanating from a number of genetically distinct sporocysts.

Table 1. Analysis of *S. leiperi* worms recovered from two 4-year-old lechwe; frequencies of two G6PDH and three MDH alleles and the observed genotypes

G6PDH	MDH-1	Lechwe A	Lechwe B
A		0.34	0.22
B		0.66	0.78
	A	0.11	0.19
	B	0.89	0.80
	C	0	0.01
		No. of worms	No. of worms
AA	AA	1	—
AA	BB	3	2
AA	AB	—	1
AB	AA	—	2
AB	BB	5	18
AB	AB	—	10
AB	BC	—	1
BB	AA	—	1
BB	BB	8	34
BB	AB	2	14
BB	BC	—	1
		19	84

The ability to identify particular genotypes by enzyme electrophoresis can also be of use in detecting multiple infections in snails. Southgate *et al.* (1980) isolated *S. bovis* from a single *B. africanus* snail from Tanzania and recovered both male and female worms from laboratory infected animals; out of seven enzymes examined, three were polymorphic. Wright & Ross (1983) found three snails shedding cercariae from about 70 *B. rohlfsi* collected from a transmission site in Ghana, and exposed hamsters separately to the cercariae from each snail. Subsequent enzyme analysis of the adult worms at two polymorphic loci, G6PDH and PGM, showed that two of the snails had been infected by at least three miracidia and the second by two. The snails had been collected over a 10 m stretch at the waters edge and it was suggested that the infected snails had been exposed to high densities of miracidia. However, it was surprising that miracidial densities could have been so high as to achieve multiple infections in two snails while the majority remained uninfected. It seemed unlikely that differences in potential susceptibility among the snail population alone could have accounted for the result.

Many studies have concentrated on using enzymes for the characterization of species and strains but no direct correlation has emerged between the enzyme profile of a parasite and the ability to develop in particular snail hosts. Whereas it is unlikely that the enzyme loci examined are of direct importance in relation to infectivity, if closely linked enzyme loci could be discovered, they would be useful as genetic markers for infectivity genes. Isolates of *S. haematobium* can display marked differences in infectivity to various species of *Bulinus*. Of particular significance is the division between those parasites that develop in *B. africanus* group snails and those that develop in tetraploid members of the *B. tropicus-truncatus* group. However, despite certain geographical trends in the distribution of enzyme types in 22 isolates of *S. haematobium* representing 13 countries, no clear enzymatic distinction was found which correlated with infectivity to snails. Similarly, isolates of *S. mansoni* from different areas do show marked differences in their ability to develop in different species and strains of *Biomphalaria* (Frandsen, 1979) and yet, despite a wide geographical range, *S. mansoni* appears to have undergone little enzymatic divergence (Fletcher *et al.*, 1981b; Boissezon & Jelnes, 1982). An interesting correlation between the frequency of certain lactate dehydrogenase (LDH) enzyme bands and infectivity to *B. glabrata* in lines of *S. mansoni* selected for different levels of infectivity to snails was reported by Fletcher *et al.* (1981a). In schistosome lines of low infectivity, frequencies of LDH-N ranged between 0.56 and 0.69, while in lines of high infectivity, LDH-N frequencies were typically 0.91 to 1.00. The inheritance of the LDH banding patterns, which appear particularly complex, has yet to be elucidated. Practical difficulties associated with crossing defined male and female schistosomes have, to date, hindered studies on the inheritance of enzyme polymorphisms. Hopefully, techniques of maintaining schistosomes by transplantation of sporocysts from snail to snail will alleviate some of these problems. Recently, Imbert-Establet, Rollinson & Ross (1984) have shown how lines of *S. mansoni* characterized by particular alleles for MDH and LDH can be selected from a polymorphic population by single miracidial infections and can be maintained in snails by transplantation.

HYBRIDIZATION AND MATING BEHAVIOUR

Within the group of schistosomes which possess a terminal spine to their egg, typified by *S. haematobium*, concepts of species based on reproductive isolation are confused due to the ability of many recognized species to hybridize. Hybridization of schistosomes has been the subject of a number of laboratory studies (Le Roux, 1954; Taylor, 1970; Wright & Southgate, 1976; Frandsen, 1978; Wright & Ross, 1980), but little is known concerning natural hybridization of schistosomes (Pitchford, 1961; Southgate, van Wijk & Wright, 1976; Wright & Ross, 1980). Recently, enzyme studies have contributed to our understanding of this phenomenon.

Hybrids between S. haematobium *and* S. mattheei

In the Eastern Transvaal, the cattle parasite *S. mattheei* has been shown to occur in man and is often associated with either or both of the normal human parasites, *S. mansoni* or *S. haematobium* (Pitchford, 1959). When *S. haematobium* and *S. mattheei* were found to occur together in the same individual, the presence of eggs intermediate in shape between those of the two species suggested that hybridization was taking place. This was later confirmed by Pitchford (1961) who selected eggs intermediate in shape, produced by mixed infections, and passaged the parasite through laboratory bred snails and rodents. The eggs produced were similar in shape to both the parental species. Wright & Ross (1980) reported the results of a study on F_1 laboratory hybrids between S. *haematobium* and S. *mattheei* and compared the enzymes of these parasites with those of suspect natural hybrids. Alleles identified for G6PDH and PGM appeared to be diagnostic for each species in the Eastern Transvaal and laboratory hybrids were readily recognized by characteristic heterozygote patterns. Parasites from two suspect hybrid infections in patients from this area were established in the laboratory. In the first sample, derived from S. *mattheei*-like eggs, all the males exhibited the G6PDH of S. *mattheei*, whereas most of the females gave heterozygote patterns. The second sample, derived from S. *mattheei*, S. *haematobium* and intermediate shaped eggs, produced G6PDH patterns characteristic of S. *mattheei*, S. *haematobium* and the hybrid. The results indicated that the shape of the eggs is not necessarily a guide to the genetic constitution of the enclosed larvae. From selected S. *mattheei*-shaped eggs produced by human infections, they recovered adult worms giving the enzyme patterns for S. *mattheei* males, S. *haematobium* males and hybrid males and females.

Most interest in the hybridization of S. *haematobium* and S. *mattheei* has focused on the possible implications for control measures, if an animal reservoir for a human pathogen exists. It has been suggested by Pitchford & Lewis (1978) that the poor response of S. *mattheei* to oxamniquine treatment may be due to hybridization with S. *haematobium* which is not susceptible to the drug. Wright & Ross (1980) extrapolated from laboratory data on some of the practical implications of hybridization in the natural situation. Laboratory hybrids tend to exhibit heterosis by their enhanced infectivity to snail hosts and experimental definitive hosts as well as increased growth rate and reproductive potential. They argued that in areas where hybridization occurs, there could be an increase in the proportion of the snail population infected and the cercariae produced will probably have a greater infectivity to man and possibly also to domestic animals. Hybridization could, therefore, lead to the establishment of greater worm loads in man with the schistosomes growing larger, maturing more rapidly and producing more eggs than either of the parental species.

Hybrids between S. haematobium *and* S. intercalatum

In a survey of 500 schoolchildren aged between 4 and 15 years, van Wijk (1969) showed that, in the late 1960s, S. *intercalatum* was the only schistosome occurring in the small town of Loum, Cameroun. S. *intercalatum* resides in the mesenteric veins of the intestine, hence, eggs are passed in the faeces. However, by 1972, a number of children in one part of the town were found to be passing eggs in their urine, and these eggs ranged in size and shape from the forms characteristic of S. *haematobium* to those of S. *intercalatum*; natural hybridization between the two species was shown to be occurring (Wright *et al.*, 1974). Therefore, some time between the late 1960s and early 1970s, S. *haematobium* became established in the town. In this area, each parasite utilizes a different snail host; S. *haematobium* develops in B. *rohlfsi* and S. *intercalatum* in B. *forskalii*. Field work in 1973 demonstrated a clear correlation between the distribution of the two snail hosts in the river Mbette and its tributaries and the distribution of schistosomes in the human population. S. *haematobium* and the hybrid parasite were only found in children inhabiting those areas where both snail hosts occurred. It was evident in 1973 that marked changes had occurred in the epidemiology of the disease over a short time and in the clinical symptoms of townspeople suffering from schistosomiasis (Southgate, van Wijk and

Wright, 1976). The situation was again monitored in 1978 and earlier predictions were confirmed by the continuing swing to urinary schistosomiasis in children between 4 and 15 years old, coupled with a marked decline in intestinal schistosomiasis (Table 2, Figs 2 and 3).

Laboratory investigations of hybrid parasites suggest that whereas the cross between male *S. haematobium* and female *S. intercalatum* is successful, the reverse cross is less so. It is the male worm which, after pairing, is believed to carry the female to the egg-laying site. Hence, it would be expected that, due to the migration of the male *S. haematobium* with female *S. intercalatum*, viable hybrid eggs should be voided in the urine and the relatively inviable eggs of the reverse mating should appear in the faeces. Examination of children passing hybrid eggs in their urine provided confirmatory evidence, as few of them were passing eggs in their faeces and those eggs which were found in faeces were not viable. Utilizing pure isolates from other areas of Cameroun, it has been possible to investigate the enzyme characters of *S. haematobium*, *S. intercalatum* and laboratory hybrids. Alleles at the PGM and G6PDH loci again appear to be diagnostic and heterozygote patterns

Table 2. Comparison of stool and urine examinations for schistosome eggs in two age groups in Loum, Cameroun, in 1968, 1973 and 1978

Year	Age Group 5–9			Age Group 10–14		
	Numbers examined	Stool + ve	Urine + ve	Numbers examined	Stool + ve	Urine + ve
1968	234	117 = 50%	0	222	122 = 55%	0
1973	164	33 = 20%	22 = 13%	61	23 = 38%	12 = 20%
1978	46	1 = 2%	12 = 26%	47	5 = 11%	24 = 51%

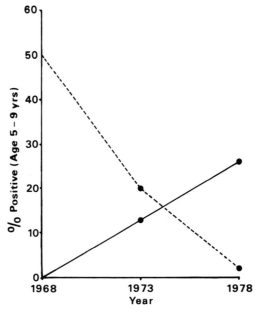

Figure 2. A comparison over 10 years of the results of stool and urine examinations for schistosome eggs in children aged 5–9 in Loum, Cameroun: ———— eggs in urine; -------- eggs in stools.

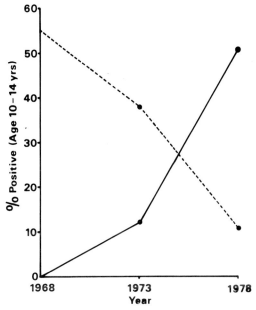

Figure 3. A comparison over 10 years of the results of stool and urine examinations for schistosome eggs in children aged 10–14 in Loum, Cameroun: ——— eggs in urine; --------- eggs in stools.

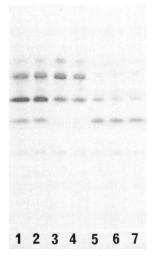

Figure 4. A phosphoglucomutase separation of extracts of *S. intercalatum* (lanes 3, 4), *S. haematobium* (lanes 5, 6, 7) and a laboratory hybrid (lanes 1, 2), run on a polyacrylamide isoelectric focusing gel.

can be identified (Fig. 4). Similar heterozygote patterns have been seen in parasites isolated from a patient passing what seemed to be *S. haematobium*-shaped eggs; the patient, a young boy, had been known to be passing hybrid eggs in 1973 and had been subsequently treated. A further indication of the results of hybridization was seen by the examination of isolates established from cercariae obtained from naturally infected snails. Laboratory studies have shown that whereas *S. haematobium* and *S. intercalatum* can only develop in *B. rohlfsi* or *B. forskalii*, respectively, the

F_1 hybrid can develop in both snail hosts. In the survey of 1978, nine snails were found to be harbouring schistosome infections: three *B. forskalii* and six *B. rohlfsi*. Of the isolates established in the laboratory, each snail yielded the expected parasite except one *B. forskalii*; the cercariae from this snail produced male schistosomes with a PGM pattern indicative of *S. haematobium*.

In laboratory hybridization studies, animals are exposed to cercariae which emanate from single sex infections within molluscs and, when there is no choice, interspecific pairing occurs. The natural situation is obviously more complex in that the definitive host may contain male and female worms of more than one species and choice of mate is possible. Southgate *et al.* (1982) looked at this problem by using enzymes to identify the male and female worm of each pair in mixed infections of *S. haematobium* and *S. intercalatum*. The results showed that there was no specific mate recognition, males and females of either species showed no preference for mates of their own species. Schistosomes within the terminal spined egg complex represent a closely related group of parasites. The absence of pre- and post-mating barriers in some cases facilitates rapid adaptation to prevailing conditions; by retaining the ability to interbreed, the freedom to evolve compatibility with local snail hosts has been maintained.

SNAILS: ENZYME VARIATION AND PARASITE SUSCEPTIBILITY

Much use has been made of enzyme electrophoresis for the identification and characterization of the intermediate hosts of schistosomes (Rollinson, 1984). In addition to providing taxonomic characters, enzyme analyses allow the study of many problems associated with population biology. Of particular significance to the understanding of schistosomiasis transmission is the possibility of using enzymes to study population structure, together with the possibility of finding linkage between observable enzyme markers and other genetically controlled characters, such as parasite susceptibility. Although much has been written concerning susceptibility of snails to schistosomes and it is appreciated that this is, at least in part, under genetic control, little is known concerning the proportion of susceptible and non-susceptible snails in natural populations. As any large-scale study of the population distribution of genes for snail susceptibility would be fraught with practical difficulties, the determination of linked enzyme markers would be a considerable advantage. With this in mind, Mulvey & Vrijenhoek (1984) conducted a study of linkage relationships of certain enzyme loci in *Biomphalaria glabrata*, a host of *S. mansoni*. Of 28 enzyme loci examined, 11 revealed interstrain differences that were further investigated, along with a pigmentation trait, by crossing experiments. Analysis of parental snails, F_1 and F_2 progeny allowed the loci to be assigned to eight linkage groups. For *Biomphalaria*, as well as *Bulinus*, the haploid chromosome number is 18. The incorporation of additional enzyme loci or other morphological characters into such analyses might eventually produce markers for the full chromosome complement. As yet, evidence to indicate close linkage between enzyme markers and genes associated with resistance or susceptibility is lacking. One interesting possibility has been suggested by the work of Michelson & Dubois (1981) who reported on the association of an acid phosphatase marker. Examination of nine laboratory populations and one field population revealed a strong correlation between the expression of particular acid phosphatase patterns and the level of snail susceptibility; the genetics of this potentially interesting observation awaits further elucidation.

Many of the planorbid snails associated with the transmission of schistosomiasis live in water bodies which undergo seasonal fluctuations due to flooding and drought. Such fluctuations have a marked influence on the size of the resident snail population during the course of a year. Certain species have the capacity to aestivate during periods of drought and to increase rapidly in number when conditions are favourable for breeding. *Biomphalaria* and *Bulinus* are both hermaphrodite and capable of self-fertilization; hence, single individuals either as survivors or colonists are able to found new populations. Under these kinds of conditions and in the absence of gene flow between populations, it is conceivable that genetic drift might lead to divergence of isolated populations, which in turn might result in populations with marked differences in compatibility to the local schistosome. Michelson & Dubois (1978) examined 17 populations of *Biomphalaria glabrata* from the state of Bahia, Brazil, with respect to their susceptibility to infection with an allopatric Puerto Rican strain of *S. mansoni*. Six of the snail strains tested proved to be completely refractory to infection with the parasite when exposed at 5–7 mm in size, whereas others exhibited infection rates ranging from 0–49%. Quite marked differences in susceptibility were seen in populations grouped in a restricted geographic region and they postulated that genetic drift might have contributed to the patchy distribution of snail susceptibility. That such a genetic structure might exist was indicated by an electrophoretic study by Mulvey & Vrijenhoek (1982) who examined seven populations of *B. glabrata* from Puerto Rico at 26 enzyme loci. Although the level of electrophoretically detectable polymorphism was surprisingly much lower (15%) than that found previously in laboratory stocks (Mulvey & Vrijenhoek, 1981a), local populations were clearly distinct. In a similar manner, Rollinson & Wright (1984) studied enzyme variation and compatibility in *Bulinus cernicus*, the intermediate host for *S. haematobium*, on the island of Mauritius. This species shows a great deal of phenotypic variation; electrophoretic analyses of 25 populations at six enzyme loci revealed regional differences in gene frequencies. Of the 22 alleles identified, five were restricted in their distribution to snails from one habitat and four were associated with snails from just two localities. The data suggested that gene flow between habitats was limited and that there was marked differentiation between some populations. Thirteen of the populations were tested for compatibility with a local isolate of *S. haematobium*; all proved susceptible, with infection rates ranging from 28.8–91.7%. In this kind of experiment, there is an underlying assumption that different susceptibilities are due to different genetic constitutions of the snails involved, and it is therefore of interest to note that no correlation was apparent between snails from known transmission sites and high or low infection rates in the laboratory.

Selection pressures that might be acting on the genes responsible for susceptibility or resistance to schistosomes in natural populations are poorly understood. It has been suggested by Michelson & Dubois (1981) that *Biomphalaria glabrata* populations may consist largely of non-susceptible snails, and they supported their hypothesis with the fact that the majority of snail surveys conducted in endemic areas of schistosomiasis reveal low infection rates. Anderson & May (1979), reviewing the literature, concluded that in cases where large samples of snails have been examined, the average incidence of infection throughout a year or over a large sampling area tends to lie in the range of 1–5%, irrespective of the species of snail or schistosome or of the geographical location. Although variability in susceptibility was acknowledged as likely to contribute to infection levels within populations of snails, emphasis was given to the role played by differential mortality between infected and uninfected snails, together with long latent periods of infection, in determining the observed patterns of prevalence. The low prevalence of snail infections in natural populations indicates that parasite selection pressure may be low. Neither snail mortality nor reduction of fecundity are immediate consequences of schistosome infection and many snail species with short generation times are likely to produce offspring and pass on sperm to other individuals before the deleterious effects of infection become apparent. Minchella & LoVerde (1981) reported that *B. glabrata* experienced an increase in egg-laying shortly after exposure to *S. mansoni*, irrespective of whether or not they became infective, hence suggesting that the snails were equipped with some compensatory mechanism.

In order to explain why non-susceptible snails are not predominant in nature, Wright (1971) suggested that insusceptibility may be associated with some disadvantageous character or physiological defect. A small amount of evidence to support this argument has been produced by Minchella & LoVerde (1983) utilizing laboratory stocks of *Biomphalaria* of known susceptibility. They concluded that non-susceptible snails had a lower reproductive output when subjected to parasite pressure and the presence of susceptible snails.

REPRODUCTIVE STRATEGIES OF SNAILS

Given that genetic variation exists within snail populations, it is interesting to examine aspects of the breeding biology which might contribute to the maintenance of heterogeneity. Utilization of genetic markers has allowed observations to be made on the occurrence of cross-fertilization, multiple insemination and sperm storage in both *Biomphalaria* and *Bulinus*. When snail samples are sufficiently large, the frequency of alleles at polymorphic loci can be tested for closeness of fit to Hardy-Weinberg expectations to establish whether the population is outcrossing. Indeed, most of the *Biomphalaria* spp. and diploid species of *Bulinus* that have been examined appear to be outcrossing in nature. Certain tetraploids such as *Bulinus truncatus* and related species show little enzyme heterogeneity (Wright & Rollinson, 1981) and populations often include a large proportion of aphallic individuals; in these species, self-fertilization, possibly parthenogenesis, is important. The tetraploid condition is not always associated with self-fertilization, as *B. permembranaceus* appears to be outbreeding in nature (Jelnes, 1977). Susceptibility to schistosomes is not confined to snails associated with particular reproductive strategies. Perhaps, more than any other group, the self-fertilizing tetraploids would seem to have the necessary prerequisites to allow the evolution of resistant populations, but records indicating that this might be so are lacking. Indeed, the tetraploid *B. truncatus* remains the major host of *S. haematobium* in North Africa.

Parent–offspring analyses in the laboratory offer a further method for studying outcrossing in natural populations. The procedure requires the isolation of adult snails immediately after collection and the monitoring of subsequent egg production. Identification of the parental genotype and comparison with those of its offspring allows an assessment as to whether cross-fertilization has taken place. The finding of alleles in the F_1 not present in the parent is indicative of that parent having received sperm from another individual and having utilized it for cross-fertilization.

Analysis of young produced over a period of time after isolation of the parent allows an insight into whether donated sperm, or fertilized eggs, can be stored.

Mulvey & Vrijenhoek (1981b) demonstrated that a population of *Biomphalaria obstructa* collected from an irrigation ditch in Florida showed little evidence of self-fertilization; genotypic frequencies at four polymorphic loci showed a close fit to Hardy-Weinberg expectations. Furthermore, 15 of 17 isolated snails produced progeny that resulted, in part, from exogenous sperm stored prior to isolation. Twelve of the 15 parents produced broods that may have been fathered, in part, by self-fertilization or by mating with an additional partner with the same genotype as 'self'. In a study of *Bulinus cernicus* from Mauritius, Rollinson & Wright (1984) noted that the frequency of alleles at polymorphic loci showed a close fit to Hardy-Weinberg expectations and isolated wild-caught snails were found to produce offspring resulting from cross-fertilization, again indicative of outbreeding. In laboratory mating experiments, it was shown by the use of enzyme markers that snails could store exogenous sperm or, possibly, fertilized eggs for up to 70 days after copulation, and that there was a preference for cross-fertilization. Similar methodology was used to study the breeding biology of four other species, *B. scalaris*, *B. tropicus*, *B. reticulatus* and *B. globosus* representing the four species groups of *Bulinus* (Rollinson, in press a). Cross-fertilization was shown to be occurring in all the populations at the time of sampling and sperm storage was common. Evidence of multiple insemination involving at least two genetically distinct donors was reported for *B. scalaris*. Therefore, evidence is accumulating to suggest that, in those species associated with ephemeral habitats, mechanisms such as cross-fertilization, sperm storage and multiple insemination might play a role in maintaining heterogeneity. Certainly, the effective gene pool of a population surviving a bottleneck phenomenon, such as a period of drought, could be increased by snails storing the sperm of one or more other individuals.

Recently, Monteiro *et al.* (1984) have made some interesting observations on sperm sharing in *Biomphalaria*. Utilizing albino markers in laboratory crossing experiments, they demonstrated that a cross-fertilized individual can share with other individuals sperm received from its previous crossmate. Hence, an individual might only act as an intermediary in sperm transfer. Acting as a female, a snail receives exogenous sperm from its male partner; when later acting as a male, it passes on a proportion of this exogenous sperm to another individual. To try and explain these intriguing results, the authors postulated that as inbreeding and kinship increase in a population, genetic differences between exogenous and endogenous spermatozoa decrease. High levels of inbreeding would tend to eliminate genetic differences between exogenous and endogenous spermatozoa, and selection pressure to differentiate between endogenous and exogenous spermatozoa might be expected to decrease. Certainly, the morphology of the reproductive tract is such that the partition of endogenous and exogenous sperm is not complete; hence, during copulation, both endogenous and exogenous sperm might be passed over. Clearly, more information is needed on the mating behaviour of snails in relation to their reproductive status.

CONCLUSIONS

The majority of experimental studies involving the genetics of schistosome and snail interactions have followed two broad interconnecting lines of research. The first has been concerned primarily with laboratory inheritance studies, utilizing well-defined stocks of parasites and snails to elucidate the genetics of compatibility between host and parasite. In some cases, these studies have attempted to mimic some of the interactions observed in nature. The second approach has been concerned with the surveillance and monitoring of natural populations and the identification of factors influencing their interaction. It is particularly encouraging that electrophoretic studies, although originally intended for detecting genetic diversity, have succeeded in forging a close link between laboratory and field observations.

It is apparent that one of the most useful applications of enzyme electrophoresis has been for the differentiation of species and strains of schistosomes and their snail hosts. This is a particularly valuable contribution as there is a growing need, from the epidemiological viewpoint, for an accurate definition of parasites, coupled with a sound knowledge of their distribution. Experimental evidence has shown that compatibility, in at least one snail host/parasite combination, that of *Biomphalaria glabrata* and *S. mansoni*, is under the control of a number of genetic factors. Further laboratory inheritance and linkage analysis studies utilizing enzyme markers promise to provide more detailed maps of genes on chromosomes and it is possible that markers for susceptibility or infectivity genes may be found. It is as yet far from clear, however, as to how these genes behave in natural populations. Data relating to the frequencies of compatibility traits in nature are virtually non-existent. Despite much speculation, it is difficult to quantify or identify the effects of selection pressures exerted by schistosomes and other parasites on snail populations. Longitudinal studies, as limited as they are, suggest that microevolutionary forces can act quickly to change parasite–snail preferences, but little is known of the corresponding evolutionary processes involved in the snail's response. *Bulinus* and *Biomphalaria* are remarkably resilient species; as a group, they appear to have a variety of reproductive strategies in their repertoire; in some ways, this must contribute to their success in terms of distribution but the importance, if any, of these strategies in relation to their parasite load awaits clarification. The study of polymorphism within snail populations, as identified by enzyme analyses, offers one possible way of looking at the behaviour of genes in natural populations.

It is within the definitive host that sexual reproduction of schistosomes occurs and this is the most stable and persistent stage within the life cycle. Estimates on the longevity of schistosomes include 3.4 years for *S. haematobium* (Wilkins *et al.*, 1984) and up to 37 years for *S. mansoni* (Vermund, Bradley & Ruiz-Tiben, 1983); a documented example of an *S. mansoni* infection continuing for 32 years was recently reported by Harris, Russell & Charters (1984). That heterogeneity exists within schistosome populations of an individual host has been indicated by the study of laboratory isolates and by analyses of worms recovered from animal infections.

Enzyme data also suggest that multiple infections in snails may be a common occurrence. One of the goals for the future is to understand more of the genetic structure of the schistosome population of a definitive host and this, in turn, may help to elucidate certain questions concerning population turnover. Some of the consequences of mingling and mixing of different schistosome genotypes have been well illustrated by studies involving hybridization of different taxa.

If future investigations continue to combine the results of field and experimental research and incorporate some of the new techniques of molecular biology, then they will surely be both exciting and rewarding. A true appreciation of the many factors involved in schistosome and snail interactions will rely heavily on the continued integration of genetic and ecological studies.

ACKNOWLEDGEMENTS

Some of the work reported herein was supported in part by the Parasitic Diseases Programme of the World Health Organization and the Wellcome Trust.

REFERENCES

ABDEL SALAM, E., ISHAAC, S. & MAHMOUD, A. A. F., 1979. Histocompatibility-linked susceptibility for hepatosplenomegaly in human schistosomiasis mansoni. *Journal of Immunology, 123:* 1829.

ANDERSON, R. M. & MAY, R. M., 1979. Prevalence of schistosome infections within molluscan populations: observed patterns and theoretical predictions. *Parasitology, 79:* 63–94.

BICKLE, Q. D., LONG, E. G., JAMES, E. R., DOENHOFF, M. J. & FESTING, M., 1980. *Schistosoma mansoni:* influence of the mouse host's sex, age and strain on resistance to reinfection. *Experimental Parasitology, 50:* 222–232.

BOISSEZON, B. & JELNES, J. E., 1982. Isozyme studies on cercariae from monoinfections and adult worms of *Schistosoma mansoni* (10 isolates) and *S. rodhaini* (one isolate) by horizontal polyacrylamide gel electrophoresis and staining of eight enzymes. *Zeitschrift für Parasitenkunde, 67:* 185–196.

CHIU, J. K., ONG, S. J., YU, J. C., KAO, C. Y. & IJIMA, T., 1981. Susceptibility of *Oncomelania hupensis formosona* recombinants and hybrids with *Oncomelania hupensis nosophora* to infection with *Schistosoma japonicum. International Journal for Parasitology, 11:* 391–397.

CLAAS, F. H. J. & DEELDER, A. M., 1979. H-2 linked immune response to murine experimental *Schistosoma mansoni* infections. *Journal of Immunogenetics, 6:* 167–175.

CLARKE, B., 1976. The ecological genetics of host–parasite relationships. *Symposia of the British Society for Parasitology, 14:* 87–103.

COLES, G. C., 1971a. Variations in malate dehydrogenase isoenzymes of *Schistosoma mansoni. Comparative Biochemistry and Physiology, 39B:* 35–42.

COLES, G. C., 1971b. Alteration of *Schistosoma mansoni* malate dehydrogenase isoenzymes on passage in the laboratory. *Comparative Biochemistry and Physiology, 40B:* 1079–1083.

COLLEY, D. G. & FREEMAN, G. L., 1980. Differences in adult *Schistosoma mansoni* worm burden requirements for the establishment of resistance to reinfection in inbred mice. 1. CBA/J and C57 B1/6. *American Journal of Tropical Medicine and Hygiene, 29:* 1279–1285.

DAVIS, G. M., 1979. The origin and evolution of the Pomatiopsidae, with emphasis on the Mekong River Triculinae. *Monograph of the Academy of Natural Sciences of Philadelphia, 20:* vii + 1–120.

DAVIS, G. M. & RUFF, M. B., 1973. *Oncomelania hupensis* (Gastropoda: Hydrobiidae) hybridisation genetics and transmission of *Schistosoma japonicum. Malacological Review, 6:* 181–197.

DEAN, D. A., BUKOWSKI, M. A. & CHEEVER, A. W., 1981. Relationship between acquired resistance, portal hypertension and lung granulomas in ten strains of mice infected with *Schistosoma mansoni. American Journal of Tropical Medicine and Hygiene, 30:* 806–814.

DEELDER, A. M., CLAAS, F. H. S. & DE VRIES, R. R. P., 1978. Influence of the mouse H-2 complex on experimental infections with *Schistosoma mansoni. Transactions of the Royal Society of Tropical Medicine and Hygiene, 72:* 321–322.

FANNING, M. M. & KAZURA, J. W., 1984. Genetic-linked variation in susceptibility of mice to *Schistosomiasis mansoni. Parasite Immunology, 6:* 95–103.

FANNING, M. M., PETERS, P. A., DAVIS, R. S., KAZURA, J. N. & MAHMOUD, A. A. F., 1981. Immunopathology of murine infection with *Schistosoma mansoni:* Relationship of genetic background to hepatosplenic disease and modulation. *Journal of Infectious Diseases, 144:* 148–153.

FLETCHER, M., LoVERDE, P. T. & RICHARDS, C. S., 1981a. *Schistosoma mansoni:* electrophoretic characterisation of strains selected for different levels of infectivity to snails. *Experimental Parasitology, 52:* 362–370.

FLETCHER, M., LoVERDE, P. T. & WOODRUFF, D. S., 1981b. Genetic variation in *Schistosoma mansoni:* enzyme polymorphisms in populations from Africa, Southwest Asia, South America and the West Indies. *American Journal of Tropical Medicine and Hygiene, 30:* 406–421.

FLETCHER, M., WOODRUFF, D. S. & LoVERDE, P. T., 1980. Genetic differentiation between *Schistosoma mekongi* and *S. japonicum:* an electrophoretic study. The Mekong Schistosome. *Malacological Review, suppl. 2:* 113–122.

FRANDSEN, F., 1978. Hybridisation between different strains of *Schistosoma intercalatum* Fisher, 1934 from Cameroun and Zaire. *Journal of Helminthology, 52:* 11–22.

FRANDSEN, F., 1979. Studies on the relationship between *Schistosoma* and their intermediate hosts. III. The genus *Biomphalaria* and *Schistosoma mansoni* from Egypt, Kenya, Sudan, Uganda, West Indies (St Lucia) and Zaire (two different strains: Katanga and Kinshasa). *Journal of Helminthology, 53:* 321–348.

HARRIS, A. R. C., RUSSELL, R. J. & CHARTERS, A. D., 1984. A review of schistosomiasis in immigrants in Western Australia, demonstrating the unusual longevity of *Schistosoma mansoni*. *Transactions of the Royal Society of Tropical Medicine and Hygiene, 78:* 385–388.

HOWARD, G. W., WRIGHT, C. A. & SOUTHGATE, V. R., 1982. Schistosome infections of lechwe and waterbuck in Zambia — a preliminary report. In M. E. Fowler (Ed.), *Wildlife Diseases of the Pacific Basin and Other Countries. Proceedings of the 4th International Conference of the Wildlife Association*: 136–138. Ames: The Association.

IAROTSKI, L. S. & DAVIS, A., 1981. The schistosomiasis problem in the world: results of a WHO questionnaire survey. *Bulletin of the World Health Organisation, 59:* 115–127.

IMBERT-ESTABLET, D., ROLLINSON, D. & ROSS, G. C., 1984. *Schistosoma mansoni*: Selection de genotypes et leurs maintenance par transplantations sporocystiques. *Comptes Rendus de l'Academie de Sciences de Paris, 299, Serie III:* 459–462.

JELNES, J. E., 1977. An electrophoretic character useful in the distinction between *Bulinus tropicus* and *B. permembranaceus* (Gastropoda, Planorbidae). *Steenstrupia, 4:* 139–141.

LE ROUX, P. L., 1954. Hybridisation of *Schistosoma mansoni* and *Schistosoma rodhaini*. *Transactions of the Royal Society of Tropical Medicine and Hygiene, 48:* 3–4.

LIE, K. J., 1982. Survival of *Schistosoma mansoni* and other trematode larvae in the snail *Biomphalaria glabrata*. A discussion of the interference theory. *Tropical and Geographical Medicine, 34:* 111–122.

LOKER, E. S., 1983. A comparative study of the life-histories of mammalian schistosomes. *Parasitology, 87:* 343–369.

LoVERDE, P. T., DEWALD, J. & MINCHELLA, D. J., 1982. Host-induced selection in *Schistosoma mansoni*. *Fifth International Congress of Parasitology. Proceedings and Abstracts Vol. II*: 105–106.

MAO, S. & SHAO, B., 1982. Schistosomiasis control in the Peoples Republic of China. *American Journal of Tropical Medicine and Hygiene, 31:* 92–99.

MICHELSON, E. A. & DUBOIS, L., 1978. Susceptibility of Bahian populations of *Biomphalaria glabrata* to an allopatric strain of *Schistosoma mansoni*. *American Journal of Tropical Medicine and Hygiene, 27:* 782–786.

MICHELSON, E. H. & DUBOIS, L., 1981. An isoenzyme marker possibly associated with the susceptibility of *Biomphalaria glabrata* populations to *Schistosoma mansoni*. *Acta Tropica, 38:* 419–426.

MINCHELLA, D. J. & LoVERDE, P. T., 1981. A cost of increased early reproductive effect in the snail *Biomphalaria glabrata*. *The American Naturalist, 118:* 876–881.

MINCHELLA, D. J. & LoVERDE, P. T., 1983. Laboratory comparison of the relative success of *Biomphalaria glabrata* stocks which are susceptible and insusceptible to infection with *Schistosoma mansoni*. *Parasitology, 86:* 335–344.

MONTEIRO, W., ALMEIDA, J. M. G., Jr. & DIAS, B. S., 1984. Sperm sharing in *Biomphalaria* snails: a new behavioural strategy in simultaneous hermaphroditism. *Nature, 308:* 727–729.

MULVEY, M. & VRIJENHOEK, R. C., 1981a. Genetic variation among laboratory strains of the planorbid snail *Biomphalaria glabrata*. *Biochemical Genetics, 19:* 1169–1181.

MULVEY, M. & VRIJENHOEK, R. C., 1981b. Multiple paternity in the hermaphroditic snail *Biomphalaria obstructa*. *Journal of Heredity, 72:* 308–312.

MULVEY, M. & VRIJENHOEK, R. C., 1982. Population structure in *Biomphalaria glabrata*: examination of an hypothesis for the patchy distribution of susceptibility to schistosomes. *American Journal of Tropical Medicine and Hygiene, 31:* 1195–1200.

MULVEY, M. & VRIJENHOEK, R. C., 1984. Genetics of *Biomphalaria glabrata*: linkage analysis and crossing compatibilities among laboratory strains. *Malacologia, 25:* 513–524.

NEWTON, W. L., 1952. The comparative tissue reaction of two strains of *Australorbis glabratus* to infection with *Schistosoma mansoni*. *Journal of Parasitology, 38:* 362–366.

NEWTON, W. L., 1953. The inheritance of susceptibility to infection with *Schistosoma mansoni* in *Australorbis glabratus*. *Experimental Parasitology, 2:* 242–257.

NEWTON, W. L., 1955. The establishment of a strain of *Australorbis glabratus* which combines albinism and high susceptibility to infection with *Schistosoma mansoni*. *Journal of Parasitology, 41:* 526–528.

PITCHFORD, R. J., 1959. Cattle schistosomiasis in man in the Eastern Transvaal. *Transactions of the Royal Society of Tropical Medicine and Hygiene, 53:* 285–290.

PITCHFORD, R. J., 1961. Observations on a possible hybrid between the two schistosomes, *S. haematobium* and *S. mattheei*. *Transactions of the Royal Society of Tropical Medicine and Hygiene, 55:* 44–51.

PITCHFORD, R. J. & LEWIS, M., 1978. Oxamniquine in the treatment of various schistosome infections in South Africa. *South African Medical Journal, 53:* 677–680.

RICHARDS, C. S., 1973. Susceptibility of adult *Biomphalaria glabrata* to *Schistosoma mansoni* infection. *American Journal of Tropical Medicine and Hygiene, 22:* 749–756.

RICHARDS, C. S., 1975a. Genetic factors in susceptibility of *Biomphalaria glabrata* for different strains of *Schistosoma mansoni*. *Parasitology, 70:* 231–241.

RICHARDS, C. S., 1975b. Genetic studies on variation in infectivity of *Schistosoma mansoni*. *Journal of Parasitology, 61:* 233–236.

RICHARDS, C. S., 1976a. Variations in infectivity for *Biomphalaria glabrata* on strains of *Schistosoma mansoni* form the same geographic area. *Bulletin of the World Health Organisation, 54:* 706–707.

RICHARDS, C. S., 1976b. Genetic aspects of host–parasite relationships. *Symposia of the British Society of Parasitology, 14:* 45–54.

RICHARDS, C. S., 1984. Influence of snail age on genetic variations in susceptibility of *Biomphalaria glabrata* for infection with *Schistosoma mansoni. Malacologia, 25:* 493–502.

ROLLINSON, D., 1984. Recent advances in the characterisation of the schistosomes of man and their intermediate hosts. *Tropical Disease Research Series WHO, 5:* 401–441.

ROLLINSON, D. in press a. Reproductive strategies of some species of *Bulinus. Proceedings of the VIII International Malacological Congress.*

ROLLINSON, D. & WRIGHT, C. A., 1984. Population studies on *Bulinus cernicus* from Mauritius. *Malacologia, 25:* 447–463.

ROLLINSON, D., ROSS, G. C. & KNOWLES, R. J., 1982. Analysis of a glucose-6-phosphate dehydrogenase polymorphism in isolates of *Schistosoma haematobium. Fifth International Congress of Parasitology:* 608.

ROSS, G. C., SOUTHGATE, V. R. & KNOWLES, R. J., 1978. Observations on some isoenzymes of strains of *Schistosoma bovis, S. mattheei, S. margrebowiei* and *S. leiperi. Zeitschrift für Parasitenkunde, 57:* 49–56.

SMITH, M. A. & CLEGG, J. A., 1979. Different levels of immunity to *Schistosoma mansoni* in the mouse: the role of variant cercariae. *Parasitology, 78:* 311–321.

SOUTHGATE, V. R., van WIJK, H. B. & WRIGHT, C. A., 1976. Schistosomiasis at Loum, Cameroun; *Schistosoma haematobium, S. intercalatum* and their natural hybrid. *Zeitschrift für Parasitenkunde, 49:* 145–159.

SOUTHGATE, V. R., ROLLINSON, D., ROSS, G. C. & KNOWLES, R. J., 1980. Observations on an isolate of *Schistosoma bovis* from Tanzania. *Zeitschrift für Parasitenkunde, 63:* 241–249.

SOUTHGATE, V. R., ROLLINSON, D., ROSS, G. C. & KNOWLES, R. J., 1982. Mating behaviour in mixed infections of *Schistosoma haematobium* and *S. intercalatum. Journal of Natural History, 16:* 491–496.

TAYLOR, M. G., 1970. Hybridisation experiments of five species of African schistosomes. *Journal of Helminthology, 44:* 253–314.

VERMUND, S. H., BRADLEY, D. J. & RUIZ-TIBEN, E., 1983. Survival of *Schistosoma mansoni* in the human host: estimates from a community-based prospective study in Puerto Rico. *American Journal of Tropical Medicine and Hygiene, 32:* 1040–1048.

WIJK, H. B. van, 1969. *Schistosoma intercalatum* — infection in school children of Loum, Cameroun. *Tropical and Geographical Medicine, 21:* 375–382.

WILKINS, H. A., GOLL, P. H., MARSHALL, T. F. de C. & MOORE, P. J., 1984. Dynamics of *Schistosoma haematobium* infection in a Gambian community. III. Acquisition and loss of infection. *Transactions of the Royal Society of Tropical Medicine and Hygiene, 78:* 227–232.

WRIGHT, C. A., 1971. Review of 'Genetics of a molluscan vector of schistosomiasis' by C. S. Richards. *Tropical Disease Bulletin 68:* 333–335.

WRIGHT, C. A., 1974. Snail susceptibility or trematode infectivity? *Journal of Natural History, 8:* 545–548.

WRIGHT, C. A. & ROLLINSON, D., 1981. Analysis of enzymes in the *Bulinus tropicus/truncatus* complex (Mollusca: Planorbidae). *Journal of Natural History, 15:* 873–885.

WRIGHT, C. A. & ROSS, G. C., 1980. Hybrids between *Schistosoma haematobium* and *S. mattheei* and their identification by isoelectric focusing of enzymes. *Transactions of the Royal Society of Tropical Medicine and Hygiene, 74:* 326–332.

WRIGHT, C. A. & ROSS, G. C., 1983. Enzymes in *Schistosoma haematobium. Bulletin of the World Health Organisation, 61:* 307–316.

WRIGHT, C. A. & SOUTHGATE, V. R., 1976. Hybridisation of schistosomes and some of its implications. *Symposia of the British Society for Parasitology, 14:* 55–86.

WRIGHT, C. A. & SOUTHGATE, V. R., 1981. Coevolution of digeneans and molluscs, with special reference to schistosomes and their intermediate hosts. In *The Evolving Biosphere, Chance, Change and Challenge:* 191–205. British Museum (Natural History)/Cambridge University Press.

WRIGHT, C. A., SOUTHGATE, V. R. & HOWARD, G. W., 1979. Observations on the life-cycle of *Schistosoma margrebowiei* and its possible interactions with *S. leiperi* in Zambia. *Journal of Natural History, 13:* 499–506.

WRIGHT, C. A., SOUTHGATE, V. R., van WIJK, H. B. & MOORE, P. J., 1974. Hybrids between *Schistosoma haematobium* and *S. intercalatum* in Cameroun. *Transactions of the Royal Society of Tropical Medicine and Hygiene, 68:* 413–414.

Experimental studies of age-intensity and age-prevalence profiles of infection: *Schistosoma mansoni* in snails and mice

R. M. ANDERSON AND J. A. CROMBIE

Department of Pure and Applied Biology
Imperial College, London University,
London SW7 2BB, U.K.

Experimental studies are described which focus on age-related changes in the average intensity and prevalence of infection with *Schistosoma mansoni* in populations of snails and inbred mice. Convex patterns of change in prevalence with snail age are shown to be determined by age-related variability in both susceptibility to infection and parasite–induced host mortality. Similar trends for average worm burdens in mice populations are thought to result from acquired resistance to infection which acts to progressively reduce parasite establishment as the intensity and duration of past exposure increases. Mathematical models are developed to aid in the interpretation of recorded trends. Observed changes with age in the intensity of infection with schistosomes in human communities are discussed with respect to acquired resistance and age-related differences in contact with infection. Herd immunity to helminth infection is examined in the context of disease control by mass chemotherapy and heterogeneity in inherent susceptibility to infection or immunological competence to resist parasite invasion. It is argued that the measurement of variability in worm loads within human communities represents an important source of information for improving both our understanding of the biological basis of the interaction between host and parasite and the design of effective long term control policies.

KEY WORDS: — Schistosomes — trickle infection — population dynamics — genetic heterogeneity — chemotherapy — acquired immunity

CONTENTS

Ecology and Genetics of Host–Parasite Interactions
ISBN: 0 12 593 690 7

INTRODUCTION

The prevalence and intensity of helminth infection often varies systematically, both among different age classes of human communities and within different cohorts of intermediate hosts. In endemic regions, host age records the duration of past exposure to infection and thus age-prevalence or age-intensity profiles reflect, in

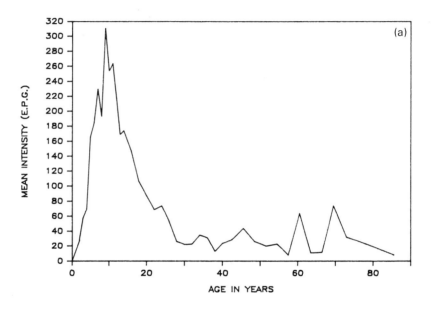

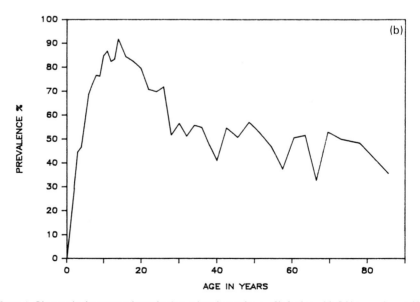

Figure 1. Changes in the average intensity (e.p.g.) and prevalence of infection with *Schistosoma haematobium* over a wide range of age classes. Graph a, Intensity; Graph b, Prevalence. (Data from Bradley & McCullough, 1973.)

part, the intensity of past and current transmission. Many factors, both physical and biological, act to determine the shape of these epidemiological profiles (whether based on horizontal or longitudinal studies) and their interpretation is beset with many practical and conceptual difficulties. A variety of different processes, for example, may be capable of generating identical patterns. Thus in the absence of additional biological or epidemiological information, difficulties arise in discriminating between alternate hypotheses as determinants of observed trends. Age-related changes in the intensity and prevalence of *Schistosoma mansoni* infection in human communities are a good example of this problem. Observed trends are invariably convex in form where average intensity and prevalence rise to a peak in the teenage groups and thereafter decline in the adult age classes (Fig. 1). Both ecological factors (age-specific exposure to infection) and immunological processes (acquired immunity), or a combination of both mechanisms, could generate these trends. Their relative significance is a matter of much current debate (Warren, 1973; Bradley & McCullough, 1973; Dalton & Poole, 1978; Anderson & May, 1985).

This paper considers a series of experiments involving *S. mansoni* infections in the intermediate snail host (*Biomphalaria glabrata*) and the mouse, aimed at improving our understanding of the factors which generate age-related changes in average intensity and prevalence of infection. Our scientific approach may be termed experimental ecology and involves both experimentation and the use of mathematical models to aid in the interpretation of observed patterns. Laboratory studies centre on the exposure of groups of hosts of known age to continual infection under defined and controlled conditions over long periods of time relative to the life expectancy of the host. Such experiments are often referred to as 'trickle' exposure studies. They are thought more closely to mimic host exposure to infection in natural environments when compared with the primary and challenge experiments (involving host exposure to large numbers of infective stages) which are a feature of much immunological research in parasitology (Anderson & Crombie, 1984; Sturrock, Cottrell & Kimani, 1984).

POPULATIONS OF SNAILS CONTINUALLY EXPOSED TO INFECTION

Many biological and physical factors are known to influence observed age-related changes in the prevalence of schistosome infections in populations of snails. They include age-related changes in snail susceptibility, temporal changes in the 'force' of infection (the per capita rate at which hosts become infected), water temperature, parasite-induced snail mortality, the ability of snails to recover from infection and snail density (Standen, 1952; De Witt, 1955; Chu, Massoud & Sabbaghian, 1966; Upatham, 1972; Sturrock & Upatham, 1973; Prah & James, 1977; Anderson, 1978; Anderson & May, 1979; Anderson, *et al.*, 1982; Carter, Anderson & Wilson, 1982). We focus on one particular aspect of this issue; namely, the interplay between the intensity of exposure to infection and age-related changes in snail demography and susceptibility to parasitic invasion. To simplify interpretation of experimental results we consider age-prevalence profiles generated under constant environmental conditions (i.e., water temperature, volume and pH).

R. M. ANDERSON AND J. A. CROMBIE

Cohort experiments

Studies of single cohorts of snails which are exposed to constant numbers of miracidia per unit of time reveal some interesting patterns (Anderson & Crombie, 1984). For high rates of exposure (30 snails of identical age, exposed to 110 miracidia/week for 30 weeks in 10 litres of water maintained at 25°C), the prevalence rises rapidly to a plateau as the duration of exposure increases (Fig. 2d). Similar patterns emerge for exposure levels of 50 and 80 miracidia per week (Fig. 2b and c) although the rate of approach to the plateau is positively associated with the intensity of exposure to infection. At very low exposure levels (10 miracidia per week), prevalence rises

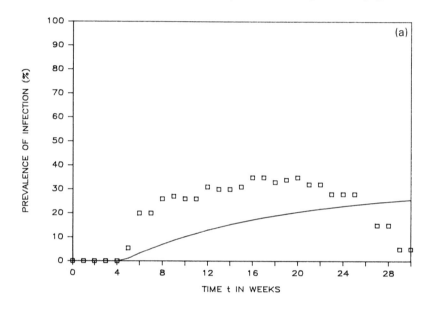

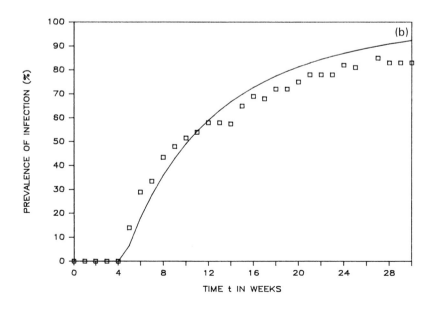

to a level of 30% and thereafter decays as duration of exposure (= age of cohort) increases (Fig. 2a). Snail mortality in these experiments was related to the intensity of exposure to infection; the death rate of infected snails shedding cercariae being approximately 12 times greater than that of uninfected hosts (Fig. 3). The average force

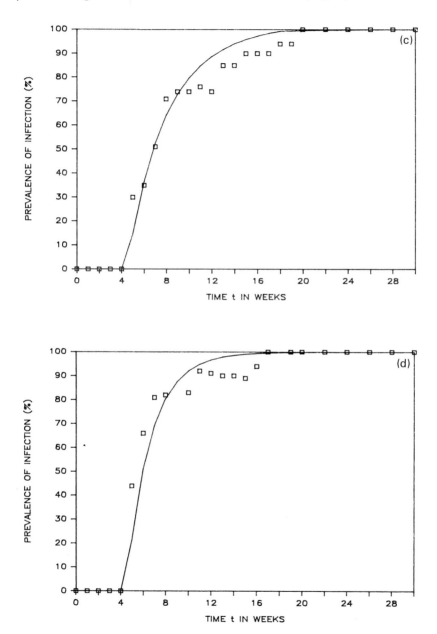

Figure 2. *(opposite and above)* Changes in the prevalence of *S. mansoni* infection in laboratory populations of *Biomphalaria glabrata.* Open squares, recorded values; solid line, predictions of the simple model defined by equations (1) to (3) in the main text. Graph (a), Parameter values $\lambda = 0.025$/week, $\mu = 0.00285$/week, $\mu'' = 0.062$/week, $\tau = 4.5$ weeks. Graph (b), $\lambda = 0.139$/week, other parameters as defined for (a). Graph (c), $\lambda = 0.308$/week, other parameters as defined for (a). Graph (d), $\lambda = 0.492$/week, other parameters as defined for (a). (After Anderson & Crombie, 1984.)

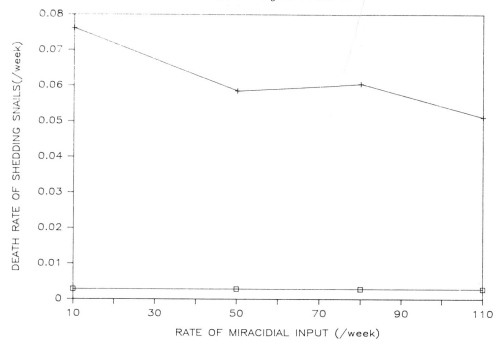

Figure 3. The average death rate of shedding snails, μ'', (top line and crosses) observed in the experiments represented in Fig. 2 in which miracidial input was 10, 50, 80 or 110/week. Bottom line and open squares, average death rate of uninfected snails, μ. (After Anderson & Crombie, 1984.)

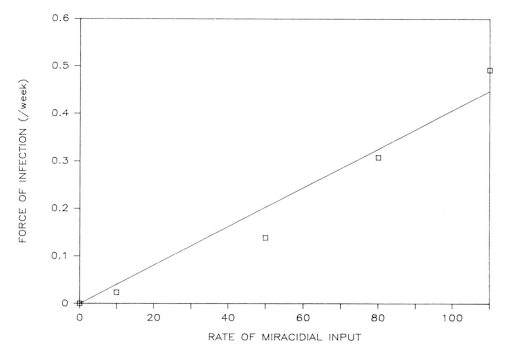

Figure 4. The relationship between the average force of infection, λ, and the rate at which miracidia were added to the experimental arenas. Open squares, observed values; solid line, best fit linear model constrained to pass via the origin with a slope of 0.004 ($r = 0.94$). (After Anderson & Crombie, 1984.)

of infection, λ, was linearly related to the rate, M, at which miracidia were added to the experimental tanks containing the cohorts of snails (Fig. 4).

Interpretation of these results is greatly facilitated by the use of simple deterministic models which mimic changes with time in the densities of uninfected, latent and shedding snails. Models of this kind (often termed catalytic models; see Muench, 1959) are of great value in evaluating the patterns of change in prevalence with time generated by various hypotheses concerning the dynamics of parasite transmission and snail survival (see Anderson & May, 1979; Anderson & Crombie, 1984). In the context of the continual infection of a cohort of snails, the members of this cohort will progress through a sequence of categories at rates dependent on the force of infection, (the per capita rate at which uninfected snails become infected) and the duration of snail latency, τ, (4.5 weeks). These categories are uninfected snails, numbering $X(t)$ at time t, infected but not releasing cercariae (latent), numbering $Z(t)$ at time t and infected and shedding cercariae, numbering $Y(t)$ at time t. We assume initially that the force of infection, λ, is constant and independent of snail age or size and define μ as the natural mortality rate of uninfected and latent snails and μ'' as the death rate of shedding snails. The model incorporating these assumptions consists of three coupled first-order differential equations denoting changes in $X(t)$, $Z(t)$ and $Y(t)$ with respect to time;

$$dX/dt = -(\lambda + \mu)X \tag{1}$$

$$dZ/dt = \lambda X - \mu Z - \lambda X(t - \tau) \exp(-\mu\tau) \, \theta(t) \tag{2}$$

$$dY/dt = \lambda X(t - \tau) \exp(-\mu\tau) \, \theta(t) - \mu'' Y \tag{3}$$

Here $\theta(t)$ is a step function; $\theta = 0$ if $t \leqslant \tau$ and $\theta = 1$ if $t > \tau$. The variables $X(t)$, $Z(t)$ and $Y(t)$ have initial values at the start of the cohort infection experiment (when $t = 0$) of $X(0) = N_0$ (the size of the cohort of snails), $Z(0) = Y(0) = 0$ (all snails uninfected at the start of the experiment). At time t the prevalence of shedding snails, $y(t)$, is simply

$$y(t) = Y(t)/[X(t) + Z(t) + Y(t)] \tag{4}$$

but this quantity underestimates the proportion of infected snails (latency and shedding) by a factor d where

$$d = 1 + [\exp(\mu\tau) - 1] \, [\mu''/\mu] \tag{5}$$

(see Barbour, 1978; Anderson & May, 1979). The model as defined in equations (1) to (3) has an exact analytical solution which is detailed in previous publications (May, 1977; Barbour, 1978; Anderson & May, 1979; Anderson & Crombie, 1984). Two aspects of this solution are relevant to the interpretation of the experimental results displayed in Fig. 2. First, estimates of λ can be obtained from a knowledge of the total density of snails at time t, $N(t)$ and the density of shedding hosts at time t, $Y(t)$ and independent estimates of the death rates μ and μ'' and the latent period, τ;

$$\lambda(t) = [\ln(N(t) - Y(t))/N_0 + \mu t]/(t - \tau) \tag{6}$$

The estimates portrayed in Fig. 4 were obtained via equation (6) and by averaging over all time periods t for each rate of input of miracidia (M) per unit of time.

Second, the relationship between the average rate $\bar{\lambda}$ and M is predicted to be approximately linear given that the life expectancy of the miracidia is short in relation to that of the snail host (this is a valid assumption since miracidia live for a few hours while snails survive for many weeks) where

$$\bar{\lambda} = AM \qquad\qquad (7)$$

and A is a constant (see Anderson & Crombie, 1984). This prediction accords with the observed trend (Fig. 4). The predictions of the simple model (equations (1) to (3)) crudely mirror observed trends in prevalence for the various levels of miracidial input (0, 10, 50, 80 and 110 miracidia per week) (Fig. 2). Discrepancies between prediction and observation are apparent, however, and these are of particular relevance with respect to changes in total snail abundance with time ($N(t)$) when compared with observed survival profiles (Fig. 5).

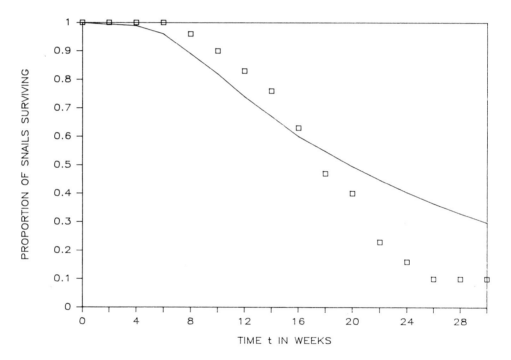

Figure 5. Decay in snail abundance with time when a cohort of snails is exposed to a constant rate of infection by miracidia. Miracidia were added to the experimental tanks at a rate of 110/week. Open squares, observed values; solid line, predictions of the model defined by equations (1) to (3) in the main text. Parameter values, $\lambda = 0.492$/week, $\mu = 0.00285$/week, $\mu'' = 0.062$/week, $\tau = 4.5$ weeks. (After Anderson & Crombie, 1984.)

A more detailed inspection and analysis of experimental results reveals two major shortcomings in the assumptions incorporated in the simple model (equations (1) to (3)). If the force of infection, λ, is estimated (via equation (6)) at a series of points in time for each of the experiments with different rates of miracidial addition, a trend is apparent as illustrated in Fig. 6. The force of infection declines as snails within the populations age, despite the fact that their rate of exposure to infection

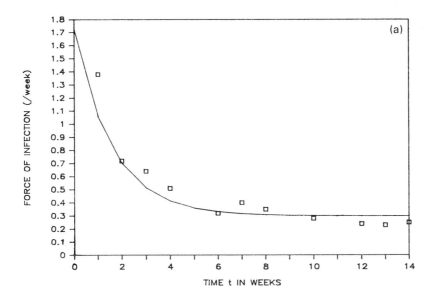

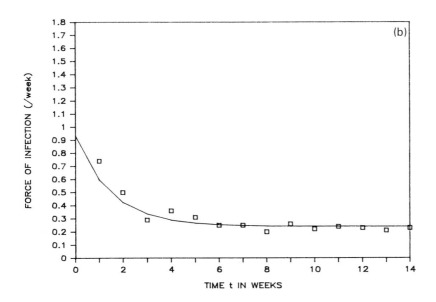

Figure 6. The dependency of the force of infection, λ, on snail age (= size) for two levels of miracidial input. Open squares are calculated values and the solid lines are the best fit model of the form $\lambda(a) = \hat{a} + b \exp(ct)$ where $\hat{a}$, b and c are constants and t denotes age in weeks. Graph (a), Miracidial input of 110/week, $\hat{a} = 0.29$, $b = 1.43$, $c = -0.63$. Graph (b), Miracidial input of 80/week, $\hat{a} = 0.24$, $b = 0.69$, $c = -0.66$. (After Anderson & Crombie, 1984.)

(the rate at which miracidia are added to the experiment tanks) is constant per unit of time and independent of host age. The relationship between λ and snail age (t) is well described empirically by a simple function of the form

$$\lambda(t) = \hat{a} + b\exp(ct) \tag{8}$$

where $\hat{a}$, b and c are constants ($c<0$). This trend is probably associated with snail growth (related to age) during the course of the experiments (Anderson & Crombie, 1984). Recent work has demonstrated that snail size, as opposed to age is the main determinant of the ability of miracidia successfully to penetrate potential snail hosts (Anderson et al., 1982). A variety of factors is involved, including physical barriers to penetration imposed by the tough and thickened epidermal body covering of older and larger snails, the efficiency of non-specific responses to invasion and the ability of the miracidia to 'locate' older snails (Chernin, 1972; Schiff, 1974; Mason, 1977; Lackie, 1980).

The second oversimplification in the assumptions incorporated in equations (1) to (3) concerns the death rate, μ'', of shedding snails. It is clear from Fig. 3 that during the latter stages of the continual infection experiments the death rate of infected snails is higher than that predicted by the simple model. Specifically the predictions of equations (1) to (3) overestimate total snail abundance from about week 20 onwards. Data from an independent short-term experiment, in which the survival of groups of shedding snails was monitored, are presented in Fig. 7. The death rate of shedding snails rises approximately exponentially from the time at which they started to release parasite infective stages. A good empirical description of the observed death rate is provided by the function;

$$\mu''(T) = \mu \exp(\gamma T) \tag{9}$$

where μ and γ are constants and the variable T denotes time (or age) from the start of cercarial shedding. The observed relationship is probably a consequence

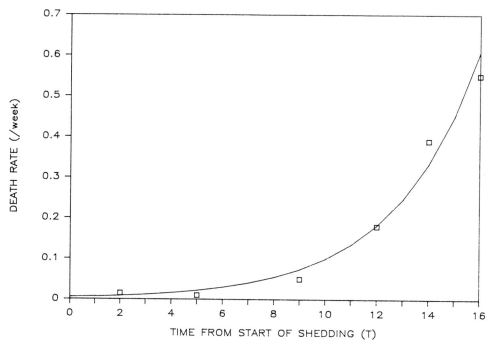

Figure 7. The relationship between the death rate of shedding snails, μ'', and the time period from the start of cercarial release (T). Open squares, observed values; solid line, best fit exponential model of the form $\mu''(T\gamma) = \mu \exp(T)$, where $\mu = 0.005$, $\gamma = 0.3$ ($r = 0.98$). (After Anderson & Crombie, 1984.)

of the accumulating stress imposed by parasite reproduction within the snail host during the life span of a shedding snail.

Continual introduction of susceptible snails

The two complications noted above, age dependency (or size dependency) in snail susceptibility to infection and time dependency (or age dependency) in the death rate of shedding snails, can be incorporated in a revised version of the simple model detailed in equations (1) to (3) (see Anderson & Crombie, 1984). For such a revision it is necessary to consider changes in the densities of susceptible, latent and infected snails both with respect to age (= size) of the snail (time t from the start of the experiment) and with respect to the duration of time (T) during which an infected snail has been shedding cercariae. We define the numbers of susceptible and latent snails at time t of age a as $X(a,t)$ and $Z(a,t)$ respectively. The number of shedding snails at time t of age a that have been shedding cercariae for T time units is denoted by the variable $Y(a,t,T)$. The rates of change of these three population variables with respect to a, t and T may be expressed as a set of coupled partial differential equations:

$$\frac{\partial x(a,t)}{\partial a} + \frac{\partial x(a,t)}{\partial t} = -(\lambda(a) + \mu)\, X(a,t) \tag{10}$$

$$\frac{\partial z(a,t)}{\partial a} + \frac{\partial z(a,t)}{\partial t} = \lambda(a)X(a,t) - \mu Z(a,t) - \lambda(a)X(a,t-\tau)\theta(t-\tau)\exp(-\mu\tau) \tag{11}$$

$$\frac{\partial y(a,t,T)}{\partial a} + \frac{\partial y(a,t,T)}{\partial t} + \frac{\partial y(a,t,T)}{\partial T} = -\mu''(T)Y(a,t,T) \tag{12}$$

Here $\lambda(a)$ denotes the age-dependent force of infection (see Fig. 6) and $\mu''(T)$ denotes the death rate of shedding snails as a function of the duration of shedding (see Fig. 7).

The initial and boundary conditions of equations (10) to (12) depend on the nature of the experiment involving continual snail exposure to miracidial infection. A good test of the model's descriptive power is provided by two additional experiments reported by Anderson & Crombie (1984). In the first of these, a cohort of snails (numbering 30 snails at time $t = 0$) was exposed to 110 miracidia per week over a 30-week period. In contrast to the experiment described earlier (see Fig. 2), however, total snail abundance was held constant throughout the 30-week period by replacing dead snails with live hosts of similar age and size. In the second experiment, a cohort of 30 snails was exposed to 80 miracidia per week over a 30-week period. Mortalities were not replaced but each week two uninfected snails (of size 4–6 mm in length) were added to the tank (an immigration-death experimental design). The recorded changes in the prevalence of shedding snails with time, for both experiments, are portrayed in Fig. 8 (mortalities replaced) and Fig. 9 (immigration-death design) as are the predictions of the revised model (equations (10) to (12) (see Anderson & Crombie, 1984)).

In both instances, model predictions well mirror observed changes. Of particular significance is the generation of convex age-prevalence curves (see Fig. 8) arising from the concomitant effects of age-related changes (= size related) in snail susceptibility to infection (Fig. 6) and duration of infection dependent changes in

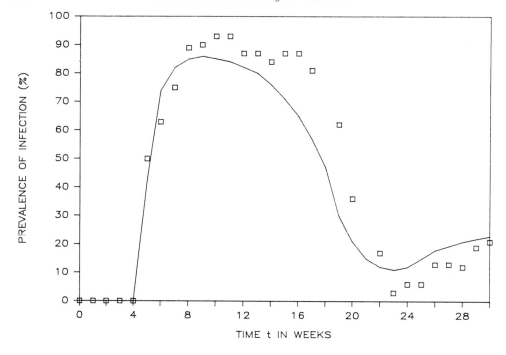

Figure 8. Changes in the prevalence of infection (% shedding) with time, within a snail population held constant in size by the replacement of dead snails with live animals of similar size and age, exposed to an input of 110 miracidia/week. Open squares, observed values; solid line predictions of the model defined by equations (10) to (12) in the main text. Parameter values, $\mu = 0.00285$, $\tau = 4.5$, $\mu'' = 0.005$, $\gamma = 0.3$, $\hat{a} = 0.29$, $b = 1.43$, $c = -0.63$ (all per week). (After Anderson & Crombie, 1984.)

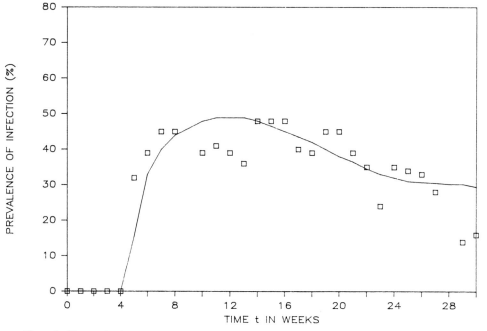

Figure 9. Changes in the prevalence of infection with time in a snail population in which susceptible hosts are added at a rate of two per week and mortalities are not replaced. Open squares, observed values; solid line, predictions of the model defined by equations (10) to (12) in the main text. Parameter values as defined in the legend of Fig. 8. (After Anderson & Crombie, 1984.)

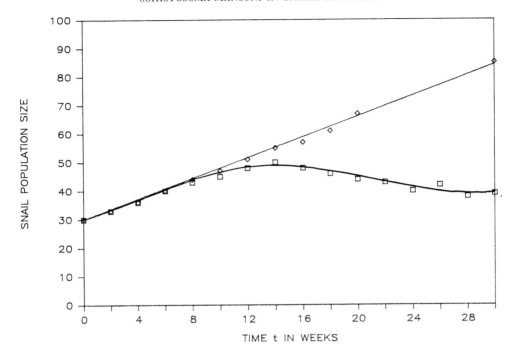

Figure 10. Changes in snail abundance with time in populations subject to an immigration rate of two susceptible snails per week. Open diamonds, observed values in control experiment with no exposure to infection; solid line, predictions of the age structured model defined by equations (10) to (12). Open squares, observed values in experiment where snail population was exposed to 80 miracidia per week; solid line, predictions of equations (10) to (12). (After Anderson & Crombie, 1984.)

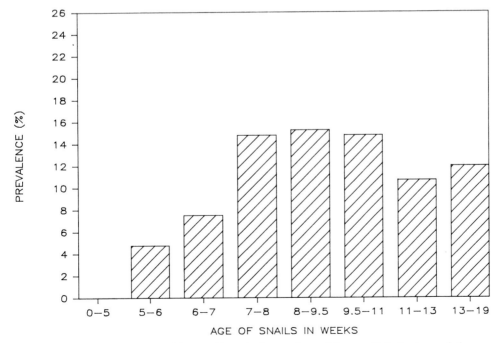

Figure 11. Observed pattern of change with age in the prevalence of *S. mansoni* infection in populations of *B. glabrata* in St. Lucia (Data from Sturrock & Webbe, 1971.)

the death rate of shedding snails (Fig. 7). The demographic impact of the parasite on snail population growth is illustrated in Fig. 10, where snail abundance through time in the immigration experiment (Fig. 9), is compared with that observed in a control experiment in which the population was not exposed to infection by *S. mansoni* miracidia. After a period of 30 weeks, the parasite has depressed snail abundance (due to the high death rate of shedding snails) by a factor of 0.5 when compared with the control population (Fig. 10). The revised model (equations (10) to (12)) again provided a good mirror of observed trends.

These experiments suggest that the complications induced by age (= size) dependent rates of host (snail) infection and by infection duration-dependent death rates of infected snails are likely to be important determinants of observed age-related changes in schistosome prevalence within natural populations of the intermediate host. The convex profiles recorded in our experiments (Fig. 8) are often observed in field studies (Fig. 11) (Sturrock & Webbe, 1971). In the latter situation the scale of the age axis is often shorter than that indicated by our experimental studies as a consequence of increased rates of host mortality in natural habitats when compared with laboratory situations (Anderson & May, 1979).

POPULATIONS OF MICE CONTINUALLY EXPOSED TO INFECTION

Knowledge of the nature and effectiveness of acquired immunity to schistosome infection in the mammalian host, under conditions of long-term exposure, is very limited at present despite its obvious relevance to the interpretation of observed epidemiological patterns in human communities (Fig. 1). Studies of the resistance of laboratory animals to schistosome infections are usually based on experimental designs involving a primary infection and subsequent challenge exposure, where large numbers of infective stages (cercariae) are administered to individual hosts on each occasion (Dean, 1983). Resistance is usually recorded as the percentage reduction in parasite establishment (and/or survival and fecundity) within challenged hosts when compared with that in naïve animals. Invariably high dose primary infections induce a marked degree of resistance on challenge, although the quantitative details of the response depend on genetic and demographic factors (i.e. the strain of the laboratory host or its age and sex) (Dean, 1983). Few studies have focused on the dynamic nature of helminth establishment and mortality, and their often presumed dependency on the rate of current exposure and past experiences of infection, within hosts repeatedly exposed to infection (Jenkins & Phillipson, 1971, 1972; Sturrock, Cottrell & Kimani, 1984).

A recent study examined the dynamics of acquired resistance to *S. mansoni* infection in inbred laboratory mice (CBA/Ca) repeatedly exposed to cercarial invasion over long periods of time (Crombie & Anderson, 1985). In this present paper we outline the main results of this experimental investigation and develop mathematical models of acquired immunity to aid in the interpretation of observed patterns. The overall aim of the experimental work is similar to that described earlier in connection with snail infection by miracidia; namely, the generation of age-intensity profiles of infection under defined conditions of host exposure to infection. Note that for snail populations we considered age-related changes in prevalence while for our mice studies we examine age-related changes in the average intensity of infection (mean worm burden per mouse).

In the absence of acquired resistance to infection, under conditions of constant exposure to infective stages, average helminth burdens per host will rise monotonically as the duration of exposure increases (as the host's age) to a stable equilibrium level. If the mean worm burden per host at time t is defined as $M(t)$ and μ and Λ are the per capita parasite death rate and host infection rate respectively then changes in $M(t)$ with time (or equivalently host age) may be defined by the simple differential equation

$$dM(t)/dt = \Lambda - \mu M(t) \tag{13}$$

If the hosts are uninfected at time (age) zero ($M(0) = 0$) then the solution of equation (13) is

$$M(t) = \frac{\Lambda}{\mu} [1 - e^{-\mu t}] \tag{14}$$

As time t increases $M(t)$ approaches an equilibrium level M^* where

$$M^* = \Lambda/\mu \atop (t \rightarrow \infty) \tag{15}$$

In other words, the plateau level of parasite burden in old hosts (under conditions of constant exposure (Λ) and constant parasite mortality (μ)) is simply the rate of infection Λ times the life expectancy of the parasite ($1/\mu$). The variable t in equation (14) is exactly equivalent to host age a and hence the simple model describes an age-intensity profile of infection. The important point illustrated by this simple example concerns the observation that average worm burdens will attain a stable plateau level in the older age classes of host populations *in the absence of acquired resistance*, provided Λ and μ are constant and independent of host age. In past work, the presence of a stable plateau in average worm load has often been interpreted incorrectly as evidence of acquired resistance to infection in older hosts (Schad & Banwell, 1984). Monotonic growth to a stable level is the basic epidemiological profile generated by constant exposure to infection, and observed patterns which differ from this trend must be interpreted in the light of this observation.

Stochastic models of immigration-death processes (equation (13)) reveal that under conditions of constant exposure and homogeneity in susceptibility to infection within the host population, the probability distribution of worm number per host will be Poisson (= random) in form. Under these circumstances, the variance equals the mean and the probability of observing i parasites in any given host at time t, $p_i(t)$ is

$$p_i(t) = \frac{M(t)^i e^{-M(t)}}{i!} \tag{16}$$

Random parasite distributions are rarely (if ever) observed in natural host populations but may arise in laboratory studies where groups of inbred mice are exposed to constant numbers of cercariae for fixed periods of time. An example is shown in Fig. 12 for inbred CBA/Ca mice exposed to *S. mansoni* cercariae. A

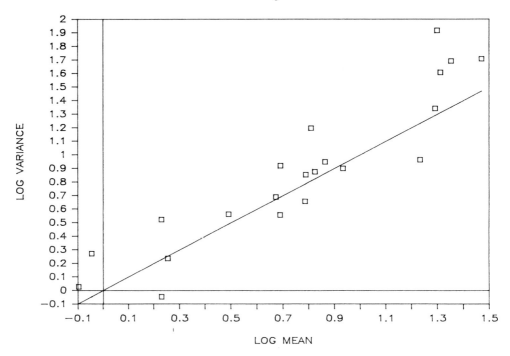

Figure 12. The relationship between the variance and mean (on $\log_{10}$ scales) of the number of adult *S. mansoni* established in groups of inbred mice (CBA/Ca) exposed to varying densities of cercariae. Open squares, observed values; solid line, Poisson prediction where the variance equals the mean.

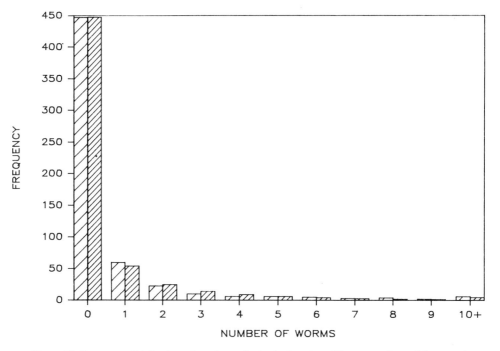

Figure 13. Frequency distribution of numbers of mice harbouring different numbers of *S. mansoni* resulting from the exposure of sentinal mice in eight field sites on St Lucia. (Data from Sturrock, 1973.) The graph portrays the observed distributions and the predictions of the best fit negative binomial model (closely hatched bars) (Mean = 0.614, k = 0.152, $X^2 = 4.1$, $N = 7$ d.f.).

plot of $\log_{10}$ variance against $\log_{10}$ mean worm burden yields a straight line with a slope little different from unity (a slope of unity implies a random distribution of worm numbers per mouse). Similar experiments with outbred mice tend to create aggregation (variance/mean) in parasite numbers per mouse. This observation illustrates the importance of genetic factors as determinants of the rate of parasite establishment within a host. Field studies of outbred mice exposed to infection in habitats containing schistosome infected snails similarly generate aggregated distributions of parasite load per host, (Sturrock, 1973) presumably as a consequence of both genetic variability between hosts and heterogeneity in the rate of exposure to cercariae (Fig. 13). For such aggregated distributions, the negative binomial probability model provides a good empirical description of observed patterns (this distribution is defined by two parameters, the mean M and a parameter k which varies inversely with the degree of parasite contagion) (Fig. 13).

Heterogeneity in the distribution of parasite numbers per host can be simply introduced into the immigration-death model (equation (13)) by treating either Λ and/or μ as random variables which adopt different values for different members of the host population (Anderson & Gordon, 1982; Anderson, 1976).

The immigration-death model serves as a starting point for the analysis of two major features of schistosome transmission in natural habitats; namely, acquired resistance to parasite establishment within the mammalian host and age-related changes in host exposure to infection (Warren, 1973). Both are believed to be of great importance in shaping the observed convex patterns in age-intensity profiles of schistosome infections in human communities (Fig. 1), although the relative significances of the two factors are poorly understood at present. We focus on one of these, namely, acquired resistance to infection.

The experimental results of Crombie & Anderson (1985) reveal monotonic growth to a stable plateau and convex age-intensity profiles within inbred mouse populations exposed to constant numbers of infective stages per unit of time. Interestingly, a convex pattern is most likely to arise if the intensity of exposure to infection is high. This point is illustrated in Fig. 14 where the results of four trickle infection experiments are recorded. Groups of 10 inbred CBA/Ca mice were exposed to either 10, 30, 100 or 300 cercariae per week for various periods of time ranging from 5 to 50 weeks. Worm burdens were counted by perfusion techniques and host dissection at intervals over the entire course of the experiment. At low intensities of exposure, the average worm burden rose monotonically to a stable plateau as predicted by the simple immigration-death model (equation (13)). At very high intensities of exposure, however, the average worm load rose rapidly but then decayed in the older age groups of mice. Such convex patterns must arise as a consequence of acquired resistance since the rate of exposure to infection was held constant throughout the course of the experiment. Separate experiments revealed that the rate of parasite establishment in previously uninfected animals following a single exposure to infection, was independent of mouse age. Juvenile worms were recovered at all time periods post-initiation of continual exposure to infection, suggesting that parasites are able to establish within mice despite long durations of past experience of infection. These results conflict with the notion that concomitant immunity to schistosome infection in mammalian hosts acts to prohibit parasite establishment (Smithers & Terry, 1969). Our observations suggest that worm burdens are determined by a dynamic interplay between parasite recruitment and mortality.

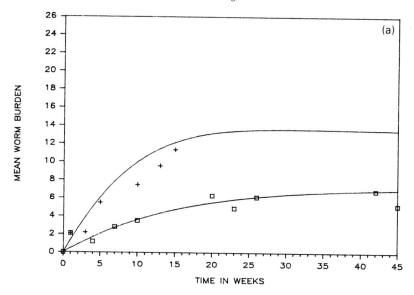

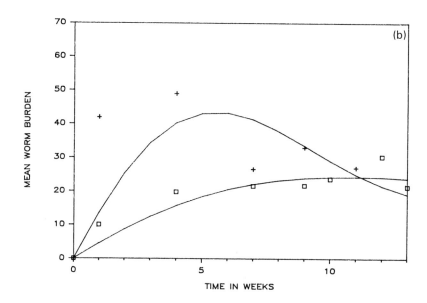

Figure 14. Mice repeatedly exposed to a constant force of infection over long periods of time (trickle infection experiments). The four graphs portray the results of different experiments in which groups of 10 mice were exposed to 10 (graph a) 30 (graph a), 100 (graph b) and 300 (graph b) cercariae per week. Open squares or crosses, observed mean worm burdens (10 mice per group); solid lines, predictions of the model defined by equations (18) and (19) in the main text. (After Crombie & Anderson, 1985.) Parameter values: $\epsilon = 0.0085$/week, $\sigma = 0.2$/week, $\mu = 0.045$/week, $\Lambda = 0.471$/week and 1.413/week (in graph a) and $\Lambda = 4.711$/week and 14.13/week (in graph b).

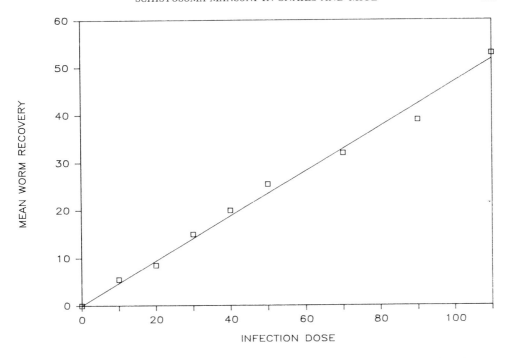

Figure 15. Worm recovery 6 weeks post-infection of naïve mice exposed to a single infection of varying intensity ((0–110) cercariae). Open squares, observed mean recoveries (10 mice); solid line, best fit linear model with slope $b = 0.4711$ ($r^2 = 0.99$). (After Crombie & Anderson, 1985.)

Acquired resistance to infection

The rate of parasite establishment in naïve hosts appears to be directly proportional to the number of cercariae to which the host is exposed. This point is clearly demonstrated in Fig. 15. This relationship, however, is unlikely to hold for mice with past experience of infection, given the observed convex form of the age-intensity curve generated by repeated exposure to high levels of infection (Fig. 14b). Current understanding of acquired resistance to *S. mansoni* infection in mice suggests that host responses primarily act to decrease the rate of establishment of adult worms (Dean, 1983). We therefore suspect that the downturn in average intensity observed in older mice repeatedly exposed to infection reflects a decline in parasite establishment (Fig. 14c). This assumption can be captured by a simple modification to the immigration-death model as follows (Anderson & May, 1985). We assume that parasite establishment decays linearly as the accumulated past experience of infection increases (Anderson & May, 1985) such that the per capita average input of parasites $\bar{\Lambda}$ takes the form

$$\bar{\Lambda}(M(a)) = \Lambda \left[1 - \epsilon \int_0^a M(a') e^{-\sigma(\delta - \delta')} da' \right] \qquad (17)$$

Here, Λ denotes the pristine per capita rate of infection in a naïve host. This rate is decreased in a linear manner (with the rate of decline defined by the parameter ϵ) as the accumulated sum of past experience of infection ($\int_0^a M(a') da'$) increases with age (= time). 'Acquired immunity' is assumed to have a duration of $1/\sigma$ units of time such that the summed experience of infection at age a' is decreased by a factor $\exp[-\sigma(a - a')]$ by age a. The parameter ϵ records the strength of acquisition of immunity and $1/\sigma$ denotes the average duration of 'immunological memory'. Equation (17) assumes that acquired immunity acts to decrease establishment as a function of *past worm burdens*. An alternative assumption would be that establishment is decreased as a function of *past exposure to infection* (i.e. $\int_0^a \Lambda e^{-\sigma(a - a')} da'$). We are unable to discriminate between these two assumptions at present (on the basis of our experimental data) and hence, for simplicity, work with the model defined in equation (17) (establishment declines as a function of past worm burdens). In essence, both are interrelated since worm burden is itself some function of the rate of exposure. A further complication arises from the choice of a linear function in equation (17). If the magnitude of the rate of acquisition of immunity (the value of ϵ) is high, this assumption would ultimately result in a *negative* input of young parasites! This is clearly unrealistic but we choose to work with this function since our experimental results (see Fig. 14) suggest that the acquisition of resistance occurs relatively slowly (i.e. the value of ϵ is very small and hence negative inputs will not be generated by the model). The linear nature of the assumption greatly facilitates analytical investigations of the properties of the acquired immunity model.

The full structure of the model takes the form (see Anderson & May, 1985),

$$\frac{dM(a)}{da} = \bar{\Lambda}[M(a)] - \mu A(a) \tag{18}$$

$$M(a) = D + \frac{\Lambda}{\lambda}\left[\frac{(p_1 + \sigma)}{p_1}e^{p_1 a} - \frac{(p_2 + \sigma)}{p_2}e^{p_2 a}\right] \tag{19}$$

where $D = \Lambda\sigma/(\sigma\mu + \epsilon\Lambda)$, $p_1 = -(\mu + \sigma - \lambda)/2$, $p_2 = -(\mu + \sigma + \lambda)/2$ and $\lambda = [(\mu - \sigma)^2 - 4\epsilon\Lambda]^{1/2}$. The model is able to generate a wide variety of patterns of change in worm burden with age, depending on the values of the parameters. These range from monotonic growth to a stable average worm burden in older age classes (if Λ and ϵ are small and σ large), convex patterns with average worm burden declining in older age classes (Λ large and σ small) to damped oscillations in intensity of infection as age increases (Λ, σ and ϵ large). A variety of these are displayed in Fig. 16. Of particular interest is the ability of the model (with no adjustable parameters other than the force of infection Λ) to reflect monotonic growth to a stable plateau in worm load for low exposures to infection (acquired resistance of little significance) and convex curves for high rates of exposure (strong acquired resistance). In human communities, the relative degree to which the intensity of infection with schistosome parasites declines in older age classes, when compared with the maximum value in the teenage groups, often appears to be positively associated with the intensity of transmission (Anderson & May, 1985) (Fig. 17). These observations, in conjunction with the patterns generated by the model defined by equation (18), support the view that convex age-intensity curves for *S. mansoni* infection in human populations may arise as a consequence of acquired immunity.

In the context of our experimental results, fitting the model to the observed age-intensity profiles depends on the estimation of four parameters (i.e. Λ, μ, ϵ and σ). Estimates of Λ and μ are available; the value of Λ is set by the experimental design (the weekly rate of exposure to cercariae; see Fig. 15) and the death rate

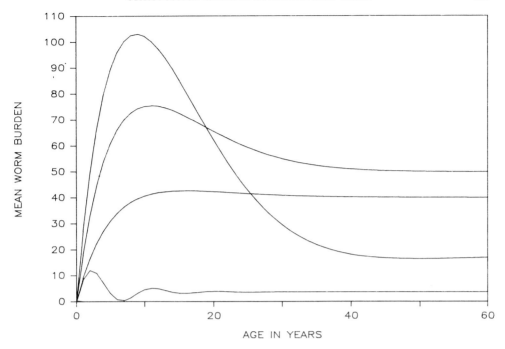

Figure 16. An illustration of the various patterns of change in average worm burden with age generated by the acquired immunity model defined by equation (19) in the main text. Parameter values: bottom line at age 10 years, $\Lambda = 10$, $\mu = 0.2$, $\epsilon = 0.05$, $\sigma = 0.2$; second bottom line at age 10 years, $\Lambda = 10$, $\mu = 0.2$, $\epsilon = 0.0005$, $\sigma = 0.1$; second top line at age 10 years $\Lambda = 20$, $\mu = 0.2$, $\epsilon = 0.0005$, $\sigma = 0.05$; top line at age 10 years, $\Lambda = 30$, $\mu = 0.2$, $\epsilon = 0.0005$, $\sigma = 0.01$ (all per year).

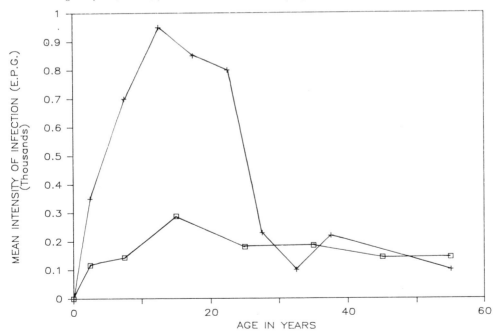

Figure 17. Observed age-average intensity of infection (e.p.g.) curves for *S. mansoni* in areas of high (top line at age 20 years, data from Abdel-Wahab *et al.*, 1980) and low (bottom line at age 20 years, data from Siongok *et al.*, 1976) transmission intensity.

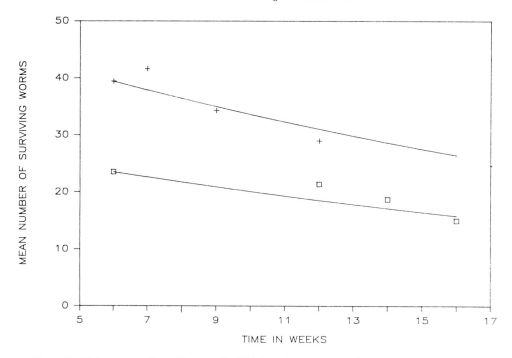

Figure 18. Adult worm survival of *S. mansoni* in CBA/Ca mice over a 10-week period post-maturation. Two examples are shown where initial adult worm densities at week 6 of infection were approximately 40 and 25 parasites per mouse. The symbols denote observed means (10 mice) and the solid lines denote the fit of an exponential decay survival model with constant death rate $\mu = 0.045$/week. (After Crombie & Anderson, 1985.)

(μ) can be crudely estimated from separate experiments which record the survival rates of cohorts of worms established in the mouse host at a fixed point in time (see Crombie & Anderson (1985) and Fig. 18). These estimates of mortality are crude, in the sense that acquired resistance in mice continually exposed to infection may well act to reduce the rates of both parasite establishment and adult parasite survival. Our estimates are based on the assumption that survival patterns of adult worms are similar in naïve and repeatedly exposed animals. A very rough estimate of ϵ is available from the observed decline in the number of juvenile worms as past exposure to infection rises (from the experiments with the highest exposure rate; 300 cercariae/week/10 mice). The slope of a plot of the number of juvenile worms (recently recruited parasites) present at time t versus the sum of past worm burden from 0 to t is approximately 0.0085/week. Our experimental design does not provide any quantitative information on the duration of immunological memory ($1/\sigma$) and hence this remains an adjustable parameter in attempts to compare model predictions with observed trends. This comparison, as presented in Fig. 14, is encouraging; the model provides a reasonable mimic of the four observed trends with a fixed value of $\sigma = 0.2$/week (i.e. an immunological memory of 5 weeks). Better fits to the data could be obtained by parameter adjustments made independently for each of the experiments with different levels of cercarial exposure. We feel this to be unjustified at present given the preliminary nature of the experimental results. Additional work is required, involving more complex experimental designs, to determine the validity of the linear assumption and the values of the parameters ϵ and σ. The model provides a useful working framework which can be modified in the light of future experimental work (whether carried out in the field or the laboratory).

Resistance following chemotherapy

Curative chemotherapy was employed in a further set of experiments to examine rates of re-infection following treatment in mice with different durations of past exposure to infection prior to drug administration. The drug 'Praziquantal' was administered to mice at a dose of 250 mg/kg divided into three applications given

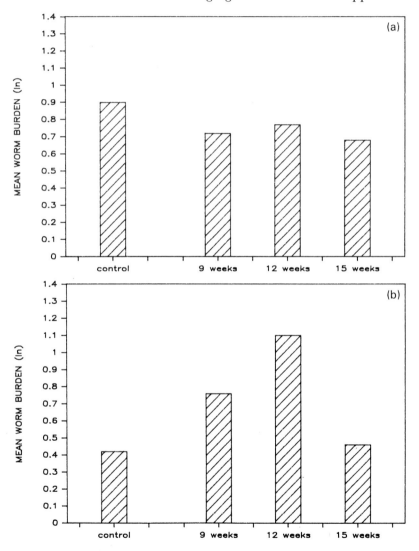

Figure 19. Worm recovery following curative chemotherapy. Graph (a), The control was exposed to infections of 10 cercariae per group of 10 mice per week for 6 weeks prior to autopsy. The experimental groups were exposed to an identical repeated infection for 9, 12 and 15 weeks prior to chemotherapy; autopsy was performed after 6 weeks of reinfection. Graph (b), As for (a) except that worm recovery was performed 9 weeks post-initial infection in the control and after 9 weeks reinfection following chemotherapy in the experimental group. (After Crombie & Anderson, 1985.)

at 4-h intervals during one 24-h period. Two different repeated exposure levels were examined, namely, 10 cercariae/week/group of 10 mice and 100 cercariae/ week/group of 10 mice (approximately 1 cercaria/mouse/week and 10 cercariae/ mouse/week respectively). For the lowest exposure level (1 cercaria/mouse/week), the duration of past exposure to infection prior to treatment was set at 9 weeks, 12 weeks and 15 weeks in three separate groups of experimental animals. In two separate sequences of experiments, reinfection following treatment at the same intensity of cercarial exposure was allowed to continue for 6 and 9 weeks before the assessment of worm burdens at autopsy. At the higher exposure level (10 cercariae/mouse/week), groups of mice were exposed to 6 weeks of trickle infection

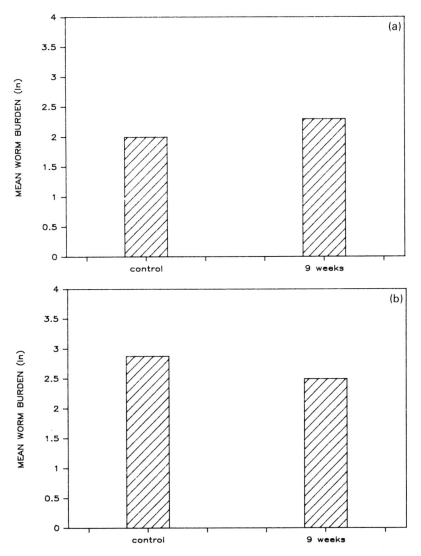

Figure 20. Similar to Fig. 19, but in graph (a) the control group was exposed to infections of 100 cercariae per group of 10 mice per week for 6 weeks prior to autopsy. The experimental group was exposed to 9 weeks infection prior to treatment and to 6 weeks reinfection post-treatment. Graph (b) is similar to (a) but with worm recovery performed 9 weeks post-initial infection in the control group and after 9 weeks reinfection in the experimental group (After Crombie & Anderson, 1985.)

and autopsied after 6 and 9 weeks of reinfection at the same intensity of cercarial exposure (Crombie & Anderson, 1985). For each design, control experiments were performed to assess average worm burdens after 6 weeks of exposure to the low and high cercarial exposure levels. The patterns of reinfection over 6 weeks after treatment in the experimental group were compared with the control groups. The results are displayed in Figs 19 and 20. One-way analyses of variance on transformed data (a square root transformation based on the observed random distributions of parasites within the different groups of inbred mice) showed no significant differences between the treated and control groups of mice, irrespective of the levels of trickle exposure or the durations of experience of infection prior to treatment (Figs 19 and 20, Crombie & Anderson, 1985). Resistance to re-infection following chemotherapy has been the subject of previous studies but the results (which were based not on trickle exposure, but on primary and single challenge experiments) have been inconclusive; residual protective immunity was apparent in some studies but not in others (Cheever et al., 1977; Scott et al., 1982). Our results from a continual exposure design tentatively suggest that the expulsion of adult worm burdens accumulated from low levels of exposure to infection eliminate the 'memory' or previous infections. In other words, treated mice with varying degrees of experience of past exposure were equally susceptible to reinfection. This is worrying if relevant to S. mansoni infections in man since it raises questions over the desirability of drug use in endemic areas among old people with many years of previous experience of infection but few symptoms of disease. It must be noted, however, that the exposure levels employed in our experimental designs were low. It is possible that residual resistance to reinfection may remain if the mouse has experienced very high levels of infection prior to treatment. Preliminary experiments suggest that this may be the case.

HERD IMMUNITY AND MASS CHEMOTHERAPY

The model defined in equations (19) and (20) can be employed to assess the likely impact of control measures on 'herd immunity' within a human community infected with schistosome parasites on the basis that our assumptions crudely capture the acquisition of resistance to reinfection. We briefly consider one problem, namely that impact of repeated mass community treatment with anthelmintic drugs, on age-related resistance to infection. Mass chemotherapy, applied at a level less than that required to eradicate the parasite, acts to reduce the overall force of transmission within the community (by reducing the average reproductive life expectancy of the adult worm). As such, it lowers the average experience of infection and hence the rate of acquisition of immunity. Mass chemotherapy can be crudely mirrored by increasing the average death rate of the parasite (μ) within the acquired immunity model defined by equation (19). The patterns generated by equation (19), resulting from various increases in μ over the 'pristine' magnitude of the parameter prior to control, represent the long term (= equilibrium) impact of repeated chemotherapy. In other words, they represent the equilibrium state to which the system would converge under the influence of the raised parasite death rate (μ). The 'pristine' rate of infection, Λ, is altered as a result of the impact of chemotherapy on the overall force of infection within the community. The new force of infection, Λ', is simply

$$\Lambda' = R_0(\mu + b)\bar{M} \tag{20}$$

where R_0 denotes the basic reproductive rate of the parasite (the average numbers of female offspring produced throughout the life span of a mature adult worm that themselves attain reproductive maturity in the absence of density-dependent constraints or acquired immunity (see Anderson, 1982) within the treated population), and $\bar{M}$ defines the overall mean worm burden under the impact of treatment (average over all age classes). Equation (20) assumes that human mortality is constant with age where life expectancy, L, is defined as $L = 1/b$. With this assumption,

$$\bar{M} = b\big|_0^\infty M'(a)\mathrm{e}^{-ba}da \tag{21}$$

where $M'(a)$ denotes the mean worm burden in age class a in the treated population.

The predicted impact of raising the death rate of adult parasites by mass treatment is displayed in Fig. 21 (by evaluating equation (19) with Λ' as defined in equation (20)). Under certain circumstances, mass chemotherapy can raise average worm burdens in the adult age classes over the levels pertaining prior to control. This

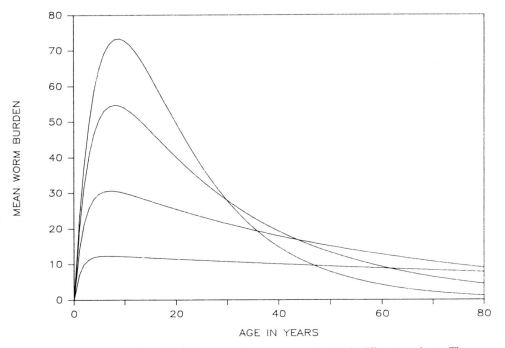

Figure 21. The impact of mass chemotherapy on the average worm burden in different age classes. The four lines denote equilibrium age-intensity profiles for the precontrol situation (top line at age 10 years) and three levels of drug application which increase the average death rate of the adult parasites within the population from $\mu = 0.25$/year (precontrol), to $\mu = 0.33$/year (second from top line at age 10 years), $\mu = 0.5$/year (second from bottom line at age 10 years) and $\mu = 0.75$ years (bottom line at age 10 years). The predictions are generated by equation (19) in the main text with parameter values, $\Lambda(\mu) = (\sigma + b)(b + \mu)[R_0 - 1]/\epsilon$, $b = 1/70$, $\mu =$ variable, $\epsilon = 0.0005$, $\sigma = 0.00001$, $R_0 = 1.44$ (when $\mu = 0.75$), $R_0 = 2.13$ (when $\mu = 0.5$), $R_0 = 3.19$ (when $\mu = 0.33$) and $R_0 = 4.16$ (when $\mu = 0.25$); all parameters defined per year. Note that an increased average parasite death rate resulting from mass treatment increases the worm load in the older age classes over that pertaining prior to control. (See Anderson & May, 1985.)

arises as a consequence of the reduced force of infection within the community, which acts to lower acquired resistance in the older age groups. These trends would be further accentuated if treatment to remove the adult worm population within an individual acted to eliminate resistance acquired from pre-treatment experience of infection. Our experimental observations on the influence of anthelmintic treatment on the rate that mice acquire infection, suggest that this may indeed be the case. This feature of mass chemotherapy has received too little attention in past research. Note, however, that our predictions are based on the assumption that older age groups in untreated populations do acquire resistance to reinfection with schistosome parasites. Our experimental observations on mice (see Fig. 14) suggest that convex age-intensity curves may arise as a result of acquired immunity but whether or not this explains similar patterns of infection in human communities is still a matter of some controversy at present (Warren, 1973; Butterworth *et al.*, 1984, 1985; Sturrock *et al.*, 1984).

GENETIC VARIABILITY IN HOST SUSCEPTIBILITY TO INFECTION

Our experimental studies and model frameworks have both been based on designs or assumptions that each host responds in a similar manner to parasite invasion and is exposed to similar levels of infection. In the context of the laboratory studies and their associated models this is correct, since inbred strains of mice and snails were employed and the experimental designs were based on the exposure on small groups of animals to constant numbers of infective stages through time. In field situations, however, host populations are likely to be heterogeneous with respect to such factors as inherent susceptibility, exposure to infection and ability to develop resistance to parasitic invasion. Much recent laboratory work on helminth infections in mice and rats clearly indicates the significance of host strain or breed as a determinant of the course of parasitic infection within an individual animal (Wakelin, 1984a,b). We examine the impact of such host-based heterogeneity on age-intensity and age-prevalence patterns.

Heterogeneity between hosts may be incorporated into our simple model of infection and parasite death (no acquired immunity) outlined in equations (13) and (14) as follows. We consider a host population consisting of a fraction, f, who are highly susceptible to infection (high force of infection Λ_1) and a fraction $(1 - f)$ who are much less susceptible (a low value of Λ_2). We further assume that the parasites are randomly distributed in any one of the two segments of the host population (Poisson distributions with means M_1 and M_2) and that the death rates of the parasites are μ_1 and μ_2, respectively, in the wormy (high Λ_1) and non-wormy (low Λ_2) hosts. At equilibrium (with respect to time), the rates of change of the mean worm burdens in each of the two segments of the population ($M_i(a)$) with respect to age, a, may be expressed as

$$dM_i(a)/da = \Lambda_i - \mu_i M_i(a) \tag{22}$$

with solution (for $i = 1$ and $i = 2$)

$$M_i(a) = \frac{\Lambda_i}{\mu_i} [1 - e^{-\mu_i a}] \tag{23}$$

The prevalences of infection at age a in the two segments (the percentage infected, $P_i(a)$) are defined as

$$P_i(a) = 100\,[\,1 - e^{-M_i(a)}\,] \qquad (24)$$

The probability generating functions (p.g.f.) for the distributions of worm numbers per host in each of the two segments of the population, $\Pi_i(Z)$, are Poisson where

$$\Pi_i(Z,a) = \exp\,[\,M_i(a)(Z-1)\,] \qquad (25)$$

The p.g.f. of the probability distribution of worms within the *total* population of age a are given by

$$\Pi(Z,a) = f\,e^{M_1(a)(Z-1)} + (1-f)e^{M_2(a)(Z-1)} \qquad (26)$$

where the overall mean in age class a, $\bar{M}(a)$, is

$$\bar{M}(a) = M_1(a)f + M_2(a)(1-f) \qquad (27)$$

and the prevalence, $\bar{P}(a)$ is

$$\bar{P}(a) = 100\,[\,fP_1(a) - (1-f)P_2(a)\,] \qquad (28)$$

Whereas the means and variance are equal for the Poisson distribution within an age class in the wormy or non-wormy segments of the population, the overall distribution with the total population of age a is aggregated or over-dispersed in form where the variance is greater than the mean. For the combined distribution, the variance, $\bar{V}(a)$, in age class a is given by

$$\bar{V}(a) = fM_1(a) + (1-f)M_2(a) + f(1-f)\,[\,M_1(a) - M_2(a)\,]^2 \qquad (29)$$

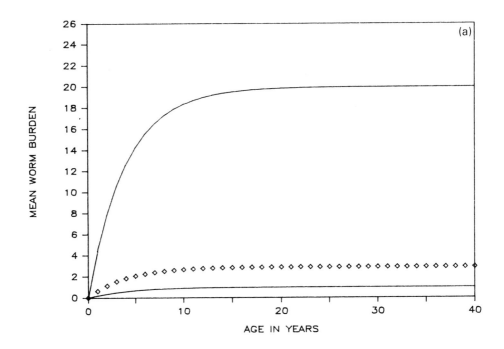

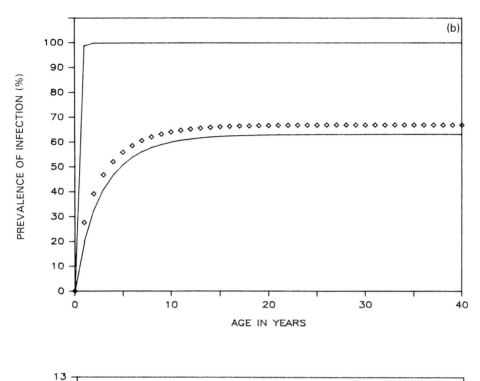

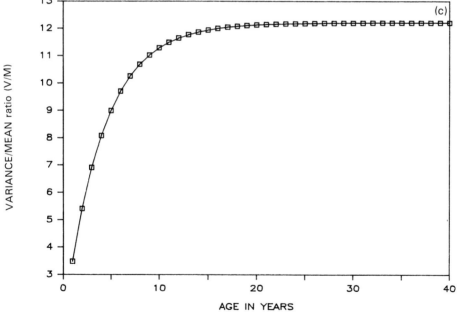

Figure 22. *(opposite and above)* Predictions of the 'heterogeneity model' defined by equations (27), (28) and (30) in the main text. Graph (a), Changes in the mean worm burdens in the 'wormy' ($M_1(a)$ — top line) and the 'non-wormy' ($M_2(a)$ — bottom line) segments of the community. The symbolled line denotes the overall mean, $\bar{M}(a)$. Graph (b), Similar to (a) but denoting changes in prevalence. Graph (c), Similar to (a) but denoting changes in the variance to mean ratio in the total population, $\bar{V}(a)/\bar{M}(a)$. Parameter values: $f_1 = 0.1$, $f_2 = 0.9$ $\Lambda_1 = 5.0$, $\Lambda_2 = 0.25$, $\mu_1 = \mu_2 = 0.25$ (all per year).

The variance to mean ratio $(\bar{V}(a)/\bar{M}(a))$ is thus defined as

$$\bar{V}(a)/\bar{M}(a) = 1 + \frac{f(1-f)[M_1(a) - M_2(a)]^2}{fM_1(a) + (1-f)M_2(a)} \tag{30}$$

which exceeds unity in value (underlying distribution is aggregated in form).

The patterns of change with age (within the total population) of the mean intensity of infection ($\bar{M}(a)$ – equation (27)), the prevalence of infection ($\bar{P}(a)$ – equation (28)) and the variability in the distribution of parasite numbers per host (as measured by $V(a)/M(a)$ – equation (29)) will depend on the relative magnitudes of both the population parameters Λ_i and μ_i and the fractions of 'wormy' (f) and 'non-wormy' ($1-f$) people. An illustrative example is presented in Fig. 22 in which the wormy people are a small percentage of the total population (usually the case in practice). An interesting feature of such models is the ability of host-based heterogeneity to generate age-related changes in the distribution of parasite numbers per host in the *absence* of age-related changes in the rates of infection or parasite mortality within either the 'wormy' or 'non-wormy' fractions of the population. In other words, heterogeneity arising from either susceptibility or immunological competence introduces a dynamic component into the distribution of worm loads between different age classes. In practice, parasite distributions are more commonly recorded for the population as a whole (not subdivided by age class). In these circumstances, it is important to note that even in the absence of heterogeneity in susceptibility within the host population the overall distribution of parasite numbers will be heterogeneous or aggregated in form. Even though the distributions are Poisson within an age class, the means of these distributions vary (as defined in equation (14)) between age classes. The overall distribution is therefore formed by compounding a series of Poisson variates. Heterogeneity between hosts within an age class acts to accentuate this degree of overdispersion or aggregation.

The simple model outlined above (equation (23)) can be generalized either to incorporate many classes of susceptibility or 'immunological competence' (as opposed to 2 classes), or to include added biological refinements such as acquired immunity. In the latter case our simple two class population model ('wormy' and 'non-wormy' people, see equation (23)) may be represented in the form

$$\frac{dM_i(a)}{da} = \Lambda_i[1 - \epsilon_i|_0^a M_i(a')e^{-\sigma_i(a-a')}da'] - \mu_i M_i(a) \tag{31}$$

Here, the subscript i denotes differences in parameter values between the two fractions of the population (f and $(1-f)$). Under these circumstances the pristine force of infection Λ_i is

$$\Lambda_i = R_{0i}(b + \sigma_i)\bar{M}(a) \tag{32}$$

where $1/b$ denotes human life expectancy, R_{0i} is the basic reproductive rate of the parasite in hosts of class i and $\bar{M}$ is the overall average worm burden in the total population:

$$\bar{M} = fb|_0^\infty M_1(a)e^{-ba}da + (1-f)b|_0^\infty M_2(a)e^{-ba}da \tag{33}$$

Models of this kind allow for heterogeneity in the abilities of different hosts, both to acquire resistance to reinfection (the parameter ϵ_i) and to 'remember' past experiences of infection (the average duration of immunological memory $1/\sigma_i$). Even simple two-class models are able to generate a wide range of patterns of change in average intensity and prevalence with age. More complex models, with many classes of susceptibility/immunological competence, demonstrate a bewildering array of possible patterns. Human communities or populations are thought to be characterized by great variability in both susceptibility to infection and 'immunological competence' to resist parasitic invasion (Cavalli-Sforza & Bodmer, 1971; Bodmer, 1980) and, as such, observed age-prevalence or age-intensity curves in endemic regions undoubtedly mask much individual variation in the present intensity and past experience of helminth infection. A simple example of how such variation can be hidden within overall average trends in the population is illustrated in Fig. 23. This example is based on a population consisting of 'wormy' and 'non-wormy' people as mirrored by the two-class acquired immunity model defined in equation (31). The majority of 'non-wormy people' (70%) have a good acquired response (high ϵ value) but this is effectively masked by the fraction (30%) of 'wormy' people (with a very low ϵ value). This example serves to illustrate the importance of recording not only prevalence and average intensity, but also some measure of variability in worm load within each age class.

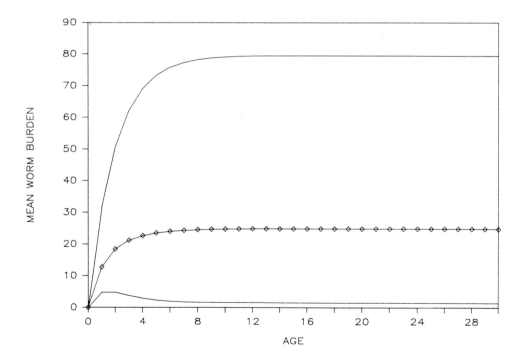

Figure 23. Predictions of the heterogeneous acquired immunity model defined by equation (31) in the main text. Changes in the mean worm burden with age in the 'wormy' fraction f_1 ($M_1(a)$), the 'non-wormy' fraction f_2 ($M_2(a)$) and the overall mean $\bar{M}(a)$. Parameter values: $\Lambda_1 = 40$, $\Lambda_2 = 10$, $\mu_1 = 0.5$, $\mu_2 = 1.5$, $\epsilon_1 = 0.00001$, $\epsilon_2 = 0.05$, $\sigma_1 = \sigma_2 = 0.1$ (all per year).

DISCUSSION

Our experimental studies have enabled us to identify, with a reasonable degree of precision, the factors that are responsible for convex patterns of change in prevalence and average intensity of infection with host age (snail or mouse) under defined and controlled laboratory conditions within inbred strains of animals. In the case of *S. mansoni* infection in snails, convexity arises from age (= size) related changes in susceptibility to parasitic invasion and age-related mortality among infected hosts. For mice, similar patterns appear to arise as a consequence of acquired resistance to infection which acts to decrease the rate of parasite establishment as the duration and intensity of past exposure increases.

Within human communities infected with schistosome parasites, age-related changes in average intensity and prevalence of infection, either recorded from horizontal or longitudinal studies, form the template of much of the past and current epidemiological research on schistosomiasis. Observed patterns (see Fig. 1) have been used, in the majority of cases, to assess the intensity of transmission within a defined locality and to identify the age groups of the community who are most at risk from infection. As mentioned earlier, the convex patterns of change of intensity with age have been a source of much controversy with respect to the relative significance of age-related contact with infection and acquired immunity as determinants of such trends. The rate of increase in average intensity over the younger age classes is clearly a reflection of the overall force of transmission within a community and, hence, is of practical value to public health scientists. Age reflects duration of past exposure and, with a relatively long-lived parasite (*S. mansoni* in man is thought to have a life span of between 3–5 years (see Goddard & Jordan, 1980)), average intensity at a given age in part records a summation of past exposures to infection. Similarly, the measurement of convexity in change of intensity or prevalence with age is also of practical significance. It helps to identify the groups of people who suffer most from disease morbidity and, as such, can aid in the design of community control programmes based on chemotherapy, hygiene, sanitation or education. Whether age-related changes in contact with infective stages or acquired immunity generates convexity, is of little significance to such practical considerations. Indeed, it is highly probable that both factors contribute to observed trends and that their relative significance differs from one community to another depending on such factors as the overall force of transmission and the prevailing social and environmental conditions. More generally, however, much information is lost by immediate recourse to average trends in intensity, or overall age-specific prevalence. Variability in worm loads within human communities is an intrinsic feature of the transmission biology of all helminth infections. As such, this variability should be regarded, not as a statistical nuisance, but as a valuable source of information, both in the context of gaining a deeper understanding of the interaction between host and parasite and with respect to the design of effective long-term control programmes. Although the sources of such heterogeneity will be many and varied it is becoming increasingly apparent that inherent host susceptibility or immunological competence to resist parasitic invasion is an extremely important component. There is an urgent need at present to pursue field investigations of the nature and sources of such variability. The longitudinal study of the intensity of infection in individual patients is one approach which can yield valuable insights. Previous work, for example, has suggested that 'wormy' people (those with high *S. mansoni* faecal egg counts) tend to remain 'wormy' through time when compared with the average egg output within the population (McCullough & Bradley, 1973). Care must obviously be exercised in the interpretation of such observations given that the duration of longitudinal study is often short in relation to the life expectancy of the reproductively mature parasite. If parasite acquisition is aggregated or clumped through time, then egg outputs will remain high following an intense exposure for the average life expectancy of the mature worms, irrespective of whether or not future rates of acquisition are high or low. More work of this nature is required where observations on individual patients (stratified according to age at the start of the study) are continued for long periods of time (10 years or more).

Evidence of predisposition to heavy infection is more easily acquired via studies of re-infection following anthelmintic treatment. Such information is of obvious relevance in the design of targeted or selected community control programmes based on chemotherapy (see Siongok *et al.*, 1976; Anderson & May, 1982; Anderson, 1985). Relative rankings, based on egg output, can be compared (within age classes) prior to treatment and following a set period of exposure to reinfection. Work of this kind on intestinal nematode infections in man has produced strong evidence for predisposition (see Anderson, 1985). The question remains open at present with respect to schistosome infections. Ideally, of course such predisposition studies (based on reinfection) should be linked with studies of behaviour related to contact with infective stages (in the case of schistosomes—water contact studies) and immunological studies of cell and antibody mediated responses to various parasite antigens. Some progress is being made in this direction (see Butterworth *et al.*, 1984, 1985) but much remains to be done to link such information with patterns of variability in the intensity of infection within different age classes in human communities. Indeed, the measurement of heterogeneity in worm loads within different segments of human populations and the interpretation of the generative sources of recorded patterns must be regarded as one of the major challenges facing epidemiological or ecological research on parasitic infections in the coming years. Such research will undoubtedly involve components of ecological and genetical work, and future progress is likely to be linked with the close integration of these two fields of study.

ACKNOWLEDGEMENTS

We are grateful to the MRC for the provision of a research studentship for J.A.C. and to the UNDP/World Bank/WHO Special Programme for Research and Training in Tropical Diseases for financial support.

REFERENCES

ABDEL-WAHAB, M. F., STRICKLAND, G. T., EL-SAHLY, A., AHMED, L., ZAKARIA, S., EL KADY, N. & MAHMOUD, S., 1980. Schistosomiasis mansoni in an Egyptian Village in the Nile Delta. *American Journal of Tropical Medicine and Hygiene, 29:* 868–874.

ANDERSON, R. M., 1976. Seasonal variation in the population dynamics of *Caryophyllaeus laticeps. Parasitology, 72:* 281–305.

ANDERSON, R. M., 1978. Population dynamics of snail infection by miracidia. *Parasitology, 77:* 201–224.

ANDERSON, R. M., 1982. Population dynamics and control of hookwork and roundwork infections. In R. M. Anderson (Ed.), *Population dynamics of infectious diseases: theory and applications.* 67–108. London: Chapman and Hall.

ANDERSON, R. M. Mathematical models for the study of the epidemiology and control of ascariasis in man. In D. W. T. Crompton (Ed.) Ascariasis and its public health significance. London: Taylor Francis, (in press).

ANDERSON, R. M. & CROMBIE, J., 1984. Experimental studies of age-prevalence curves for *Schistosoma mansoni* infections in populations of *Biomphalaria glabrata. Parasitology, 89:* 79–104.

ANDERSON, R. M. & GORDON, D. M., 1982. Processes influencing the distribution of parasite numbers within host populations with special emphasis on parasite-induced host mortalities. *Parasitology, 85:* 373–398.

ANDERSON, R. M. & MAY, R. M., 1979. Prevalence of schistosome infections with molluscan populations: observed patterns and theoretical predictions. *Parasitology, 79:* 63–94.

ANDERSON, R. M. & MAY, R. M., 1982. Population dynamics of human helminth infections: control by chemotherapy. *Nature 297:* 557–563.

ANDERSON, R. M. & MAY, R. M., 1985. Helminth infections of humans: mathematical models, population dynamics and control. *Advances in Parasitology, 24:* 1–101.

ANDERSON, R. M. & MAY, R. M., 1985. Herd immunity to helminth infection: implications for parasite control. *Nature,* in press.

ANDERSON, R. M., MERCER, J. G., WILSON, R. A. & CARTER, N. P., 1982. Transmission of *Schistosoma mansoni* from man to snail: experimental studies of miracidial survival and infectivity in relation to larval age, water temperature, host size and host age. *Parasitology, 85:* 339–360.

BARBOUR, A. D., 1978. Macdonald's Model and the transmission of bilharzia. *Transactions of the Royal Society of Tropical Medicine and Hygiene, 77:* 6–15.

BODMER, W. F., 1980. The HLA system and diseases. *Journal of the Royal College of Physicians London,* 43–50.

BRADLEY, D. J. & McCULLOUGH, F. S., 1973. Egg output and stability and the epidemiology of *Schistosoma haematobium* Part II. An analysis of the epidemiology of endemic *S. haematobium. Transactions of the Royal Society of Tropical Medicine and Hygiene, 67:* 491–500.

BUTTERWORTH, A. E., DALTON, P. R., DUNNE, D. W., MUGAMBI, M., OUMA, J. H., RICHARDSON, B. A., ARAP SIONGOK, T. K. & STURROCK, R. F., 1984. Immunity after treatment of human *schistosomiasis mansoni* I. Study design, pretreatment observations and the results of treatment. *Transactions of the Royal Society of Tropical Medicine and Hygiene, 78:* 108–123.

BUTTERWORTH, A. E., CAPRON, M., DALTON, P. R., DUNNE, D. W., KARIVKE, H. C., KOECH, D., MUGAMBI, M., OUMA, J. H., PRENTICE, M. A., RICHARDSON, B. A., ARAP SIONGOK, T. K., STURROCK, R. F. & TAYLOR, D. W., Immunity after treatment of *schistosomiasis mansoni* II. Identification of resistant individuals and analysis of their immune responses. *Transactions of the Royal Society of Tropical Medicine and Hygiene,* (in press).

CARTER, N. P., ANDERSON, R. M. & WILSON, R. A., 1982. Transmission of *Schistosoma mansoni* from man to snail: laboratory studies on the influence of snail and miracidial densities on transmission success. *Parasitology, 85:* 361–372.

CAVALLI-SFORZA, L. & BODMER, W. F., 1971. *The Genetics of Human Population.* San Francisco: Freeman.

CHEEVER, A. W., KAMEL, J. A., ELWI, A. M., MUSIMAN, J. E. & DANNER, R., 1977. *Schistosoma mansoni* and *S. haematobium* infections in Egypt. II. Quantitative parasitological findings at necropsy. *American Journal of Tropical Medicine and Hygiene, 26:* 702–716.

CHERNIN, E., 1972. Penetrative activity of *Schistosoma mansoni* miracidia stimulated by exposure to snail conditioned water. *Journal of Parasitology, 58:* 209–212.

CHU, K. Y., MASSOUD, J. & SABBAGHIAN, H., 1966. Host parasite relationship of *Bulinus truncatus* and *Schistosoma haematobium* in Iran. I. Effect of the age of *B. truncatus* on the development of *S. haematobium. Bulletin of the World Health Organisation, 34:* 113–119.

CROMBIE, J. A. & ANDERSON, R. M., 1985. Repeated infection of mice with *Schistosoma mansoni:* population dynamics and acquired immunity. *Nature,* in press.

DALTON, P. R. & POOLE, D., 1978. Water contact patterns in relation to *Schistosoma haematobium* infection. *Bulletin of the World Health Organisation, 56:* 417–426.

DEAN, D. A., 1983. A Review. *Schistosoma* and related genera: acquired resistance in mice. *Experimental Parasitology, 55:* 1–104.

DE WITT, W. B., 1955. Influence of temperature on penetration of snail hosts by *S. mansoni* miracidia. *Experimental Parasitology, 4:* 271–276.

GODDARD, M. J. & JORDAN, P., 1980. On the longevity of *Schistosoma mansoni* in man on St. Lucas, West Indies. *Transactions of the Royal Society of Tropical Medicine and Hygiene, 74:* 185.

JENKINS, D. C. & PHILLIPSON, R. F., 1971. The kinetics of repeated low level infections of *Nippostrongylus braziliensis* in the laboratory rat. *Parasitology, 62:* 457–465.

JENKINS, D. C. & PHILLIPSON, R. F., 1972. Increased establishment and longevity of *Nippostrongylus braziliensis* in immune rats given repeated small infections. *International Journal of Parasitology, 2:* 105–111.

LACKIE, A. M., 1980. Invertebrate immunity. *Parasitology, 80:* 393–412.

McCULLOUGH, F. S. & BRADLEY, D. J., 1973. Egg output and stability and the epidemiology of *Schistosoma haematobium.* Part I. Variation and stability in *Schistosoma haematobium* egg counts. *Transactions of the Royal Society of Tropical Medicine and Hygiene, 67:* 475–490.

MASON, P. R., 1977. Stimulation of the activity of *Schistosoma mansoni* miracidia by snail — conditioned water. *Parasitology, 75:* 325–338.

MAY, R. M., 1977. Togetherness among schistosomes: its effects on the dynamics of infection. *Mathematical Biosciences, 35:* 301–343.

MUENCH, H., 1959. *Catalytic models in epidemiology.* Cambridge, Massachusetts: Harvard University Press.

PRAH, S. K. & JAMES, C., 1977. The influence of physical factors on the survival and infectivity of miracidia of *Schistosoma mansoni* and *S. haematobium.* I. Effect of temperature and ultra-violet light. *Journal of Hygiene, 51:* 73–85.

SCHAD, G. A. & BANWELL, J. G., 1984. Hookworms. In K. S. Warren & A. A. F. Mahmoud (Eds) *Tropical and Geographical Medicine*, 358–372. New York: McGraw-Hill.

SCHIFF, C. J., 1974. Seasonal factors influencing the location of *Bulinus (physopsis) globosus* by miracidia of *Schistosoma haematobium* in nature. *Journal of Parasitology, 60:* 578–583.

SCOTT, D., SENKER, K. & ENGLAND, E. C., 1982. Epidemiology of human *Schistosoma haematobium* infection around Volta Lake, Ghana, 1973–5. *Bulletin of the World Health Organisation, 60:* 89–100.

SIONGOK, T. K. A., MAHMOUD, A. A. F., OUMA, J. H., WARREN, K. S., MULLER, A. S., HANDY, A. K. & HOUSER, H. B., 1976. Morbidity in schistosomiasis mansoni in relation to intensity of infection: study of a community in Machakos, Kenya. *American Journal of Tropical Medicine and Hygiene, 25:* 273–284.

SMITHERS, S. R. & TERRY, R. J., 1969. Immunity in schistosomiasis. *Annals of the New York Academy of Sciences, 160:* 826–840.

STANDEN, O. D., 1952. Experimental infection of *Australorbis glabratus* with *Schistosoma mansoni.* I. Individual and mass infection of snails, and the relationship to temperature and season. *Annals of Tropical Medicine and Parasitology, 46:* 48–53.

STURROCK, R. F., 1973. Field studies on the transmission of *Schistosoma mansoni* and on the bionomics of its intermediate host *Biomphalaria glabrata* on St. Lucia, West Indies. *International Journal of Parasitology, 3:* 175–194.

STURROCK, R. F. & WEBBE, G., 1971. The application of catalytic models to schistosomiasis in snails. *Journal of Helminthology, 45:* 189–200.

STURROCK, R. F. & UPATHAM, E. S., 1973. An investigation of the interaction of some factors influencing the infectivity of *Schistosoma mansoni* miracidia to *Biomphalaria glabrata. International Journal of Parasitology, 3:* 35–41.

STURROCK, R. F., COTTRELL, B. J. & KIMANI, R., 1984. Observations on the ability of repeated light exposures to *Schistosoma mansoni* cercariae to induce resistance to reinfection in Kenyan baboons *(Papio anubis). Parasitology, 88:* 505–514.

UPATHAM, E. S., 1972. Effects of some physico-chemical factors on the infection of *Biomphalaria glabrata* by miracidia of *Schistosoma mansoni* in St. Lucia, West Indies. *Journal of Helminthology, 46:* 307–315.

WAKELIN, D., 1984a. *Immunity to parasites,* London: Edward Arnold.

WAKELIN, D., 1984b. Evasion of the immune response: survival within low responder individuals of the host population. *Parasitology, 88:* 639–658.

WARREN, K. S., 1973. Regulation of the prevalence and intensity of schistosomiasis in man: immunology or ecology? *Journal of Infectious Diseases, 127:* 593–609.

A murine model of genetically controlled host responses to leishmaniasis

JENEFER M. BLACKWELL

Department of Tropical Hygiene, London School of Hygiene and Tropical Medicine, Keppel Street, London WC1E 7HT, U.K.

In recent years, the use of inbred and other genetically manipulated strains of mice has allowed precise identification of the genes and mechanisms which control the spectrum of disease profiles observed both within one *Leishmania* species and between different species. Interestingly, many of the single genes identified and mapped thus far have been shown to have a profound effect upon the course of infection for one *Leishmania* species while having little or no effect on others. There is also clear separation between genes controlling different phases of the host response. Hence, the *Lsh* gene located on mouse chromosome 1 plays a vital role in the early course of infection with *L. donovani* and with such phylogenetically distinct species as *Salmonella typhimurium*, *Mycobacterium bovis*, and *M. lepraemurium*, but has no effect on *L. major* or *L. mexicana mexicana* infection. The *Scl* gene located on chromosome 8 has a profound effect upon *L. major* and, to a lesser extent, *L. m. mexicana* but plays no role in *L. donovani* infection. These results are more interesting when it is considered that both genes are thought to operate at the macrophage level early in infection. A similar dichotomy is observed for the effect of *H-2* on the later phase of visceral infection (*L. donovani*) versus cutaneous (*L. major*, *L. m. mexicana*) infections. For *L. donovani*, different *H-2* haplotypes on both B10 and BALB genetic backgrounds produce widely different disease profiles. For *L. major* and *L. m. mexicana*, the same *H-2* haplotypes on the same genetic backgrounds produce only minor differences in the host response. The action of different genes does not, however, always follow the division between visceral versus cutaneous forms of the disease. Recent studies with B10.129(10M) mice have, for example, demonstrated an *H-11*-linked gene which causes a similar alteration in disease profiles compared with the congenic BIO strain for both *L. donovani* and *L. major*, but exerts little effect on *L. m. mexicana*. These studies provide very clear evidence that genetically controlled differences in the host response are important in determining why some individuals may be more susceptible to infection than others. They also serve to remind us, however, that the final outcome of an infection is likely to be the result of a complex interplay between genes exerting their influence at different stages during the course of an infection. This, in turn, may have important implications for the study of genetically controlled host responses to infection in natural populations.

KEY WORDS:—Mouse model—immunogenetics—host response—infection—*Leishmania*

CONTENTS

Ecology and Genetics of Host–Parasite Interactions
ISBN: 0 12 593 690 7

INTRODUCTION

In leishmanial infections in man and reservoir hosts, a broad spectrum of disease profiles has been observed (Turk & Bryceson, 1971; Bryceson, 1985). While these are controlled to some extent by the particular tissue tropisms of the different *Leishmania* species, environmentally and genetically controlled variations in the host response also play a role. Hence, the broad distinction between cutaneous and visceral forms of the disease is largely influenced by the species of parasite but, within each species, a range of infections from subclinical to fatal visceral disease or from self-healing to disseminated cutaneous lesions may occur. In our laboratory, our particular interest has been in examining the genetically controlled component of this variability in the host response.

In this paper, the individual effects of just four host genes on the courses of infection with three distinct *Leishmania* species will be examined in genetically defined inbred mouse strains. It should be stated quite clearly at the outset that, although rodents have been shown to act as reservoir hosts for various leishmanial species (Lainson & Strangways-Dixon, 1964; Camerlynck, Rangue & Quilici, 1967; Hoogstraal *et al.*, 1963; Lainson & Shaw, 1973; Haile & Lemma, 1977; Bettini, Gradoni and Pozio, 1978; Dedet *et al.*, 1979), naturally infected *Mus musculus* have never been reported. Our laboratory models do not in any way attempt to mimic natural infection. The routes, doses and stages of the parasite used for inoculation frequently bear little or no relation to those employed by the sandfly vector. The strains of mice used are highly inbred and are frequently manipulated genetically and immunologically still further to suit our purposes in determining the immunological mechanisms associated with the action of each gene. In effect, what we are doing is using the mice as the 'test-tubes' in which we vary both the composition of genes and the efficiency of various immunoregulatory cell populations, add the parasite and determine the outcome of the infection. By altering just one gene at a time, we can then determine the relative contributions of each gene to the overall response of the host.

The natural resistance gene Lsh

The first gene to be identified for its effect in controlling the early response of mice to visceral infection following intravenous inoculation of *L. donovani* amastigotes was the *Lsh* gene located between *Idh*-1 and *ln* on mouse chromosome 1 (Bradley, 1974, 1977; Bradley *et al.*, 1979). In 1975, we embarked on a breeding program which would allow us to transpose the resistant allele for the *Lsh* gene from C57L mice onto the genetic background of C57BL/10ScSn (or B1O) mice which normally carry the *Lsh* susceptible allele. F1 mice were backcrossed to B1O mice and, in each successive generation, the heterozygous progeny were selected and backcrossed again to the homozygous *Lsh*^{s} B1O parental strain. With each successive generation, the background genes from the original C57L parent were diluted out. In 1981, after 10 generations of backcrossing, heterozygous mice were crossed with each other and the homozygous resistant progeny (determined by further test crosses to B1O mice) mated together to obtain a homozygous *Lsh*^{r} line on the B1O genetic background. This is the standard protocol for production of congenic strains (Bartlett

& Haldane, 1935) and is relatively simple, for example, for loci which can be typed in live mice but is a longwinded and laborious process in the case of a disease resistance gene where the typing for each new generation must be carried out retrospectively. At the tenth generation we could, however, expect to have diluted out all the background genes to a distance within 0.1 map units on either side of the selected locus (Bartlett & Haldane, 1935). Typing for the closest known genes, *Idh*-1 and *ln*, for which the two original strains carried alternative alleles, confirmed that the C57L alleles had been replaced by B1O alleles. The congenic strain, designated B1O.LL*sh*^{r}, has proved to be invaluable not only in studying expression of the gene for *L. donovani*, but also in determining its action for other intracellular pathogens.

Detailed studies carried out in our own and other laboratories (Plant *et al.*, 1982; Skamene *et al.*, 1982) had already indicated that the *Lsh* gene was indistinguishable on immunogenetic grounds from the genes *Ity* and *Bcg* which control the early responses of mice to *Salmonella typhimurium* and *Mycobacterium bovis* (Montreal strain), respectively. The congenic B1O.LL*sh*^{r} strain also types as *Ity*^{r} and *Bcg*^{r}. Functional studies also suggest that the three genes are identical. Studies with all three pathogens have shown that expression of resistance does not require a functional T cell population (Bradley & Kirkley, 1972; O'Brien & Metcalf, 1982; Gros *et al.*, 1983), can be transferred along with the donor haematopoietic system in reciprocal radiation bone marrow chimaeras (Hormaeche, 1979; Gros *et al.*, 1983; Crocker, Blackwell & Bradley, 1984a), and correlates with a reduction in the rate of proliferation of each micro-organism in liver or spleen *in vivo* (Bradley, 1979; Hormaeche, 1980; Crocker, Blackwell & Bradley, 1984b) or in peritoneal macrophages *in vitro* (Stach *et al.*, 1984).

Studies examining the action of the gene against growth of *L. donovani in vitro* in liver macrophage populations isolated from mice infected *in vivo* (Crocker *et al.*, 1984b) proved interesting since they revealed that the naïve state of macrophages from both B1O and B1O.LL*sh*^{r} mice was 'susceptible' and that 2–3 days were required before *Lsh* gene activity was expressed. Although we do not, as yet, fully understand the mechanism of *Lsh* gene activity, our most recent observations (Blackwell, Crocker & Channon, 1984a; Crocker *et al.*, 1984b) suggest that the gene controls some form of T cell-independent macrophage 'activation' process which appears to be triggered by 'LPS-like' molecules in the parasite surface and does not involve production of reactive oxygen intermediates as the effector mechanism for resistance.

Studies *in vivo* (Crocker *et al.*, 1984b) and *in vitro* (Blackwell *et al.*, 1984a; Crocker *et al.*, in prep.) have confirmed that the *Lsh* gene is expressed at the level of the infected resident liver macrophage independently of other cell types. What is perhaps most interesting is that, despite its action against such phylogenetically distinct micro-organisms as *S. typhimurium* (Plant *et al.*, 1982), *M. bovis* (Skamene *et al.*, 1982) and *M. lepraemurium* (Brown *et al.*, 1982; Skamene *et al.*, 1984), the gene does not appear to exert any influence *in vivo* on *L. major* or *L. mexicana mexicana*, at least when these species are inoculated subcutaneously and even when controlling for the influence of background genes by the use of the congenic strains (Blackwell & Alexander, 1984). To what extent this represents differences between macrophage subpopulations in the viscera versus the skin, or differences in the ability of the parasite (surface) to trigger the action of the gene, remains to be determined.

The influence of H-2 on L. donovani infection

Studies in our laboratory have shown that some homozygous recessive Lsh^s mouse strains may ultimately self-cure from intravenous *L. donovani* amastigote infection (Bradley & Kirkley, 1977; Blackwell *et al.*, 1980). Cure in these strains is T cell-mediated (Skov & Twohy, 1974) and correlates with a positive delayed-type hypersensitivity response (DeTolla *et al.*, 1980; Rezai *et al.*, 1980) and with the lymphokine-generating capacity of spleen cells from curing mice (Murray *et al.*, 1982). Other strains of inbred mice maintain immense parasite loads for up to 2 years involving mononuclear phagocytes throughout the body (Bradley & Kirkley, 1977). On B1O and BALB genetic backgrounds, this difference in long-term response (measured as liver or spleen parasite load over 130 days of infection) is controlled by genes mapping to IE and a subregion to its left (presumed to be IA) in the K end of the major histocompatibility complex (MHC) *H-2* (Blackwell *et al.*, 1980; Blackwell, 1982, 1983).

Using parasite inocula of 5×10^5 and greater (Blackwell, Freeman & Bradley, 1980; Ulczak & Blackwell, 1983), three *H-2*-controlled phenotypic patterns of long-term response to infection are observed: early cure (s and r haplotypes), cure (b haplotype) and non-cure (d, f and q haplotypes), with non-cure haplotypes varying in their degree of dominance over cure haplotypes according to the particular heterozygote combination (Blackwell, 1983). At these higher inoculation doses, non-cure in $H\text{-}2^d$ mice is accompanied by the generation of a potent Lyt-1^+2^- suppressor T cell (T_s) population during infection (Blackwell & Ulczak, 1984), which can be abrogated by 550 rad sublethal whole body irradiation prior to infection (Ulczak & Blackwell, 1983). When injected with parasite doses of 5×10^4 or lower (Ulczak & Blackwell, 1983), B1O D2/n ($H\text{-}2^d$) non-cure mice present a cure profile.

Hence, at least for *L. donovani* infection in B1O *H-2* congenic strains, there appear to be two determinants for the development of T_s cells, a sufficiently high antigenic load and the type of class II MHC molecule (Ia antigen) presented by antigen presenting cells (dendritic cells and/or macrophages) in association with parasite antigen. It is not yet known whether the Lyt-1^+2^- T^s cell interacts directly with MHC class II molecules nor whether they are the T_s effector cells or some other element (e.g. T_s inducer) in a more complex suppressor pathway. It seems clear, however, that under certain circumstances, polymorphism for loci of the MHC may be important in determining the balance between different T cell subsets and, hence, whether non-cure or cure phenotypes predominate.

The importance of the Scl gene relative to H-2 in L. major infection

The demonstration of Lyt-1^+2^- T_s cells (Blackwell & Ulczak, 1984) and the prophylactic effect of 550 rad sublethal irradiation (Ulczak & Blackwell, 1983) for *L. donovani* infection in genetically determined non-cure strains was interesting because it was reminiscent of the earlier observations of Howard and colleagues (Howard, Hale & Liew, 1981; Liew, Hale & Howard, 1982) for subcutaneous *L. major* infection in the non-healing BALB/c strain. In the latter case, however, reduction of the parasite inoculum to as low as 20 parasites (Howard, Hale & Chan-Liew, 1980a) still resulted in progressive lesion development and fatal disease. Examination of congenic strains carrying different *H-2* haplotypes on BALB and

B1O genetic backgrounds demonstrated only a very minor influence of *H-2* on the course of infection (Howard *et al.*, 1980a). In fact, the overriding genetic determinant for the outcome of *L. major* infection in inbred mouse strains is another gene (Howard *et al.*, 1980a; DeTolla, Scott & Farrell, 1981), *Scl*, which, on current evidence, maps to mouse chromosome 8 (Blackwell *et al.*, 1984c).

Resistance and susceptibility controlled by the *Scl* gene is again determined by descendents of the donor haematopoietic cells in reciprocal radiation bone marrow chimaeras (Howard *et al.*, 1980b). The generation of T_s cells during *L. major* infection in non-healing strains is, therefore, thought to be the secondary effect of the high antigenic load resulting from an *Scl*-controlled primary macrophage defect (Howard *et al.*, 1980b). Studies *in vitro* (Gorczynski & MacRae, 1982) have indeed shown that skin macrophages from susceptible mice support greater multiplication of the parasites than macrophages from resistant mice. Expression of Ia and antigen presenting function also differs in skin macrophages isolated from resistant and susceptible mice (Gorczynski & MacRae, 1982). However, no formal linkage between either of these functions and the *Scl* gene has yet been made. Studies with peritoneal macrophage populations also suggest that there is a correlation between susceptibility to *L. major* infection *in vivo* and both quantitative (Behin, Mauel & Sordat, 1979) and qualitative (Nacy *et al.*, 1983) responses to lymphokine activation *in vitro*.

The *Scl* gene may also exert some influence over subcutaneous *L. m. mexicana* infection in BALB/c and SWR mice (Blackwell & Alexander, 1985). Its influence, along with the very minor influence of *H-2* differences on a B1O genetic background (Alexander & Blackwell, 1984), appears to be secondary to other genetic influence which cause all mouse strains except DBA/2 to display progressive and ultimately fatal lesion development in response to *L. m. mexicana* infection (Blackwell & Alexander, 1985).

The influence of H-11 or an H-11-linked gene on L. donovani and L. major infection

Each of the genes examined thus far has been shown to have a profound effect upon the course of infection produced by one particular species of *Leishmania* while having little or no effect on other species. This separate action of distinct genes at various stages during the course of infection with different species of *Leishmania* may, to some extent, be explained by the different routes of infection employed, the different stages of the parasite inoculated, and the growth of the parasite at separate sites in the host. In recent studies (Blackwell *et al.*, 1984b), a characteristically different *H-11* (or closely linked gene)-controlled non-cure/non-healing phenotype, first documented for *L. donovani* (De Tolla *et al.*, 1980; Blackwell, 1982), has been shown to act in a parallel manner for both intravenous infection with *L. donovani* amastigotes and subcutaneous infection with *L. major* promastigotes. It appears to have little effect, however, on primary lesion growth following subcutaneous inoculation of *L. m. mexicana* amastigote (Blackwell & Alexander, 1984), although it does affect metastatic lesion growth and visceralization of the parasite (unpublished observation).

The characteristics of the *H-11*-linked non-cure/non-healing phenotype are a curious mixture of those observed for other genes. The non-cure/non-healing phenotype is again determined by descendents of the donor haematopoietic cells in radiation bone marrow chimaeras (Blackwell *et al.*, 1984c) but prior sublethal irradiation has only a weak and transient prophylactic effect. Interestingly, and in contrast to the previously described H-2-controlled non-cure phenotype for *L. donovani*, low parasite inocula result in progressive disease for both parasite species.

The influence of *H-11* or an *H-11*-linked gene on *L. donovani* and *L. major* infection was again determined by the use of congenic mouse strains. In this case, B1O.129(1OM) mice, originally produced by backcrossing and selection for the *H-11*[b] allele from 129 mice onto the B1O genetic background (Snell & Bunker, 1965), were used. As with the B1O.LL*sh*[r] strain, alleles for closely linked polymorphic loci may also have been carried across along with the selected *H-11*[b] allele. *H-11* itself remains unmapped. Irrespective of whether it is the *H-11* locus itself or some linked genetic locus which controls the response of B1O.129(1OM) mice, it is clear that further elucidation of its mode of action may provide us with some important new insight into the common events involved in the development of the cell-mediated immune response to both cutaneous and visceral forms of leishmaniasis.

CONCLUSIONS

In this paper, we have compared the roles of just four host genes in controlling the severity of the diseases caused by three different species of *Leishmania*. These studies provide very clear evidence that genetically controlled differences in the host response may play a major role in determining the severity of infection in individuals. They also serve to remind us, however, that the interplay between host genes and parasite populations at various stages during the course of infection is complex. Whilst we can manipulate the mouse genome with comparative ease to determine the effect of single genes, the outcome of a natural infection in a natural host is likely to reflect the action of many genes during the course of infection. In fact, some explanation for the difficulties experienced in obtaining firm evidence for association between particular genetic markers and susceptibility phenotypes in human populations (reviewed by Fine, 1981; Blackwell, 1985) can be obtained by closer consideration of the mouse model of leishmaniasis. For the long-term response of B1O mice to *L. donovani* infection, for example, genetic manipulation altering the allele at just one other locus (*H-11*) or tight linkage group in the B1O.129(1OM) strain transformed the normally *H-2*[b]-controlled self-curing phenotype into a severe non-curing response. This does not mean that *H-2* may not, given the chance, perform its normal immunoregulatory function. Indeed, the role of class II molecules of the MHC in antigen presentation and the proliferation of different T cell subsets could provide a key point in the overall immunoregulatory process where progression of the disease could be controlled, and may be even more important in determining vaccination protocols. In the case of B1O.129(1OM) mice, however, the action of *H-11* (or an *H-11*-linked gene) presumably precedes and/or overrides the action of *H-2*.

Such findings in mice cast some real doubt on the value of attempting to look for gross correlations between particular genetic markers and susceptibility phenotypes at the population level. Experience has shown, in fact, that such studies rarely bear fruit (Fine, 1981; Blackwell, 1985). As in the mouse, for example, not all people carrying a particular HLA haplotype may have a self-limiting infection. It may, nevertheless, be true that this same haplotype is a prerequisite to self cure. Family linkage analyses (e.g. De Vries *et al.*, 1976; Fine *et al.*, 1979; Van Eden *et al.*, 1980) may provide firmer evidence for such associations but these too can be expensive in terms of manpower, equipment and time and may give minimum return for effort. The prospective worker in this area is certainly well advised to study in detail the constraints of such analyses in terms of the minimum number of families required and the numbers of infected versus uninfected offspring per family, before proceeding with what might predictably be an inconclusive study. In the case of leishmaniasis, we have yet to find a population where all the criteria are met and which might prove tractable to such analyses. For leprosy, earlier (De Vries *et al.*, 1976; Fine *et al.*, 1979; Van Eden *et al.*, 1980) family studies carried out in Surinam and India all demonstrated an association between HLA and tuberculoid forms of leprosy, but only the more recent (Van Eden *et al.*, 1985) study in China was successful in extending this association to the lepromatous form of the disease. With the application of modern technology, it may eventually be possible to bypass such procedures. The production, for example, of DNA probes for the various resistance genes identified in mice should enable us to cross the species barrier in determining whether homologous genes occur in man or in possible reservoir hosts. *In vitro* culture procedures and the use of monoclonal antibodies may also provide a more direct assessment of the role of MHC encoded class I and class II molecules in the immunoregulation of human disease. It is hoped that some of these modern procedures may indeed provide the ultimate answers in determining the functional links between susceptibility phenotypes and the genes which control them in human populations.

ACKNOWLEDGEMENTS

Work carried out at the LSHTM on the mouse models of *L. donovani*, *L. major* and *L. m. mexicana* is supported by grants from the Medical Research Council and the Wellcome Trust. Collaborative studies on *L. major* and *L. m. mexicana* are also carried out with Drs James Howard and Eddy Liew at the Wellcome Research Laboratories, Beckenham, Kent, and with Dr James Alexander at the Imperial College Field Station, Silwood Park, Ascot, Berks, respectively. J. Blackwell holds a Wellcome Trust Senior Lecturership.

REFERENCES

BARTLETT, M. S. & HALDANE, J. B. S., 1935. The theory of inbreeding with forced heterozygosis. *Journal of Genetics, 31:* 327–340.

BEHIN, R., MAUEL, J. & SORDAT, B., 1979. *Leishmania tropica*: pathogenicity and *in vitro* macrophage function in strains of inbred mice. *Experimental Parasitology, 48:* 81–91.

BETTINI, S., GRADONI, L. & POZIO, E., 1978. Isolation of *Leishmania* strains from *Rattus rattus* in Italy. *Transactions of the Royal Society of Tropical Medicine and Hygiene, 72:* 441–442.

BLACKWELL, J. M., 1982. Genetic control of recovery from visceral leishmaniasis. *Transactions of the Royal Society of Tropical Medicine and Hygiene, 76:* 147–151.

BLACKWELL, J. M., 1983. *Leishmania donovani* infection in heterozygous and recombinant *H-2* haplotype mice. *Immunogenetics, 18:* 101–109.

BLACKWELL, J. M., 1985. Host genetics and tropical diseases. *Rivista di Immunologia ed Immunofarmacologia, v*(i): 3–7.

BLACKWELL, J. M. & ALEXANDER, J., 1985. Different host genes recognise and control infection with taxonomically distinct *Leishmania* species. *Annales de Parasitologie (Paris)*, in press.

BLACKWELL, J. M. & ULCZAK, O. M., 1984. Immunoregulation of genetically controlled acquired responses to *Leishmania donovani* infection in mice: demonstration and characterisation of suppressor T cells in noncure mice. *Infection and Immunity, 44:* 97–102.

BLACKWELL, J. M., FREEMAN, J. C. & BRADLEY, D. J., 1980. Influence of *H-2* complex on acquired resistance to *Leishmania donovani* infection in mice. *Nature (London), 283:* 72–74.

BLACKWELL, J. M., CROCKER, P. R. & CHANNON, J. Y., 1984a. The role of the macrophage in genetically controlled resistance and susceptibility to leishmaniasis. In R. van Furth (Ed.), *Proceedings of the Fourth Leiden Conference on Mononuclear Phagocytes*: in press. The Hague, Martinus Nijhoff Publishers BV.

BLACKWELL, J. M., HALE, C., ROBERTS, M. B., ULCZAK, O. M., LIEW, F. Y. & HOWARD, J. G., 1984b. An *H-11*-linked gene has a parallel effect on *Leishmania major* and *L. donovani* infection in mice. *Immunogenetics*, in press.

BLACKWELL, J. M., HOWARD, J. G., LIEW, F. Y. & HALE, C., 1984c. Mapping of the gene controlling susceptibility to cutaneous leishmaniasis. *Mouse News Letter, 70:* 86.

BRADLEY, D. J., 1974. Genetic control of natural resistance to *Leishmania donovani. Nature (London), 250:* 353–354.

BRADLEY, D. J., 1977. Regulation of *Leishmania* populations within the host. II. Genetic control of acute susceptibility of mice to *Leishmania donovani* infection. *Clinical and Experimental Immunology, 30:* 130–140.

BRADLEY, D. J., 1979. Regulation of *Leishmania* populations within the host. IV. Parasite and host cell kinetics studied by radioisotope labelling. *Acta Tropica, 36:* 171–179.

BRADLEY, D. J. & KIRKLEY, J., 1972. Variation in susceptibility of mouse strains to *Leishmania donovani* infection. *Transactions of the Royal Society of Tropical Medicine and Hygiene, 66:* 527–528.

BRADLEY, D. J. & KIRKLEY, J., 1977. Regulation of *Leishmania* populations within the host. I. The variable course of *Leishmania donovani* infections in mice. *Clinical and Experimental Immunology, 30:* 119–129.

BRADLEY, D. J., TAYLOR, B. A., BLACKWELL, J. M., EVANS, E. P. & FREEMAN, J., 1979. Regulation of *Leishmania* populations within the host. III. Mapping of the locus controlling susceptibility to visceral leishmaniasis in the mouse. *Clinical and Experimental Immunology, 37:* 7–14.

BROWN, I. N., GLYNN, A. A. & PLANT, J., 1982. Inbred mouse strain resistance to *Mycobacterium lepraemurium* follows the *Ity/Lsh* pattern. *Immunology, 47:* 149–156.

BRYCESON, A. D. M., 1985. Clinical variations associated with various species of *Leishmania. Annales de Parasitologie (Paris)*, in press.

CAMERLYNCK, P., RANQUE, Ph. & QUILICI, M., 1967. Intérêt des cultures systematiques et des subcultures dans la recherche des reservoirs de virus naturels de la leishmaniose cutanée. A propos de l'isolement de cinq souches de *Leishmania* chez *Arvicanthus niloticus. Medecine Tropicale, 27:* 89–92.

CROCKER, P. R., BLACKWELL, J. M. & BRADLEY, D. J., 1984a. Transfer of innate resistance and susceptibility to *Leishmania donovani* infection in mouse radiation bone marrow chimaeras. *Immunology, 52:* 417–422.

CROCKER, P. R., BLACKWELL, J. M. & BRADLEY, D. J., 1984b. Expression of the natural resistance gene *Lsh* in resident liver macrophages. *Infection and Immunity, 43:* 1033–1040.

DEDET, J. P., DEROUIN, F., HUBERT, B., SCHNUR, L. F. & CHANCE, M. L., 1979. Isolation of *Leishmania (tropica) major* from *Mastomys erythroleucus* and *Tatera gambiana* in Senegal (West Africa). *Annals of Tropical Medicine and Parasitology, 73:* 433–437.

DE TOLLA, L. J., SEMPREVIVO, L. H., PALCZUK, N. C. & PASSMORE, H. C., 1980. Genetic control of acquired resistance to visceral leishmaniasis in mice. *Immunogenetics, 10:* 353–361.

DE TOLLA, L. J., SCOTT, P. A. & FARRELL, J. P., 1981. Single gene control of resistance to cutaneous leishmaniasis in mice. *Immunogenetics, 14:* 29–39.

DE VRIES, R. R. P., LAI, A., FAT, R. F. M., NIJENHUIS, L. E. & VAN ROOD, J. J., 1976. HLA-linked control of host response to *Mycobacterium leprae. Lancet, 2:* 1328–1330.

FINE, P. E. M., 1981. Immunogenetics of susceptibility to leprosy, tuberculosis, and leishmaniasis. An epidemiological perspective. *International Journal of Leprosy, 49:* 437–454.

FINE, P. E. M., WOLF, E., PRITCHARD, J., WATSON, B., BRADLEY, D. J., FESTENSTEIN, H. & CHACKO, C. J. G., 1979. HLA-linked genes and leprosy: a family study in Karigiri, South India. *Journal of Infectious Diseases, 140:* 152–162.

GORCZYNSKI, R. M. & MACRAE, S., 1982. Analysis of subpopulations of glass-adherent mouse skin cells controlling resistance/susceptibility to infection with *Leishmania tropica*, and correlation with the development of independent proliferative signals to $Lyt-1^+2^+$ T lymphocytes. *Cellular Immunology, 67:* 74–89.

GROS, P., SKAMENE, E. & FORGET, A., 1983. Cellular mechanisms of genetically controlled host resistance to *Mycobacterium bovis* (BCG). *Journal of Immunology, 131:* 1966–1972.

HAILE, T. T. & LEMMA, A., 1977. Isolation of *Leishmania* parasites from *Arvicanthus* in Ethiopia. *Transactions of the Royal Society of Tropical Medicine and Hygiene, 71:* 180–181.

HOOGSTRAAL, H., VAN PEENEN, P. F. D., REID, T. P. & DIETLEIN, D. R., 1963. Leishmaniasis in the Sudan Republic. 10. Natural infections in rodents. *American Journal of Tropical Medicine and Hygiene, 12:* 175–178.

HORMAECHE, C. E., 1979. The natural resistance of radiation chimaeras to *S. typhimurium. Immunology, 37:* 329–332.

HORMAECHE, C. E., 1980. The *in vivo* division and death rates of *Salmonella typhimurium* in the spleen of naturally resistant and susceptible mice measured by the super-infecting phage technique of Meyell. *Immunology, 41:* 973–979.

HOWARD, J. G., HALE, C. & CHAN-LIEW, W. L., 1980a. Immunological regulation of experimental cutaneous leishmaniasis. I. Immunogenetic aspects of susceptibility to *Leishmania tropica* in mice. *Parasite Immunology, 2:* 303–314.

HOWARD, J. G., HALE, C. & LIEW, F. Y., 1980b. Genetically determined susceptibility to *Leishmania tropica* infection is expressed by haematopoietic donor cells in mouse radiation chimaeras. *Nature (London), 288:* 161–162.

HOWARD, J. G., HALE, C. & LIEW, F. Y., 1981. Immunological regulation of experimental cutaneous leishmaniasis. IV. Prophylactic effect of sublethal irradiation as a result of abrogation of suppressor T cell generation in mice genetically susceptible to *Leishmania tropica*. *Journal of Experimental Medicine, 153:* 557–568.

LAINSON, R. & SHAW, J. J., 1973. Leishmanias and leishmaniasis of the New World, with particular reference to Brazil. *Paho Bulletin, VII:* 1–19.

LAINSON, R. & STRANGWAYS-DIXON, J., 1964. The epidemiology of dermal leishmaniasis in British Honduras: II. Reservoir-hosts of *Leishmania mexicana* among the forest rodents. *Transactions of the Royal Society of Tropical Medicine and Hygiene, 58:* 136–153.

LIEW, F. Y., HALE, C. & HOWARD, J. G., 1982. Immunological regulation of experimental cutaneous leishmaniasis. V. Characterization of effector and specific suppressor T cells. *Journal of Immunology, 128:* 1917–1922.

MURRAY, H. W., MASUR, H. & KEITHLY, J. S., 1982. Cell-mediated immune responses in experimental visceral leishmaniasis. I. Correlation between resistance to *Leishmania donovani* and lymphokine-generating capacity. *Journal of Immunology, 129:* 344–350.

NACY, C. A., FORTIER, A. H., PAPPAS, M. G. & HENRY, R. R., 1983. Susceptibility of inbred mice to *Leishmania tropica* infection: correlation of susceptibility with *in vitro* defective macrophage microbiocidal activities. *Cellular Immunology, 77:* 298–307.

O'BRIEN, A. D. & METCALF, E. S., 1982. Control of early *Salmonella typhimurium* growth in innately *Salmonella*-resistant mice does not require functional T lymphocytes. *Journal of Immunology, 129:* 1349–1351.

PLANT, J. E., BLACKWELL, J. M., O'BRIEN, A. D., BRADLEY, D. J. & GLYNN, A. A., 1982. Are the disease resistance genes *Lsh* and *Ity* at one locus on mouse chromosome 1. *Nature (London), 297:* 510–511.

REZAI, H. R., FARRELL, J. & SOULSBY, E. L., 1980. Immunological responses of *Leishmania donovani* infection in mice and significance of T cell in resistance to experimental leishmaniasis. *Clinical and Experimental Immunology, 40:* 508–514.

SKAMENE, E., GROS, P., FORGET, A., KONGSHAVN, P. A. L., ST CHARLES, C. & TAYLOR, B. A., 1982. Genetic regulation of resistance to intracellular pathogens. *Nature (London), 297:* 506–509.

SKAMENE, E., GROS, P., FORGET, A., PATEL, P. J. & NESBITT, M. N., 1984. Regulation of resistance to leprosy by chromosome 1 locus in the mouse. *Immunogenetics, 19:* 117–124.

SKOV, C. B. & TWOHY, D. W., 1974. Cellular immunity to *Leishmania donovani*. I. The effect of T cell depletion on resistance to *L. donovani* in mice. *Journal of Immunology, 113:* 2004–2011.

SNELL, G. D. & BUNKER, H. P., 1965. Histocompatibility genes of mice. V. Five new histocompatibility loci identified by congenic resistant lines on a C57BL/10 background. *Transplantation, 3:* 235–252.

STACH, J-L., GROS, P., FORGET, A. & SKAMENE, E., 1984. Phenotypic expression of genetically-controlled natural resistance to *Mycobacterium bovis* (BCG). *Journal of Immunology, 132:* 888–892.

TURK, J. L. & BRYCESON, A. D. M., 1971. Immunological phenomenon in leprosy and related diseases. *Advances in Immunology, 13:* 200–266.

ULCZAK, O. M. & BLACKWELL, J. M., 1983. Immunoregulation of genetically controlled acquired responses to *Leishmania donovani* infection in mice: the effects of parasite dose, cyclophosphamide and sublethal irradiation. *Parasite Immunology, 5:* 449–463.

VAN EDEN, W., DE VRIES, R. R. P., MEHRA, N. H., VAIDYA, M. C., D'AMARO, J. & VAN ROOD, J. J., 1980. HLA segregation of tuberculoid leprosy: confirmation of the DR2 marker. *Journal of Infectious Diseases, 141:* 693–701.

VAN EDEN, W., GONZALES, N. M., DE VRIES, R. R. P., CONVIT, J. & VAN ROOD, J. J., 1985. HLA-linked control of predisposition to lepromatous leprosy. *Journal of Infectious Diseases, 151:* 9–14.

Ecological and evolutionary dynamics of parasites: The case of *Trypanosoma diemyctyli* in the red-spotted newt *Notophthalmus viridescens*

DOUGLAS E. GILL AND BEVERLY A. MOCK*

*Department of Zoology,
The University of Maryland,
College Park, MD 20742, U.S.A.*

Parasites often are alleged to have no effect on the fitness of their hosts, and thereby act more as commensals than true parasites. If true, this claim raises at least two general ecological and evolutionary questions: do parasites and hosts mutually regulate one another's population density, and does natural selection favour decreasing virulence in the parasites? This paper discusses the conceptual problems of both questions and offers a general evolutionary model by which the parasite's inherent reproductive rate and pathogenicity to the host are lowered by individual selection. The results of a long-term study of the demography and population regulation of trypanosomes in populations of red-spotted newts showed no significant influence of trypanosomiasis on newt survival and minimal effects on reproduction. We rule out the possibility of reciprocal population regulation, apply our model to the interaction between trypanosomes and juvenile efts, and explain the evolutionary origin of the current apathogenic relationship between trypanosomes and newts.

KEYWORDS: — Apathogenicity — demography — evolution — natural selection — *Notophthalmus viridescens* — parasite ecology — population regulation — red-spotted newt — *Trypanosoma diemyctyli* — trypanosomiasis.

CONTENTS

Ecology and Genetics of Host–Parasite Interactions
ISBN: 0 12 593 690 7

*Present address: Department of Immunology, Walter Reed Army Institute of Research, Washington, D.C. 20307, USA

INTRODUCTION

The ecology and evolution of parasite–host interactions is currently replete with unsolved conceptual problems. Contrary to their very definition, many parasites appear to be living in a commensal relationship with their natural hosts and induce no detectable pathologies (Dubos, 1965; Alexander, 1981; Noble & Noble, 1976). While the devastating effects of such communicable diseases as bubonic plague in 15th century Europe, smallpox on Amerindians in 18th century North America, and scarlet fever and measles in 19th century America are legend (Dubos, 1965; Pereira, 1982), it is hard to point to the extinction of any species or population where the agent of destruction was without question a parasite (G. Vermeij, pers. comm.).

In addition, there exist few examples of natural parasite–host interactions where it has been clearly shown that the participants mutually regulate one another's population growth (Crofton, 1971a,b; Holmes, 1982). In general, the significance of infectious parasites on the ecology of their hosts, especially the demography, population size or distribution of natural animal and human populations, is not known (Hassell, 1982).

Many notions about the evolutionary relationship of parasites and their hosts exist in the parasitological, literature. Authorities have claimed that parasites evolve to become commensals with their hosts (e.g. Alexander, 1981; Hoeprich, 1977), that parasites can stabilize at intermediate pathogenicities (e.g. Anderson & May, 1981; Levin & Pimentel, 1981) and that parasites become increasingly virulent with time (Levine, 1972; Ewald, 1983). Although the assertion that parasites evolve to be commensals is particularly widespread, its proponents have consistently failed to present an internally logical theory of how the conventional process of natural selection of individuals favours that direction. May & Anderson (e.g. 1983a,b) have repeatedly pointed out that several evolutionarily stable outcomes of parasite–host interactions are theoretically possible, and no particular one should be expected *a priori*.

If the prevalent pattern of parasite–host interactions is one of peaceful co-existence and stable commensalism, then two paths of evolution to that state can be envisioned: 1) the parasites themselves evolve in the direction of decreasing virulence, and 2) the hosts rapidly evolve resistance or immunity that renders them unharmed irrespective of parasite evolution.

The first path implies that parasites induce highly virulent pathology in new interactions with their hosts while historically older parasites do no measurable harm to their hosts. The graded patterns of pathogenicity by trypanosomes and other protozoan parasites of humans and ungulates in Africa are often cited as supporting evidence of this evolutionary path. *Trypanosoma brucei rhodesiense* is highly pathogenic to humans and clearly derived from *T. b. brucei*, which is native to African ruminants and is not infectious to humans (Baker, 1963; Chandler & Read, 1961). Several species of *Trypanosoma* and *Theileria* show parallel patterns of inducing chronically mild infections in native wild ruminants, more severe morbidity and mortality in endemic or domesticated cattle, and lethal infections in exotic species or breeds of cattle (Allison, 1982). Malarial infections multiply more rapidly in unnatural monkey hosts than natural ones (Cohen, 1979). Attenuation of virulence of pathogens in the laboratory is also well known. Both measles virus and the BCG strain of tuberculosis bacteria have been rendered avirulent after many repeated subcultures in artificial culture medium (Hoeprich, 1977). Thus, there is some evidence that some old relationships are co-adapted and benign while the young interactions are virulent. However, the precise mechanism of evolution in these cases remains unspecified.

Surprisingly, there appear to be only two unequivocal demonstrations of decreases in virulence in natural parasites under field conditions: myxoma virus in both Australia and Britain (Fenner, 1965; Fenner & Ratcliffe, 1965) and chestnut blight in the United States and Europe (Anagnostakis, 1982; Fulbright, Weidlich, & Hart, 1982). Part of a man-directed bio-control program, the myxoma virus underwent genuine genetic diversification after three epizootics and has independently stabilized around genotypes of intermediate virulence in both localities (May & Anderson, 1983b). In contrast, hypo-virulent strains of *Endothia parasitica* appeared spontaneously in native stands of chestnut trees in Italy after 13 years and in the United States 72 years after the first fungal infections were found (Anagnostakis, 1982). But the hypo-virulence of the chestnut blight is caused by a cytoplasmically transmitted virus that renders the fungus non-fatal to the chestnuts. Thus, it appears to be a case of hyper-parasitism rather than a genetic change in the focal parasite itself.

Parenthetically, it is inaccurate to assert that all initial contacts between a parasite and a host are necessarily virulent. Infective stages of many parasitic species are widespread and many potential hosts may be exposed to them. But most such 'transmissible' stages fail to invade or reach maturity in such species because the would-be hosts are in fact unsuitable (Holmes, Hobbs & Leong, 1977). In our discussion about the evolutionary destination of parasite–host interactions, we assume that the parasite is established in a set of hosts through which it can complete its life cycle and we focus on the subsequent evolutionary processes in the interaction.

The second major path to benign interactions between parasite and host is the rapid acquisition of immunity and/or evolution of resistance in the host. Genetic variation for resistance in native and domesticated mammals is well documented (Wakelin, 1978). Indeed, experimental infections under controlled conditions showed that the graded series of responses in the various ruminants in Africa were in fact attributable to variation in host resistance rather than intrinsic variation in pathogenicity of the parasite (Allison, 1982). Sickle-cells mediate the pathology of malaria (Friedman, 1978, 1979). If parasites evolve more slowly than their hosts, as Manter's Rule dictates (Eichler, 1941a,b; Mitter & Brooks, 1983), then the evolution of resistance by the host may be the general answer rather than the evolution of avirulence in the parasite. However, as argued by Levin (1982) and discussed below, many parasites have shorter generation times than their host and are expected to have faster rates of evolution.

Parasite–host interactions are often claimed to be intensely co-evolutionary (Price, 1977; 1980). Many cases, such as the intimate morphological and hormonal interactions of some helminths and their vertebrate hosts (Holmes, 1983), are offered as examples of co-evolution, but very few actually meet the criteria of co-evolution (*sensu stricto* Futuyma & Slatkin, 1983) where evolutionary changes in both parasites *and* host have been demonstrated. The famous myxoma virus — Australian rabbit interaction (Fenner, 1965; Fenner & Ratcliffe, 1965; Levin, 1982) is perhaps the best known example. The gene-for-gene interactions of cereal grasses and their fungal pests (Person, 1967; Flor, 1971; Barrett, 1983), and the defensive egg mimicry of the Passifloraceae to their *Heliconius* butterfly pests (Gilbert, 1983) also provide persuasive examples of co-evolutionary interactions in parasite–host systems. But these are rare gems among hundreds of imperfect, roughcut claims of co-evolution between parasites and hosts (Futuyma & Slatkin, 1983).

One reason for our current lack of understanding of these major issues is that the ability of population biologists to measure survival rates or reproductive performance of hosts under parasitized and unparasitized conditions for a generation or more is very limited. Long-term studies of the dynamics of natural parasite–host interactions in which the time course of infection in marked individuals has been followed are rare in the literature. Data which are quantitatively rigorous, demographically accurate and critically analysed are simply not available to evaluate the issues of population regulation and evolutionary trends in most natural parasite systems.

This paper first presents a general argument why natural selection of individual parasites favours those which have higher reproductive rates and are more virulent. After pointing out some common misconceptions about evolution in parasites and discussing Lewontin's (1970) assertion that the only mechanism by which apathogenicity can evolve in the parasite is interdemal selection, we offer a model of the evolution of apathogenicity in parasites by natural selection of individual (genotypes or isogenic clones). We then summarize the results of a long-term study of the population dynamics of a trypanosome specific to natural populations of red-spotted newts. The lack of significant parasite-induced mortality and the minimal suppression of reproductive performance in the salamanders are discussed in light of the issue of population regulation and the evolutionary model of apathogenicity.

EVOLUTIONARY CHANGES IN PARASITE PATHOGENICITY

Natural selection and evolutionary increases in parasite pathogenicity

One evolutionary theory argues strongly that, in general, individual selection should favour parasite phenotypes of greater pathogenicity over more benign individuals. Consider the outcome of competition between two or more parasite genotypes within one host individual. Suppose one genotype is relatively non-pathogenic because it has a low reproductive rate and damages the host minimally; the other genotype is highly pathogenic because it aggressively converts host energy into its progeny or induces severe protective (e.g. inflammatory) responses by the host. Whether the parasite multiplies asexually by fission or reproduces sexually by eggs, the release of progeny to the outside environment per unit time will be greater by the aggressive, more pathogenic genotype than by the slower reproducing individual. If transmission occurs at all, its rate should be proportional to the number of extruded propagules. Hence, the basic reproductive rate R_0, or the rate at which secondary infections are produced (Anderson, 1980; 1982), of the aggressive parasite is expected to be greater than the R_0 of the less productive genotype.

This argument makes three critical assumptions: 1) higher short-term transmission rates in parasites are achieved by higher reproductive rates; 2) pathogenicity is directly linked to the reproductive activities of the parasite; and 3) competition among parasite genotypes within hosts favours the most virulent one. All three assumptions are valid but require discussion.

In general, those parasite individuals that have higher effective fecundities are more successful at transmitting progeny to secondary hosts than parasite individuals with lower rates of reproduction. Strains of *T. brucei* that have higher rates of division mount a higher parasitaemia during the first peak (Clayton, 1978; Sacks *et al.*, 1980) and are expected to transmit more trypanosomes to biting flies during that time than will strains with slower rates of division. The more rapidly dividing genotype of two or more clones of *Plasmodium vivax* occurring together in the same host should mount a greater parasitaemia, produce larger numbers of gametocytes per unit time, and have a greater probability of transmission to mosquitoes (Coatney *et al.*, 1971). In general, the parasitaemias of microparasites that reproduce by fission must pass a threshold for effective transmission (Chandler & Read, 1961), and that parasite which can pass that threshold sooner with its progeny will be transmitted at a faster rate.

Evidence that directly links individual fecundity of helminths to transmission rates is absent from the literature. However, there is some indirect evidence that supports the expectation of a positive relationship. In some helminthic parasitisms, e.g. schistosomes (Warren, 1978; Cheever, Duvall & Minker, 1980a,b; Cheever *et al.*, 1980c) and hookworms (Sangster *et al.*, 1979), experimental infections reveal a high linear correlation of the number of eggs shed in faeces with the number of reproducing adult worms. Were it measurable, the same proportionality should obtain among conspecific individuals that vary in their intrinsic fecundities: more eggs should be shed with host faeces from a female *S. mansoni* that is producing 310 eggs/day than from a female shedding only 300 eggs/day. It follows by inductive reasoning that natural selection among clones of microparasites and infrapopulations (*sensu* Esch, Gibbons & Borque, 1975) of macroparasites within individual hosts will favour that parasite genotype or individual with the highest transmission rate, i.e. the greatest number of infective progeny produced per unit time.

There are several arguments supporting the generality of the second assumption, i.e. severity of host pathology is correlated with parasite reproductive activity. In general, severity is related to the burden or number of parasites in a host. The larger the parasite burden the greater the harm to the host for any one of several reasons: 1) depletion of host resources (Calow & Jennings, 1974; Cornford & Huot, 1981); 2) damage or destruction of host tissues (Warren, 1978); 3) production of toxins (Boreham & Wright, 1976); 4) suppression of host-immune response, rendering susceptibility to other damaging pathogens (Sacks *et al.*, 1980; Ewald, 1980), etc.

For microparasites (as for any organism with exponential growth) the parasitaemia of a monoclonal infection at any time is primarily determined by the rate of replication and the time since inoculation. Among strains of *T. brucei*, those that mount a higher parasitaemia faster during the first peak not only cause greater morbidity but also cause earlier death (Clayton, 1978; Sacks *et al.*, 1980). The rhythmic chills and fevers in tertian malaria (caused by *P. vivax* which produces 15–20 merozoites every 48 h) are more severe than those in quartan malaria (caused by *P. malariae* which produces only 6–12 merozoites every 72 h). Severity of the cyclic fevers is apparently proportional to the number of infected eythrocytes and the rate of schizogony (Coatney *et al.*, 1971). In general, the intensities of viral influenzas and poxes, bacterial infections, etc. are all proportional to the density of the microparasites.

In contrast to microparasites, infrapopulation numbers of helminths are not the products of replication but, rather, are strictly determined by the accumulation of independent infections minus losses due to age-dependent mortality in the parasite and/or mounting physiological resistance by the host. Yet, it is usually the reproductive activity of the macroparasite that causes the harm (Kelly *et al.*, 1978). In his discussion of the pathogenesis of schistosomiasis, Warren (1978) stated so categorically. Within each type of human schistosomiasis, the major disease syndromes of hepatosplenic and obstructive urinary tract disease are due to the hypersensitivity reactions of the host to schistosome eggs trapped in host tissues (Miyake, 1971). Modulated by the age and location of the flukes (Cheever *et al.*, 1980a) *within* both Japanese and Philippine strains of *Schistosoma japonicum*, the number of eggs passed in the faeces of experimental rabbits was a good measure of the number of eggs deposited in the tissues and the severity of hepatic fibrosis (Cheever *et al.*, 1980b Cheever *et al.*, 1980c). In general, it is expected that intraspecific genotypes with higher reproductive rates cause more severe acute pathologies.

A common rebuttal to this assumption is that there exist pairs of parasite species in which the species with the lower rate of reproduction is more pathogenic. For example, in human malaria *P. falciparum* has a slower rate of schizogony but is much more dangerous than *P. vivax* (Chandler & Read, 1961). Comparing the two mesenteric species in human schistosomiasis, *S. mansoni* produces one-tenth the number of eggs/day than *S. japonicum* but induces the more severe pathology. Comparing *S. mansoni* with *S. haematobium*, which inhabits the urinary tract, the former causes a much more severe disease than the latter, but *S. mansoni* lays far fewer eggs than does *haematobium*. There are cases of slow replicating bacteria that are more toxic than other faster reproducing species.

However, interspecific comparisons do not fairly challenge the generality of a positive association between parasite reproduction and disease because the mechanisms of pathogenesis in the various species may be extremely different. Just as it is pointless to compare hepatitis with influenza, or malaria with trypanosomiasis, so it may be misleading to compare the diseases caused by congeners if their aetiologies are fundamentally different. In *falciparum* malaria, the dangerous pathology results from clumps of erythrocytes clogging capillaries and causing serious thromboses (Friedman, 1978, 1979). The other malarias do not have this pathology, and require higher parasitaemias for pathogenesis. A positive association of parasite density and pathology does appear to hold within each kind of malaria: the more schizonts there are, the more serious are the malarial symptoms. In the case of both *mansoni* and *japonicum* schistosomiasis, the debilitating symptoms are primarily the result of hepatic granulomas and internal haemorrhage caused by errant eggs from older worms. *Schistosoma haematobium* causes totally unrelated diseases of the urinary tract (Warren, 1978). Thus, comparison of *haematobium* schistosomiasis with the mesenteric schistosomiases is irrelevant.

Differences in site location of the worms may also appear to reverse the numerical effect. For example, more eggs of the Philippine strain of *S. japonicum* lodge in tissue and cause more severe symptoms and fewer are passed in faeces than by the Japanese strain of the same species (Cheever *et al.*, 1980b). But, within each strain, there are good correlations of disease severity, worm burden, reproductive activity and number of faecal eggs (Cheever *et al.*, 1980b; see also Olveda *et al.*, 1983). Thus, indirect evidence supports the claim that pathogenicity of helminthic parasites is positively correlated with individual reproductive activity.

The third assumption states that competition among genotypes when present together in the same individual host favours the most virulent. The pathology manifest in the host is caused by the most pathogenic genotype of parasite. If the pathology is lethal, then the most pathogenic genotype will cause death in the shortest time. The most pathogenic strain gains the short-term advantage in transmission by the time all the genotypes perish with the host individual if transmission is continuously and readily possible. There is no opportunity for compensatory reproductive gains by the slower reproducing genotypes at a later time. This point is illustrated well by the several strains of *T. brucei* studied by Clayton (1978) and Sacks *et al.* (1980), where the net parasitaemias of the fastest reproducing and most virulent strain were greatest by the time the host died.

The expectation of evolutionary increases in virulence by natural selection is supported by many examples (Ball, 1943; Garnham, 1971; Levine, 1972; Anderson & May, 1982). The cases of rapid evolution of strains of parasites resistant to prophylactic pharmaceuticals, such as chloroquine-resistant *Plasmodium falciparum* (Peters, 1974; Smith, 1982), sheep trichostrongylids resistant to benzimidazole (Sangster *et al.*, 1979), and gonorrhea bacteria resistant to penicillin (Holmes & Stilwell, 1977; Yorke *et al.*, 1978), are interpretable as simulating how parasites evolve in response to natural resistance in hosts. In a recent review of human infectious diseases, Ewald (1983) concluded that among vector-transmitted parasites of humans, severity of disease is *positively* associated with the degree to which the parasite has been associated with man.

Misconceptions about evolution in parasites

Because many parasites seem harmless to their hosts, many people believe that the natural evolutionary cycle of the interaction is a virulent beginning and benign end (Ball, 1943; Chandler & Read, 1961; Sprent, 1963; Dubos, 1965; Hoeprich, 1977; Noble & Noble, 1976). A very common but erroneous corollary states that parasites as species ought not destroy their hosts so that they themselves do not become extinct. Such misconceptions are stated explicitly in Swellengrebel's (1940) invalid hypothesis of 'efficient parasites' and in several recent authoritative reviews (Dubos, 1965: 165, 188; Hoeprich, 1977: 34; Alexander, 1981: 114–115). Like Slobodkin's (1968, 1974) 'prudent predator', such misconceptions invoke the discredited group selection arguments that evolution works for the best interests of the species rather than the individual (Williams, 1966). Elementary evolutionary theory instructs that it is the suite of heritable traits that confers a reproductive advantage to individuals that spreads through populations by natural selection (Lewontin, 1970). To ask parasites to save hosts for future infections by themselves or their progeny is requesting an act of altruism that is impossible to evolve by any known mechanism of evolution. See Williams (1966) for a full discussion of this important point.

In the face of the strong expectation that natural selection of individual parasites should favour those with higher reproductive rates and greater pathogenicities, what evolutionary explanations can account for the observations of benign parasite–host relationships? Attenuation of virulence requires a sophisticated evolutionary explanation to be compatible with modern theory. The principle alternative to date is the interdemal selection hypothesis offered by Lewontin (1970). Its importance requires reiteration.

Interdemal selection and evolutionary decreases in parasite pathogenicity

In his seminal paper on the units of selection, Lewontin (1970) made the astonishing assertion that patterns of decreasing pathogenicity in parasites were not consistent with the principles of individual selection. With particular reference to the case history of myxomatosis in Australian rabbits, he said that the reduction in virulence in the myxoma virus could not be explained by individual selection. Lewontin (1970) argued that the only mechanism available to explain the observed evolution of avirulent strains of the myxoma virus in the wild was selection at the polygenotypic or population level, i.e. interdemal selection of Wright (1931). His assertion was tacitly assumed by Levin and Pimentel (1981) in their mathematical model of the myxoma case.

Lewontin's (1970) assertion is internally consistent. He assumed that by harbouring many genotypes of viruses, each infected rabbit possessed a random frequency distribution of virulent phenotypes. He then postulated that when rabbits infected with one or more highly virulent strains died during each epizootic, the process was in fact the extinction of demes of viruses, and only rabbits (= demes of viruses) with low virulent strains survived. Hence, interdemal selection favoured avirulent strains because effective transmission of their genotypes was greater. Thus, the characteristic strain of myxoma virus was moderate relative to the original hypervirulent strain after three epizootics.

In order that interdemal selection plays the major role in the evolution of reduced virulence, it is necessary that the turnover rate of hosts (= parasite demes) be greater than the rate of competitive displacement of parasite genotypes within each host. In the myxoma virus case, the Australian rabbits did indeed turn over rapidly enough for Lewontin's hypothesis to work.

It is important to point out the distinction between Lewontin's (1970) hypothesis and the popular one that claims it is in the parasite's best interest not to harm its host. Lewontin argues that competition among parasites residing *within* the same host individual consistently favours the most virulent genotype because it outreproduces all other genotypes within the host. His hypothesis of interdemal selection *among* virus demes is proposed as the only mechanism operating on the parasite that counteracts this trend within parasite demes. In contrast, the popular notion implies that individual selection among individual parasite genotypes favours altruistic traits of harmlessness so that resources are preserved for future generations. This notion requires advanced planning and foresight, neither of which are permissible in the contemporary definition of natural selection of individuals (Williams, 1966; Lewontin, 1970).

A MODEL OF THE EVOLUTION OF APATHOGENICITY
IN PARASITES BY NATURAL SELECTION

The question asked here is whether Lewontin's assertion that evolutionary declines in virulence are antithetical to natural selection is correct. Our answer is no. There exists at least one common circumstance in which natural selection will favour lower rates of reproduction in parasites and apathogenic effects on their hosts. Transmission of parasites among hosts is not always enhanced by maximization of rates of parasitic reproduction within individual hosts.

Whenever there is a prolonged intra- or epihost stage in the life cycle of the parasite in which transmission to the next host is impossible, there will be no short-term advantage to rapid and prolific reproduction. Until the host engages in a new activity in which transmission is possible, reproduction by all its parasites, whether aggressive or benign, is futile. If the host dies prior to that new activity, especially as a consequence of the pathology induced by the most virulent genotype among the clones it carries, all the parasites are losers; none are favoured by selection as our earlier argument and that of Lewontin (1970) had envisioned.

For the purposes of our model, we are explicitly relegating to the background all other conditions impinging on the host, including the presence of other parasite species. This is proper because the full set of such unspecified conditions is the backdrop of the stage upon which our focal parasite is playing. If an individual host is killed by a storm, a predator or another species of parasite before the pathogenicity of our focal parasite is expressed, then that host is an irrelevant stage for the evolutionary play about pathogenicity in our parasite.

Living in or on a host during a period of prolonged isolation from possible transmission submerges parasites in an environment that obligately selects against any virulent parasite genotype that decreases the probability of its host surviving through that period. Only those parasite genotypes which impose no deficit on host survival during the period of isolation will be transmitted and survive by virtue of completing their life cycles.

Under these conditions, it is likely that those apathogenic parasites in monogenotypic (= monoclonal in microparasites) infections are the individuals most favoured by natural selection. Consider the ranking of the following parasite individuals: 1) benign genotype living alone in a host (= monogenotypic infection); 2) benign parasite living together with other genotypes in the same host (= polygenotypic infection); 3) virulent genotype occurring in a monogenotypic infection; and 4) virulent genotype occurring in any polygenotypic infection. Suppose the virulent genotype kills the host before the period of impossible transmission ends. Then parasite individuals 3 and 4 are absolutely selected against with equivalent vigour. It makes no difference whether the virulent death of the host is soon after entry into the transmission-free period or moments before it ends, the net impact on highly virulent and moderately virulent parasite genotypes is the same, i.e. zero fitness. In addition, there is a finite probability that parasite individuals 2 and 4 occur in the same polygenotypic infection. As a consequence, individual 2 is expected to fail to complete its life cycle more often than parasite individual 1. Hence, parasite individual 1, a benign genotype in monogenotypic infection, is most likely to be represented in future generations.

Comparing parasite individual 2 with individual 4 under these conditions, we observe that natural selection favours individual 2, because it is more likely to complete its life cycle whenever it co-occurs with other benign genotypes in the same host. This comparison is the same interdemal model of Lewontin (1970) discussed above. Thus, our model argues that individual and interdemal selection operate in the same direction; both favour the benign parasite as the one most likely to get through the period of impossible transmission.

The distinctions between our model and the popular notion as expressed by (Alexander, 1981) and the interdemal selection hypothesis of Lewontin (1970) are subtle but important. The popular notion places total emphasis on survival of the species through altruism of individuals, and is a direct outgrowth of the discredited concepts of epideictic behaviour proposed by Wynne-Edwards (1962). Our hypothesis focuses attention only on the process of differential mortality of individual parasites during that life stage bridging a large gulf between transmission opportunities. In specifying that the competition among parasites in polygenotypic infections favours the more virulent genotype, Lewontin (1970) assumed that transmission was at least sometimes possible and competitive advantage could result in a reproductive (= selective) advantage through transmission. Our hypothesis specifies that absolutely no transmission occurs during an extended period of isolation, competitive advantage by the more virulent parasite genotype does not translate into reproductive advantage during that period, and the parasite genotypes most likely to survive to the transmission opportunity are those which are apathogenic and in monogenotypic infections.

The condition of prolonged containment without the possibility of transmission is quite possibly a common feature in parasite–host interactions. Examples that come to mind include parasites with transovarial transmission, feather ectoparasites of birds, and endemic parasites linked to migratory hosts. Processes that force parasites through episodes of sparse distributions in their hosts include external interferences with transmission and catastrophic reductions in host population densities.

We illustrate our model with the following excerpts of a detailed, long-term investigation of the interaction of trypanosomes in natural populations of red-spotted newts (Mock, 1983; Gill, Berven & Mock, 1983). Although Wenyon (1926, 1965) said nearly all cases of trypanosomiasis in natural, non-human or wild animals were avirulent, we knew of no rigorous, quantitative, demographic data that supported his statement. Before we began our studies, we did not know whether the interaction between trypanosomes and newts was pathogenic or benign.

THE CASE OF TRYPANOSOMES IN THE RED-SPOTTED NEWT

In order to learn about the ecological and evolutionary dynamics of a natural parasite population, we investigated the interaction between the blood protozoan *Trypanosoma diemyctyli* Tobey and its vertebrate host, the red-spotted newt *Notophthalmus viridescens* (Rafinesque). Our studies took advantage of the long-term demographic studies of the red-spotted newt already in progress in the Shenandoah Mountains of Virginia, U.S.A. (Gill, 1978a,b,c, 1979, 1984; Gill *et al.*, 1983). Since 1974, over 9000 adult newts have been individually marked and their activities monitored. Repeated samples of blood from nearly 6000 known individuals over a 6-year period permitted the thorough assessment of the dynamics of trypanosomiasis in these natural salamander populations (Mock & Gill, 1984). Details of the study of newt trypanosomiasis are in Mock (1983).

In this study, we asked two general questions: 1) do trypanosomes and newts mutually regulate one another's population density; and 2) can the characteristics of pathogenicity in the interaction between trypanosomes and newts be explained by natural selection of individual clones of trypanosomes.

The demography and ecology of the red-spotted newt

The life cycle of the red-spotted newt in a constellation of small ponds constructed between 8 and 100 + years ago in the Shenandoah Mountains, Virginia, U.S.A.

study area has been documented (see Gill, 1978a; Gill *et al.*, 1983 for details). Adult newts hibernated in the forest and returned every year *en masse* to the same breeding ponds in mid-March. Each year, the breeding stock of adult newts was composed of approximately 50% new recruits, which were breeding for the first time, and declining proportions of veterans in their second to tenth (plus) adult years. The majority of male and female newts bred every year, but a minority did skip a variable number of breeding opportunities (Gill, 1984). Courtship and oviposition behaviours persisted from March through June, and adults left the ponds on rainy days in August and September. Adult male newts had a constant annual survival rate of 73% while adult females survived at the rate of 67% per year; both sexes had a median life expectancy after maturity of approximately three breeding seasons.

Larvae were present in the ponds throughout summer, but post-metamorphic juveniles (efts) departed at a mean length of 17 mm in September through October. The boom-or-bust pattern of post-metamorphic production, with numbers ranging from 0 to over 2500 juveniles per pond, showed no regularity among ponds and between successive years (Gill *et al.*, 1983). Bright orange-red in colour and deadly with tetrodotoxin, the sexually immature efts were strictly terrestrial until they reached adult size. Recovery of marked juveniles as breeding adults has confirmed that most newts returned to their natal ponds for breeding, and that maturity took an astonishing average of 6.2 years (range 4–9 years) in this area. Therefore, generation time was approximately 9 years in these montane Virginia populations of red-spotted newts.

The ponds also supported breeding populations of several other species of amphibians, of which wood frogs (*Rana sylvatica*), Jefferson's salamanders (*Ambystoma jeffersonianum*), and spotted salamanders (*Ambystoma maculatum*) were most common. None of these species or any other amphibian in the study area revealed the presence of trypanosomes in their peripheral blood. Yet all are attacked by the amphibian leech, *Batrachobdella picta* Verrill, which is the only known vector of transmission of trypanosomes to newts (Barrow, 1953; Mock & Gill, 1984).

Life cycle of the trypanosome

The specificity of a large, morphologically distinctive trypanosome in the red-spotted newt and its failure to complete its life cycle in other syntopic amphibian populations suggests the trypanosome–newt relationship is evolutionarily old. Barrow (1958) described the life cycle of *T. diemyctyli* as revolving between the red-spotted newt and the amphibian leech. Complex reproductive stages of trypanosomes, including crithidial and leptomonal forms, in the leech were studied in detail by Barrow (1953). Leeches transmit metacyclic forms of the trypanosomes to both larval and adult newts; only trypomastigotes, which are said to undergo fission, have been observed in newt blood (Nigrelli, 1929; Barrow, 1954; Mock, 1983). The dynamics of a trypanosome suprapopulation in a pond depends in part on the dynamics (rates of recruitment, births, deaths and emigration) of its host populations. Important epidemiological aspects of trypanosome population dynamics occur when new ponds are created and colonized by infected newts and leeches, and when older ponds fill in or are otherwise destroyed as viable habitats.

Methods

Twice weekly throughout each year from February through November, newts were captured by the technique of drift fences and pitfall traps at each of the study ponds (Gill, 1984). The efficiency of capture was routinely 95% per year (Gill, 1984). Individual newts were identified by the unique pattern (number and arrangement) of vermilion spots on the dorsum. Blood samples were taken from free-swimming, experimentally caged, and laboratory housed newts according to standardized protocols (Mock & Gill, 1984).

Prevalence and intensity of trypanosomes in the
red-spotted newt

Trypanosomes were conspicuous in all the life stages of the red-spotted newt in the Shenandoah Mountains but not in any other amphibian in the study area (Mock & Gill, 1984; Gill, 1978c). The prevalence of infection ranged from 6–70% in post-metamorphic juveniles from ponds known to have infected adults and leeches, 42% in the red efts, and 10–35% in transforming adults. By June of the first breeding season, prevalences became nearly 100% and were characteristically high in all adult age groups (Fig. 1A). Adults in their fourth adult year or older had significantly lower prevalences than younger adults (Mock & Gill, 1984).

The intensity of infection (number of trypanosomes/ml blood) rose sharply in all new adults within a few weeks after entering breeding ponds that harboured infected leeches (Fig. 1B). Intensities of 300 to 400 thousand tryps/ml were routinely observed in first- and second-year adults in mid summer, but parasitaemias in older adults were significantly lower. No oscillations on a daily or weekly time scale were observed in adult newts during their first two breeding seasons. However, in older adults, annual cycles with mid-summer highs and early spring lows corresponded with each year's challenges of leeches and new infections in the pond and departures to hibernacula on land.

We have inferred that individual newts are capable of carrying infections throughout their 6-year period of efthood. The incidence of trypanosomiasis in post-metamorphic juveniles confirms that newt larvae are attacked by leeches and many newts acquire their primary infections during that stage. Given the minute size of the newt larvae (19–24 mg), and the comparable or larger sizes (6–80 mg) of aggressive leeches, it is unlikely that larval newts survive more than one attack by an adult leech. Thus, we speculate that most of the primary infections contracted by larval newts, and hence those observed in red efts in the forests and transforming adults arriving at ponds for their first breeding, may be monoclonal in origin.

We surmise that polyclonal infections must be common in adult newts. Although we have no proof that infected newts do not have premunition against secondary infections, those transforming efts that enter ponds with a primary infection experience secondary inoculations that are separated from their primary infections by 4 to 9 years. The sharp rises in intensities in uninfected and previously infected new recruits during their first breeding season are identical, suggesting equivalent susceptibility to the new challenges. Similarly, as adult newts re-enter the same pond each year, they are rechallenged by dozens to hundreds of leeches from a new generation. We have little doubt that each adult newt is infected with many clones of trypanosomes in its life time.

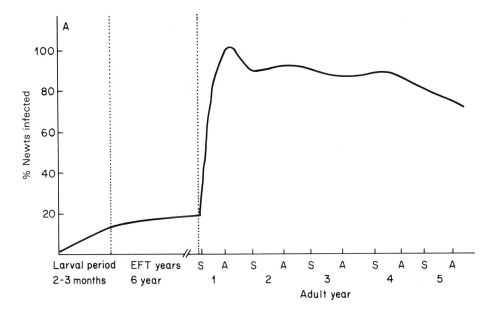

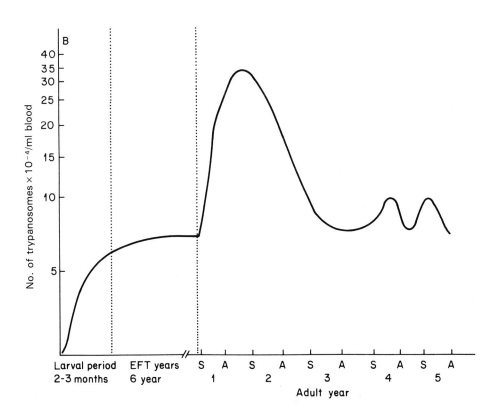

Figure 1. Summary of the change in prevalence (A) and intensity (B) of trypanosomiasis in red-spotted newts (from Mock, 1983).

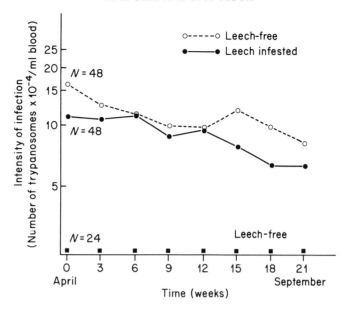

Figure 2. Time course of infection of trypanosomiasis in older (three or four breeding seasons) adult male red-spotted newts in leech-infested and leech-free ponds. Circles, infected newts originating from a leech-infested pond; Squares, uninfected newts from a leech-free pond acting as controls.

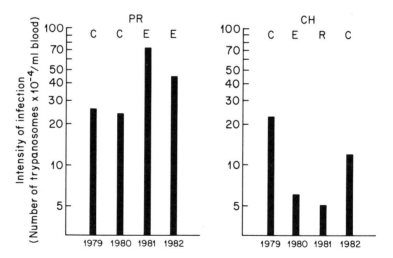

Figure 3. Changes in levels of infection of trypanosomiasis in adult newts in ponds where the population size of the leech vector was lowered by removal of its blood meal supply from wood frogs and ambystomatid salamanders. PR, Pond Ridge Pond; CH, Cline's Hacking Pond; C, control year (no manipulation); E, experimental year (frogs and salamanders removed); R, replacement and amplification year (numbers of frogs and salamanders doubled).

Long-term monitors of known individuals confirmed that most adults sustained infections throughout their lives and parasitaemias can remain extremely high for several years. About 15% of infected adults in their first breeding year lose detectable infections by their second year, but 10% of those regained infections by their third year (Mock, 1983). In one experiment, the placement of infected newts in leech-free ponds showed that the maintenance of high, stationary levels of infection did not depend on transmission (Fig. 2). In another set of experiments, wood frogs and ambystomatid salamanders were excluded from Cline's Hacking Pond (CH) and Pond Ridge Pond (PR) and this manipulation successfully induced a collapse in the leech populations (Mock, 1983). While the intensities of trypanosomiasis dropped correspondingly in pond CH, they rose in PR (Fig. 3). The results of these two experiments confirmed that transmission was not a significant factor in sustaining the high levels of infection in adult newts.

Impact of trypanosomiasis on the fitness of red-spotted newts

Trypanosomiasis could influence the fitness of newts in three ways: 1) lower survivorship, 2) interfere with breeding cycles, and 3) reduce fecundity. We evaluated all three in our studies (Mock, 1983).

Mock & Gill (1984) concluded that trypanosomiasis was not a significant factor in the survivorship schedules of adult red-spotted newts. They reached this conclusion by observing that the significant declines in prevalence and intensity of infection with age of adult newt did not correspond to a change in the annual survival rates of adults. If infection levels elevated mortality significantly above non-infected levels, then adults in their first and second years of breeding should have suffered lower survival rates than adults in their fourth and fifth years. This should have been evident in age-specific survivorship curves as a reversed J-shape, or Type III survivorship curve (Deevey, 1947). It was not. Adult newt survivorship was straightline, constant across age classes, and Type II (Fig. 4; Gill et al., 1983; Gill, 1984). Crude calculations of Anderson & May's (1979) alpha, the parasite–induced mortality rate, revealed values as small as 10^{-7} (Mock, 1983). These results are consistent with those of Dorney (1969) who reported from very small sample sizes that trypanosomiasis had no detectable influence on the survivorship of red squirrels and eastern chipmunks.

Mock & Gill (1984) and Gill et al. (1983) did report an intriguing relationship between levels of infection and frequency of breeding in females. Females that had a history of skipping breeding seasons had significantly higher levels of infection than those females which were known to have been breeding in the ponds every year. Moreover, there was a significant positive correlation of number of years skipped with levels of infection. We had speculated that newts which acquired exceptionally severe infections in their first breeding season were so stressed that their ability to breed in subsequent years was significantly impaired.

Analyses of large cohorts over longer periods of time have failed to confirm the original correlation or to support the speculation of parasite-induced interference to breeding schedules. Infected and uninfected adult newts have equivalent survivorships after maturity (Mock, 1983). Careful monitoring of marked individuals revealed that adult females that were uninfected at the end of their first year failed to return to breed in their second year as often as infected females (Fig. 5a). Similarly, there was no difference in absenteeism between those females that had high infections ($\geq 10^5$ trypanosomes/ml) and those that had low infections (0 to 10^4 tryps/ml) in their first breeding season (Fig. 5b). Thus, we must refute our earlier conclusion and report that trypanosomiasis does not have a detectable impact on breeding frequency in female red-spotted newts.

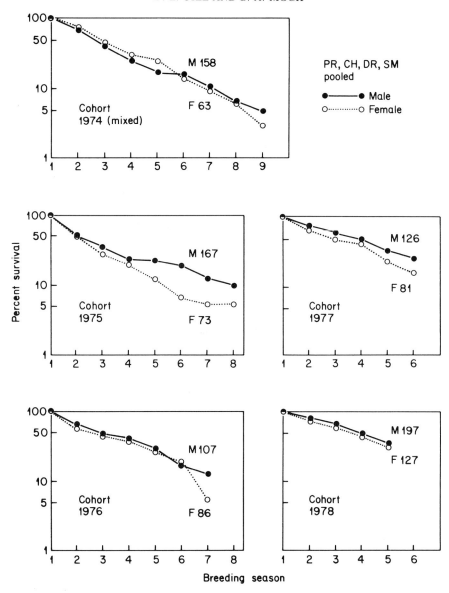

Figure 4. Age-specific survivorship after maturity in cohorts of adult red-spotted newts. The year-cohorts at four breeding ponds were pooled; the sexes are shown separately. Type II survivorships of Deevey (1947), indicating constant survivorship rates across all age classes, are evident.

Infected female newts in their first and second breeding seasons did have significantly lower body weights and fewer ovulated eggs than did uninfected females (Mock, 1983). There was also a significant negative correlation between levels of infection and female body weight, but this was due to the fact that uninfected females had more eggs. These newts were captured before they had entered the water at Dictum Ridge Pond or laid any eggs. The difference therefore represented a significant difference in fecundity. However, egg weights on a per egg basis were equivalent. In addition, there was no significant difference in body weight between infected and uninfected post-metamorphic efts as they left the pond.

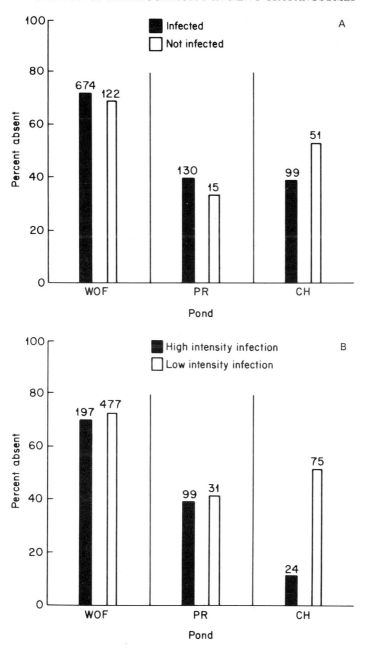

Figure 5. Frequency of skipping the second breeding season by female red-spotted newts in three ponds. WOF, White Oak Flat Pond; PR, Pond Ridge Pond; CH, Cline's Hacking Pond. A, Comparison of infected and uninfected first-year adults. No significant difference was found between the two groups. B, Comparison of first-year adults with high and low infections (see text). No significant difference was found between the two groups.

The significant effect on fecundity is the only indication of any negative impact of trypanosomiasis on the fitness of red-spotted newts. But, the studies do not establish cause and effect of disease and reproductive performance. Those females with high parasitaemias and low body weights could have had fewer eggs for other reasons (e.g. poor nutrition). Hence, we cautiously offer the negative correlation as tentative evidence of an impact of trypanosomes on the *potential* growth rate of newt populations.

Moreover, the differences in fecundity in gravid females were not manifest as significantly different numbers of either eggs oviposited in experimental tanks in the field or metamorphosing efts emerging from the study ponds themselves. On the contrary, more (but not significantly) eggs (10.2 ± 3.4 eggs *vs* 6.8 ± 2.9 eggs) were recovered from tanks housing breeding females with high infections than from tanks containing females with low infections. Similarly, in those years at WOF when infection levels were highest, the number of metamorphosing efts was also highest (Mock, 1983). Thus, we have only one significant relationship between infections by trypanosomiasis and pre-ovipositional fecundity in young adult females from one pond, but that difference failed to materialize in empirical or experimental correlations of infection and per capita post-ovipositional egg or juvenile production.

Thus, we conclude that there is no significant impact of trypanosomiasis on the survival of red-spotted newts, and minimal and ambiguous effects on newt reproductive performance. The current state of the relationship between *T. diemyctyli* and *N. viridescens* is demonstrably apathogenic.

Discussion

The results of our studies on the demography of the red-spotted newt and the interaction of trypanosomes and newts have significance with respect to both the question of mutual population regulation of parasites and hosts and the question of the evolution of pathogenicity in parasite–host relationships.

Mutual population regulation

The answer to the question of mutual population regulation requires examining both sides of the coin: do trypanosomes regulate the population growth of newts and do newts regulate the population growth of trypanosomes? Based on the empirical and experimental data on the survivorship and reproduction of red-spotted newts obtained in the field under natural conditions, the answer to the first question is no. Despite intensities of infection ranging from zero to 500 000ml blood, no influence of trypanosomiasis on newt survivorship was detectable. The significant correlation of infection with pre-ovipositional fecundity was not apparent in the numbers of young actually produced under either experimental or empirical conditions and is therefore judged an insignificant factor in newt reproduction. Therefore, trypanosomiasis cannot be a significant factor in the regulation of newt population densities.

To answer the reciprocal question about the factors regulating the population growth of the trypanosomes, we have employed the classification of parasite population regulation proposed by Bradley (1972, 1974).

Type I concerns density independent interference of transmission rates. Our experiments showed conclusively that leeches are essential for the acquisition of infections, and that many adult newts which lose infections can reacquire infections after re-exposure to leeches. They also proved that intensities of infection once acquired were not influenced by variation in transmission rates from leeches. We deliberately interfered with transmission by significantly reducing the population sizes of the vector, but that failed to produce a significant change in the levels of infection of trypanosomiasis in the newts. We conclude that at least with respect to the circulation of trypanosomes between adult newts and leeches in infected ponds, transmission rates are high and cannot regulate the parasite population growth.

In the other stages of the newt, low transmission rates may be significant. The juveniles emerging from infected ponds in some years had very low prevalences of infection. This observation suggests ineffective transmission of trypanosomes to larval newts, but we do not know the reasons. Our data also strongly indicate that efts in their long terrestrial life are not exposed to any transmitting vectors for 4–9 years. Our fragmentary data on this stage hint at losses of infections.

Type II Regulation (Bradley, 1972, 1974) concerns the parasite–induced elimination of heavily infected hosts and the production of permanently immune hosts. Our failure to detect *any* effect of trypanosomes on mortality schedules, irrespective of high intensities, rules out differential mortality of heavily infected hosts as a significant mode of regulation of trypanosome population growth by newts. Although Mock & Gill (1984) reported a significant inverse relationship between intensity of infection and frequency of breeding in females that was consistent with Type II Regulation, our present data fail to confirm that relationship.

Trypanosomiasis in red-spotted newts routinely persisted for years in adults, and we surmise it does for 4–9 years in the eft stage. The apparent rate of loss of infections is low, and many adults have records of reacquiring infections. Thus, our data indicate that most newts do not develop a permanent immunity or become refractory to secondary infections of trypanosomiasis. We conclude that Type II mechanisms of regulation of trypanosomes are not present in the red-spotted newt.

Type III Regulation (Bradley, 1972, 1974) concerns the control of parasite burdens in every infected host by immunological mechanisms and the premunition of secondary infections. The dynamics of trypanosome infections in adult newts clearly indicates some upper limit to intensities. Rather than exploding to infinity, the intensity of trypanosomes in first-year adults levels off to an average of approximately 4×10^5 tryps/ml blood. We do not know whether this carrying capacity is determined by density dependent mechanisms in the trypanosome population itself, or by some kind of physiological control by the newt, but we can speculate on some possibilities.

It is implausible that trypanosomes severely deplete host resources in a way that suppresses their own reproduction or elevates mortality within clones without inducing some symptoms of illness in the newts. Trypanosomes derive their nutrition (carbohydrate, glycoproteins, etc.) from sources in the blood, and depletion of these nutrients would surely have a negative impact on the host. It is possible that trypanosomes have a mechanism of autoregulation, such as contact inhibition, that operates in a density-dependent manner and independent of nutritional requirements, but that possibility has not been demonstrated. Intracellular forms of *T. diemyctyli* are not known in the newt (perhaps they will be discovered), so speculation about density dependent regulation anywhere other than among trypomastigotes in newt blood is unwarranted.

The possible mechanisms by which newts can control the growth of trypanosome infrapopulations (clones) seem limited. The persistence of high intensity infections for years and the absence of any kind of short-term cyclicity in adult newts are features of this trypanosome–newt interaction that are unlike the dynamics of the more familiar mammalian trypanosomes *T. brucei, T. rhodesiense, T. gambiense, T. lewisi,* or *T. musculi* (Allison, 1982). Our data suggest that most newts do not have an effective immune response system that can eliminate trypanosomes once they are established in the peripheral blood. The significant decline in the peak levels of infection in old adult newts does suggest a host response that may increase in effectiveness with age or prior experience with infections. Perhaps newt blood does become increasingly inhospitable to trypanosomes, but whether the mechanism is an active immunological response by the newt or a passive consequence of aging is unknown.

The results discussed above lead to the conclusion that trypanosomes and newts do not mutually regulate each other's population growth. The densities of both species in this interaction are regulated by factors independent of the parasite–host interaction.

The origin of apathogenicity in the trypanosome–newt interaction

Our results indicate that the current interaction between trypanosomes and the red-spotted newt is a commensalism: trypanosomes benefit from living in newts but do no harm to the newts in turn. Earlier in the paper we pointed out that the origin (and maintenance) of an apathogenic interaction such as this can derive from only two paths: either the newts have evolved mechanisms of resistance so effective that trypanosomes are incapacitated or the trypanosomes themselves have evolved characteristics of harmlessness.

We concluded above that most red-spotted newts do not seem to have a specific mechanism of regulation of their trypanosome infections. That newts have not evolved an effective mechanism of resistance against trypanosomiasis is not surprising when one considers the disparity between the generation times of trypanosomes and newts. Behaving as haploids and reproducing asexually very rapidly in both newts and leeches (Barrow, 1953), *T. diemyctyli* has a generation time that is measured on the time scale of hours or days. In contrast, we know that the red-spotted newt in our system has a generation time of 9 years. Moreover, some trypanosomes play games with their antigenic surfaces as they escape surveillance by vertebrate antibodies (Vickerman, 1978; Bloom, 1979; Turner, 1980). Because they are capable of doing so very rapidly, we would expect that any antagonistic biochemical weapon deployed by the newt against their trypanosomes would be quickly countered by an immunosuppressive mechanism in the trypanosome. As Levin (1982) argued, the issue of co-evolution in host–parasite systems with great disparity in generation times can justifiably focus on the evolutionary processes in the parasite alone.

Therefore, our attention turns to the processes of evolution by which apathogenicity could have evolved in *T. diemyctyli*. Earlier, we identified three processes pertaining to the evolution of pathogenicity in parasites in general: 1) natural selection favouring increasing pathogenicity when alternative genotypes simultaneously infect a host; 2) interdemal selection by which hosts with highly virulent genotypes die more rapidly than hosts with a random collection of avirulent forms; and 3) our model in which natural selection favours apathogenic genotypes when parasite individuals are distributed sparsely among host individuals and endure a prolonged life stage in a host without any prospects of transmission. We can comment on each process as they apply to the trypanosome–newt interaction.

The interaction of adult newts and leeches in the breeding ponds seems very favourable to the evolution of highly virulent forms of trypanosomes. Adult newts are continuously exposed to attacking leeches for nearly 6 months every year. Every year, approximately 40–50% of the breeding population of newts are new recruits (transforming efts) apparently susceptible to new or secondary infections. Prevalence becomes nearly 100% by June and intensities of infection in most newts reach over 330 000 by summer. These observations confirm that transmission rates are high and that the time it takes for a trypanosome to complete one cycle from leech–newt–leech is one summer or less.

We reason that under these conditions natural selection would favour trypanosome genotypes of ever increasing replication rate and, as a consequence, virulence. If there were to appear a mutation in a trypanosome that accelerated replication rate, its rate of transmission in both directions (leech to adult newt and adult newt to leech) would be greater than its parental genotype. The multiplicative dynamics of transmission in such an endemic setting should lead to rapid fixation. Inductively, every time such a mutation arose in a resident population of trypanosomes and newts, natural selection would favour it. This repeated process would generate a trend of ever increasing replication rates in the trypanosome. Because pathology is positively linked to the density of trypanosomes in the blood, we expect evolutionary increases in pathogenicity with time.

Only if the mechanisms of density dependence in the trypanosome were antagonistic to the trait of rapid replication (high intrinsic rate of natural increase r) could there be any limit to the intensities of infection attained by the trypanosomes in newts or leeches (Gill, 1974, 1978d; Esch, Hazen & Aho, 1977). Investigations into the possible mechanisms of density dependence in trypanosomes would be valuable.

The possibility of interdemal selection counteracting the effects of natural selection among adult newts and leeches in the pond seems remote. At the very least, the antagonistic tension of individual selection favouring pathogenicity and interdemal selection against it should have produced pathogenicities of intermediate intensity if their strengths were comparable. Such did occur in the myxoma virus cases (May & Anderson, 1983b).

In addition, the speed at which natural selection would favour a virulent trypanosome genotype accelerates because of the multiplicative process of transmission. In contrast, the rate of interdemal selection against pathogenic trypanosomes is only additive because it is determined by the rate at which single lethal mutations appear in any one parasite per host. We conclude that the observed apathogenicity in the trypanosome–newt system could not have evolved by interdemal selection overpowering individual selection for increasing virulence in ponds.

Our hypothesis that natural selection of individual parasites can favour apathogenic genotypes when the parasites reside in a host for a long period without any possibility of transmission is satisfactorily fulfilled in the eft stage of the red-spotted newt. We surmised from the low prevalences and the probable mechanisms of transmission of trypanosomes to larval newts that post-metamorphic juveniles are likely to harbour only a monoclonal infection of trypanosomiasis as they leave ponds. Prevalence levels of trypanosomes in red efts in the forest were also low. These observations suggest that clones of trypanosomes are in fact distributed sparsely among newts at this stage.

Because efts are not in contact with leeches until they reach maturity, and because the time between their departure as post-metamorphs and re-entry as adults is

4–9 years, there is an absolute selective premium on traits of trypanosomes that keep their host efts alive until they become adult newts. Any trypanosome that kills an eft (or increases the probability of death) before it re-enters a pond and rejoins the cycle between newts and leeches is absolutely selected against. It makes no difference whether the lethal effect occurs 1 years or 5 years 6 months after metamorphosis: both are genetic deaths for the injurious trypanosomes. Hence, highly pathogenic as well as mildly pathogenic genotypes of trypanosomes are strongly selected against by natural selection during the long eft stage in these populations of the red-spotted newt. Even if the infections in the red eft were polyclonal, the action of interdemal selection would be in the same direction as that of monoclonal selection, and the two could not be distinguished.

As a consequence of the selection during the eft stage, we argue that at the time of transformation to adulthood, those efts that are infected with trypanosomes carry only apathogenic forms. Such efts have two interesting futures: either they enter a pond that has an active infection cycling between leeches and older adult newts, or they colonize a new pond that has no current infection.

Because 50% of the breeding stock of newts in every pond is composed of new recruits each year, and that 10–35% of them carry primary infections when they enter, the genetic structure of the trypanosome suprapopulation is strongly influenced by an immigration rate of apathogenic genotypes of approximately 5–18% per year. This would suppress significantly the evolutionary propulsion towards increasing virulence in the trypanosome cycle in the pond driven by the interaction between adult newts and leeches. At the very least, a polymorphism of trypanosome genotypes might be maintained in the pond if the rate of immigration of the apathogenic strains was equal to the endemic rate of individual selection of the virulent strains in the pond.

The other future of the transforming efts, namely colonization of new ponds, generates a very interesting epidemiology of trypanosomiasis in red-spotted newts. All new demes of *T. diemyctyli* that become established by founder cohorts of efts begin in a totally apathogenic state. If efts are regularly colonizing new ponds, as hypothesized by Gill (1978a), then the age distribution of ponds themselves in a large forest determines the characteristics of pathogenicity in trypanosome populations on a larger, metapopulation scale. If most ponds in a region are young and recently colonized by efts, then most populations of newt trypanosomes will be apathogenic; if most water bodies are ancient geologic structures, such as glacial lakes, then most newt trypanosome populations in the region could be characteristically virulent.

Our study ponds are all young: none are of geological age and most are only 20–30 years old. They all have been recently colonized by efts that experienced the putative process of selection against virulent clones of trypanosomes. Hence, the reason why we failed to detect any significant pathology in newts from their trypanosomiasis is because we came upon the system when all the trypanosome–newt–leech interactions had just recently been initiated in every pond. Our studies have occurred during the process of intense selection for apathogenicity in the eft stage and before virulent strains have arisen within any pond. We predict that virulent forms will arise independently in each pond and increase in frequency by natural selection.

In a curious way, our conclusion that young trypanosome–newt interactions are benign and older interactions are virulent both supports and contradicts the assertion of Ewald (1983) that new parasite–host interactions are less pathogenic than older ones. At the newt deme (individual pond) level, the hypothesis is supported. We propose that as new newt breeding populations get started through colonization and new apathogenic trypanosomes are brought in by transforming efts, initial interactions between the two are benign. As the interaction ages in the pond, the interaction should become more virulent. On the other hand, our conclusions that the interaction between trypanosomes and newts is old and specialized and yet apathogenic seems to contradict Ewald (1983). We suggest that it is the epidemiological dynamics of the interaction, with many recent colonizations of ponds by newts throughout the Shenandoah Mountains, that has established the large, global façade of apathogenicity in this interaction.

Superficially, our trypanosome–newt system also seems to contradict Anderson's (1978) assertion that parasites which cause little damage to their hosts generate unstable equilibria. The sizes of the breeding newt populations have shown stationary dynamics for 10 years (Gill *et al.*, 1983) and the prevalence and frequency distribution of trypanosomes in newts has shown little change over 4 years (Mock, 1983). The ecological patterns in both newts and trypanosomes have been highly predictable.

Over a longer time span, the epidemiological dynamics of the trypanosome–newt interaction may be consistent with Anderson's (1978) assertion. We are suggesting that trypanosomes in endemic communities of newts and leeches go through a natural cycle of apathogenic origins and virulent ends. There may be a long lag in the apathogenic stage before there arises a novel mutation which confers higher replication rates and greater pathogenicity. However, once such a mutation arises the trypanosomes will move rapidly away from the original, unstable, apathogenic equilibrium along a path of increasing pathogenicity. Concomitant lowering of adult newt survivorship and shortening of newt longevity should ensue. Whether the system will ever equilibrate at a position of low host density and intermediate pathogenicity in the trypanosomes as hypothesized by Anderson & May (1979) may be difficult to demonstrate.

CONCLUSIONS

We accept the theoretical argument that natural selection among competing genotypes of parasites co-occurring in individual hosts should favour the one with the highest reproductive rate and the greatest pathogenicity whenever transmission is opportune. In order to explain trends of decreasing pathogenicity observed in some parasites, we offer a model in which natural selection favours avirulent parasite genotypes whenever the parasites are sparsely distributed among host individuals, and the parasites reside in a host for a prolonged period of time without any possibility of transmission. During that period any virulent genotype of the parasite will fail to be transmitted, and only apathogenic forms will be represented in future generations. Individual selection and interdemal selection are expected to favour the same individuals under these conditions, and promote apathogenicity together.

We present a summary of long-term studies of the demography of red-spotted newts in Virginia and the impact of an infection of trypanosomiasis that they carry. Empirical and experimental results demonstrate that the trypanosomes have no impact on the survival of newts and minimal effect of their net reproduction. We conclude the current interaction is apathogenic. Most newts have no effective mechanism of resistance against trypanosomiasis. We reason that rapidly dividing, highly virulent forms of trypanosomes should be favoured by selection in the adult newt–trypanosome–leech interaction in breeding ponds. We hypothesize that the absence of pathogenic trypanosomes from this system is due to natural selection against virulent trypanosome clones in the long eft stage during which no transmission is possible. Selection strongly favours those trypanosome genotypes that permit their eft hosts to reach maturity and re-enter an endemic cycle between adult newts and amphibian leeches in a pond. We suggest that the epidemiology of efts colonizing new ponds with apathogenic strains of trypanosomes persistently resets the evolutionary clock to avirulence in the interaction. We conclude that our study system is at a young stage, prior to the appearance of virulence mutations in the trypanosomes.

ACKNOWLEDGEMENTS

This work was supported by National Science Foundation grants DEB 77-04817, DEB 78-10832, and DEB 80-05080 to DEG, and Sigma XI and University of Maryland Research grants to BAM. The paper benefited from discussions with K. A. Berven, G. Borgia, J. Coyne, D. J. Futuyma, W. Haber, P. Hamel, J. C. Holmes, A. Kuris, R. M. May, N. G. Hairston, Sr., J. R. Ott, G. Otto, S. J. Smith-Gill, G. J. Vermeij, D. S. Wilson, the students in the 84-1 and 84-3 OTS courses in Costa Rica, and two anonymous reviewers of an earlier version.

REFERENCES

ALEXANDER, M., 1981. Why microbial predators and parasites do not eliminate their prey and hosts. *Annual Review Microbiology, 35:* 113–133.
ALLISON, A. C., 1982. Co-evolution between hosts and infectious disease agents and its effects on virulence. In R. M. Anderson & R. M. May (Eds) *Population Biology of Infectious Diseases*. Life Sciences Research Report 25: 245–267. Berlin: Dahlem Konferenzen.
ANAGNOSTAKIS, S. L., 1982. Biological control of chestnut blight. *Science, 215:* 466–471.
ANDERSON, R. M., 1978. The regulation of host population growth by parasitic species. *Parasitology, 76:* 119–157.
ANDERSON, R. M., 1981. Population ecology of infectious disease agents. In R. M. May (Ed.) *Theoretical Ecology 2nd Ed.:* 318–355. Oxford: Blackwell Scientific Publications.
ANDERSON, R. M., 1982. Transmission dynamics and control of infectious disease agents. In. R. M. Anderson & R. M. May (Eds) *Population Biology of Infectious Diseases:* 149–176. Life Sciences Report 25 Berlin: Dahlem Konferenzen.
ANDERSON, R. M. & MAY, R. M., 1979. Population biology of infectious diseases: Part I. *Nature, 280:* 361–367.
ANDERSON, R. M. & MAY, R. M, 1981. The population dynamics of microparasites and their invertebrate hosts. *Philosophical Transactions of the Royal Society B, 291:* 451–524.
ANDERSON, R. M. & MAY, R. M., 1982. Coevolution of hosts and parasites. *Parasitology, 85:* 411–426.
BAKER, J. R., 1963. Speculations on the evolution of the Family Trypanosomatidae Doflein, 1901. *Experimental Parasitology, 13:* 219–233.
BALL, G. H., 1943. Parasitism and evolution. *American Naturalist, 77:* 345–364.
BARRETT, J. A., 1983. Plant-fungus symbioses, In D. J. Futuyma & M. Slatkin, (Eds) *Coevolution:* 137–160. Sunderland, Mass: Sinauer Associates.
BARROW, J. H., 1953. The biology of *Trypanosoma diemyctyli (Tobey).* I. *Trypanosoma diemyctyli* in the leech, *Batrachobdella picta* (Verrill). *Transactions of the American Microscopical Society, 72:* 197–216.
BARROW, J. H., 1954. The biology of *Trypanosoma diemyctyli* (Tobey). II. Cytology and morphology of *Trypanosoma diemyctyli* in the vertebrate host, *Triturus v. viridescens. Transaction of the American Microscopical Society, 73:* 242–257.
BARROW, J. H., 1958. The biology of *Trypanosoma diemyctyli* (Tobey). III. Factors influencing the cycle of *Trypanosoma diemyctyli* in the vertebrate host *Triturus v. viridescens. Journal of Protozoology, 5:* 161–170.

BLOOM, B. R., 1979. Games parasites play: how parasites evade immune surveillance. *Nature, 279:* 21–26.

BOREHAM, P. F. L. & WRIGHT, I. G., 1976. The release of pharmacologically active substances in parasitic infections. *Progress in Medical Chemistry, 13:* 159–204.

BRADLEY, D. J., 1972. Regulation of parasite populations. A general theory of the epidemiology and control of parasitic infections. *Transactions of the Royal Society of Tropical Medicine and Hygiene, 66:* 697–708.

BRADLEY, D. J., 1974. Stability in host–parasite systems. In M. B. Usher & M. H. Williamson (Eds) *Ecological Stability:* 71–87. London: Chapman and Hall.

CALOW, P. & JENNINGS, J. B., 1974. Calorific values in the phylum Platyhelminthes: the relationship between potential energy, mode of life and the evolution of entoparasitism. *Biological Bulletin, 147:* 81–94.

CHANDLER, A. C. & READ, C. P., 1961. *Introduction to Parasitology:* 822 pp. New York: John Wiley & Sons.

CHEEVER, A. W., DUVALL, R. H., MINKER, R. G., 1980a. Quantitative parasitologic findings in rabbits infected with Japanese and Philippine strains of *Schistosoma japonicum. American Journal of Tropical Medicine and Hygiene, 29:* 1307–1315.

CHEEVER, A. W., DUVALL, R. H. & MINKER, R. G., 1980b. Extrahepatic pathology in rabbits infected with Japanese and Philippine strains of *Schistosoma japonicum,* and the relation of intestinal lesions to passage of eggs in the feces. *American Journal of Tropical Medicine and Hygiene, 29:* 1316–1328.

CHEEVER, A. W., DUVALL, R. H., MINKER, R. G. & NASH. T., 1980c. Hepatic fibrosis in rabbits infected with Japanese and Philippine strains of *Schistosoma japonicum. American Journal of Tropical Medicine and Hygiene, 29:* 1327–1339.

CLAYTON, C. E., 1978. *Trypanosoma brucei:* influence of host strain and antigenic type in infections in mice. *Experimental Parasitology, 44:* 202–208.

COATNEY, G. R., COLLINS, W. E., McWILSON, W. & CONTACOS, P. G., 1971. *The Prime Malarias:* 366 pp. Washington, D.C.: USGPO.

COHEN, S., 1979. Review lecture. Immunity to malaria. *Proceedings of the Royal Society of London, Series B, 203:* 323–345.

COLE, L. C., 1954. The population consequences of life history phenomena. *Quarterly Review of Biology, 29:* 103–137.

CORNFORD, E. M. & HUOT, M. E., 1981. Glucose transfer from male to female schistosomes. *Science, 213:* 1269–1271.

CROFTON, H. D., 1971a. A quantitative approach to parasitism. *Parasitology, 62:* 179–193.

CROFTON, H. D., 1971b. A model of host parasite relationships. *Parasitology, 63:* 343–364.

DEEVEY, E. S., Jr., 1947. Life tables for natural populations of animals. *Quarterly Review of Biology, 22:* 283–314.

DORNEY, R. S., 1969. Epizootiology of trypanosomes in red squirrels and eastern chipmunks. *Ecology, 50:* 817–824.

DUBOS, R., 1965. *Man Adapting:* 527 pp. New Haven: Yale University Press.

EICHLER, W., 1941a. Wirtsspezifität und stammesgeschichtliche Gleichläufigkeit (Fahrenholz Regel) bei Parasiten im allgemeinen und bei Mallophagen im besonderen. *Zool. Anzeiger, 132:* 254–292.

EICHLER, W., 1941b. Korrelation in der Stammesentwicklung von Wirten und Parasiten. *Zeitschrift für Parasitenunde, 19:* 24.

ESCH, G. W., GIBBONS, J. W. & BOURQUE, J. E., 1975. An analysis of the relationship between stress and parasitism. *American Midland Naturalist, 93:* 339–353.

ESCH, G. W., HAZEN, T. C., AHO, J. M., 1977. Parasitism and r- and K-selection. In G. W. Esch (Ed.) *Regulation of Parasite Populations:* 9–62. New York and London: Academic Press.

EWALD, P. W., 1980. Evolutionary biology and the treatment of signs and symptoms of infectious disease. *Journal of Theoretical Biology, 86:* 169–176.

EWALD, P. W., 1983. Host–parasite relations, vectors, and the evolution of disease severity. *Annual Review of Ecology and Systematics, 14:* 465–485.

FENNER, F., 1965. Myxoma virus and *Oryctolagus.* In H. G. Baker & G. L. Stebbins (Eds), *The Genetics of Colonizing Species:* 485–501. New York and London: Academic Press.

FENNER, F. & RATCLIFFE, F. N., 1965. *Myxomatosis.* Cambridge: Cambridge University Press.

FLOR, H. H., 1971. Current status of the gene-for-gene concept. *Annual Review of Phytopathology, 9:* 275–296.

FRIEDMAN, M. H., 1978. Erythrocytic mechanisms of sickle-cell resistance to malaria. *Proceedings of the National Academy of Science, USA, 75:* 1994–1997.

FRIEDMAN, M. J., 1979. Oxidant damage mediates variant red-cell resistance to malaria. *Nature, 280:* 245–247.

FULBRIGHT, D. W., WEIDLICH, W. H. & HART, J. H., 1982. Abnormal cankers on American Chestnut (*Castanea dentata*) trees and hypovirulent strains of *Endothia parasitica* in Michigan (USA). *Phytopathology, 72:* 929.

FUTUYMA, D. J. & SLATKIN, M., 1983. *Coevolution:* 555 pp. Sunderland, Mass: Sinauer Associates.

GARNHAM, P. C. C., 1971. *Progress in Parasitology:* 224 pp. London: Athlone Press.

GILBERT, L. E., 1983. Coevolution and mimicry. In D. J. Futuyma & M. Slatkin (Eds), *Coevolution:* 263–281. Sunderland, Mass: Sinauer Associates.

GILL, D. E., 1974. Intrinsic rate of increase, saturation density, and competitive ability. II. The evolution of competitive ability. *American Naturalist, 108:* 103–116.

GILL, D. E., 1978a. The metapopulation ecology of the red-spotted newt, *Notophthalmus viridescens* (Rafinesque). *Ecological Monographs, 48:* 145–166.

GILL, D. E., 1978b. Effective population size and interdemic migration rates in a metapopulation of the red-spotted newt, *Notophthalmus viridescens* (Rafinesque). *Evolution, 32:* 839–849.

GILL, D.E., 1978c. Occurrence of trypanosomiasis in the red eft stage of the red-spotted newt, *Notophthalmus viridescens. Journal of Parasitology, 64:* 930–931.

GILL, D. E., 1978d. On selection at high population density. *Ecology, 59:* 1289–1291.

GILL, D. E., 1979. Density dependence and homing behavior in adult red-spotted newts, *Notophthalmus viridescens* (Rafinesque). *Ecology, 60:* 800–813.

GILL, D. E., 1984. Interpreting breeding patterns from census data: a solution to the Husting dilemma. *Ecology, 60:* 344–354.

GILL, D. E., BERVEN, K. A. & MOCK, B. A., 1983. The environmental component of evolutionary biology. In C. A. King & P. S. Dawson (Eds), *Population Biology: Retrospect and Prospect:* 1–36. New York: Columbia University Press.

HASSELL, M. P., 1982. Impact of infectious diseases on host populations. In R. M. Anderson & R. M. May (Eds), Population Biology of Infectious Diseases: 15–35. Life Sciences Research Report 25. Berlin: Dahlem Konferenzen.

HOEPRICH, P. D., 1977. Host-parasite relationships and the pathogenesis of infectious disease. In P. D. Hoeprich (Ed.), *Infectious Diseases:* 34–45. New York: Harper and Row.

HOLMES, J. C., 1982. Impact of infectious disease agents on the population growth and geographical distribution of animals. In R. M. Anderson and R. M. May (Eds), *Population Biology of Infectious Diseases:* 37–51. Life Science Research Report 25. Berlin: Dahlem Konferenzen.

HOLMES, J. C., 1983. Evolutionary relationships between parasitic helminths and their hosts. In D. J. Futuyma & M. Slatkin (Eds), *Coevolution:* 161–185. Sunderland, MA: Sinauer Associates.

HOLMES, K. K. & STILWELL, G. A., 1977. Gonococcal Infection. In P. D. Hoeprich (Ed.), *Infectious Diseases:* 491–506. New York: Harper and Row.

HOLMES, J. C., HOBBS, R. P. & LEONG, T. S., 1977. Populations in perspective: community organization and regulation of parasite populations. In G. W. Esch (Ed.), *Regulation of Parasite Populations:* 209–245. New York and London: Academic Press.

KELLY, J. D., WHITLOCK, H. V., THOMPSON, H. G., HALL, C. A., MARTIN, I. C. A. & LeJAMBRE, L. F., 1978. Physiological characteristics of free-living and parasitic stages of *Haemonchus contortus*, susceptible or resistant to benzimidazole anthelmintics. *Research in Veterinary Science, 25:* 376–385.

LEVIN, B. R., 1982. Evolution of parasites and hosts. In R. M. Anderson & R. M. May (Eds), *Population Biology of Infectious Diseases*: 213–243, Life Sciences Research Report 25, Berlin: Dahlem Konferenzen.

LEVIN, S. A. & PIMENTEL, D., 1981. Selection of intermediate rates of increase in parasite–host systems. *American Naturalist, 117:* 308–315.

LEVINE, N. D., 1972. Relationship between certain protozoa and other animals. *Research in Protozoology, 4:* 291–350.

LEWONTIN, R. C., 1970. The units of selection. *Annual Review of Ecology and Systematics, 1:* 1–18.

MAY, R. M. & ANDERSON, R. M. 1983a. Epidemiology and genetics in the coevolution of parasites and hosts. *Proceedings of the Royal Society of London B, 219:* 281–313.

MAY, R. M. & ANDERSON, R. M., 1983b. Parasite–host coevolution. In D. J. Futuyma & M. Slatkin (Eds), *Coevolution:* 186–206. Sunderland, MA, Sinauer Associates.

MITTER, C. & BROOKS, D. R., 1983. Phylogenetic aspects of coevolution. In D. J. Futuyma & M. Slatkin (Eds), *Coevolution:* 65–98. Sunderland, Mass: Sinauer Associates.

MIYAKE, M., 1971. Schistosomiasis *japonicum.* In R. A. Marcial-Rojas (Ed.), *Pathology of Protozoal and Helminthic Diseases:* 414–433. Baltimore: William & Wilkins.

MOCK, B. A., 1983. *The population biology of* Trypanosoma diemyctyli. Ph.D. Dissertation, University of Maryland.

MOCK, B. A. & GILL, D. E., 1984. The infrapopulation dynamics of trypanosomes in red-spotted newts. *Parasitology, 88:* 267–282.

NIGRELLI, R. F., 1929. On the cytology and life-history of *Trypanosoma diemyctli* and the polynuclear count of infected newts (*Triturus viridescens*). *Transactions of the American Microscopical Society, 68:* 366–387.

NOBLE, E. R. & NOBLE, G. A., 1976. *Parasitology* (4th edition): 566 pp. Philadelphia: Lea & Febiger.

OLVEDA, R. M., TIU, E., FEVIDAL, P., Jr., DE VEYRA, F., Jr., ICATLO, F. C. Jr., & DOMINGO, E. O., 1983. Relationship of prevalence and intensity of infection to morbidity in schistosomiasis japonica: a study of three communities in Leyte, Philippines. *American Journal of Tropical Medicine & Hygiene, 32:* 1312–1321.

PEREIRA, M. S., 1982. The impact of infectious diseases on human demography today. In R. M. Anderson & R. M. May (Eds), *Population Biology of Infectious Diseases:* 53–64. Life Sciences Research Report 25. Berlin: Dahlem Konferenzen.

PERSON, C., 1967. Genetic aspects of parasitism. *Canadian Journal of Botany, 45:* 1193–1204.

PETERS, W., 1974. Recent advances in antimalarial chemotherapy and drug resistance. *Advances in Parasitology, 12:* 69–114.

PRICE, P. W., 1977. General concepts on the evolutionary biology of parasites. *Evolutionary, 31:* 405–420.

PRICE, P. W., 1980. *Evolutionary Biology of Parasites.* Princeton, NJ: Princeton University Press.

SACKS, D. L., SELKIRK, M., OGILVIE, B. M. & ASKONAS, B. A., 1980. Intrinsic immunosuppressive activity of different trypanosome strains varies with parasite virulence. *Nature, 283:* 476–478.

SANGSTER, N. C., WHITLOCK, H. V., KELLY, J. D., GUNAWAN, M. & HALL, C. A., 1979. The effect of single and divided dose administration on the efficacy of fenbendazole against adult stages of benzimidazole resistant sheep trichostrongylids. *Research in Veterinary Science, 26:* 85–89.

SLOBODKIN, L. B., 1968. How to be a predator. *American Zoologist, 8:* 43–51.

SLOBODKIN, L. B., 1974. Prudent predation does not require group selection. *American Naturalist, 108:* 665–678.

SMITH, C. E. G., 1982. Practical problems in the control of infectious diseases. In R. M. Anderson & R. M. May (Eds), *Population Biology of Infectious Diseases:* 177–190. Life Sciences Research Report 25. Berlin: Dahlem Konferenzen.

SPRENT, J. F. A., 1963. *Parasitism.* Baltimore: Williams & Wilkins.

SWELLENGREBEL, N. H., 1940. The efficient parasite. *Proceedings of the Third International Congress of Microbiology:* 119–127. Baltimore: Waverly Press.

TURNER, M., 1980. How trypanosomes change coats. *Nature, 284:* 13–14.

VICKERMAN, K., 1978. Antigenic variation in trypanosomes. *Nature, 273:* 613–617.

WAKELIN, D., 1978. Genetic control of susceptibility and resistance to parasitic infection. *Advances in Parasitology, 16:* 219–309.

WARREN, K. S., 1978. The pathogenicity, pathobiology and pathogenesis of schistosomiasis. *Nature, 273:* 609–612.

WENYON, C. M., 1926. *Protozoology. I. A Manual for Medical Men, Veterinarians and Zoologists:* 442–607. New York: William Wood & Co.

WENYON, C. M., 1965. *Protozoology. II:* 1039–1041. New York: Hafner Publishing Co.

WILLIAMS, G. C., 1966. *Adaptation and Natural Selection:* 307 pp. Princeton, New Jersey: Princeton University Press.

WRIGHT, S., 1931. Evolution in Mendelian populations. *Genetics, 16:* 97–159.

WYNNE-EDWARDS, V. C., 1962. *Animal Dispersion in Relation to Social Behaviour.* Edinburgh: Oliver and Boyd.

YORKE, J. A., HEATHCOTE, H. W. & NOLD, A., 1978. Dynamics and control of the transmission of gonorrhea. *Sexually Transmitted Diseases, 5:* 51–56.

Genetics of protein variation in populations of parasitic protozoa

A. TAIT

Department of Genetics, University of Edinburgh,
West Mains Road, Edinburgh EH9 3JN, U.K.

Protein variation has been examined by use of electrophoretic techniques in a considerable number of parasitic protozoa, particularly those causing disease in man. This paper attempts to examine the rationale of such studies both in terms of what information protein electrophoretic data can give about genetic diversity and what questions can be examined by this technique. By considering a hypothetical parasite, the importance of the nature and source of the parasite material examined is discussed and these points are illustrated by reference to specific examples using studies on protein variation in *Plasmodium* and *Trypanosoma*. Using these examples, the contribution of electrophoretic protein variation studies to our knowledge of the genetics and ploidy, the delineation of populations, subspecies and species and the relationship between disease, host and parasite genotype is discussed.

KEY WORDS: — Genetics — parasitic protozoa — protein variation

CONTENTS

INTRODUCTION

The initial impetus for the study of protein variation in parasitic protozoa has come from the need to define morphologically very similar or identical organisms in relation to the diseases they cause and the hosts that they infect rather than from any idea that this group of organisms is either experimentally very suitable for protein variation studies or that it has unique properties likely to advance our basic understanding of protein variation. In many instances, parasitic protozoa have considerable disadvantages as experimental organisms for the study of protein

Ecology and Genetics of Host–Parasite Interactions
ISBN: 0 12 593 690 7

variation. Thus the main rationale for studying protein variation in parasitic protozoa is the use of such variation to gain information about the basic biology, genetics, epidemiology and speciation of these organisms.

A considerable body of information is now available on protein variation in *Plasmodium* (Walliker, 1983b), *Trypanosoma* (Miles *et al.*, 1980; Gibson, Marshall & Godfrey, 1980; Mehlitz *et al.*, 1982; Tait, Babiker, LeRay, 1985; Tait *et al.*, 1984b) and *Leishmania* (Miles *et al.*, 1981b; Kreutzer *et al.*, 1983) and to a lesser extent in *Coccidia* (Shirley & Rollinson, 1979). This paper is aimed at outlining the main questions that can (and have) been examined using protein variation analysis as a research tool, discussing the strategies needed to examine these questions and, by reference to specific examples, illustrating how knowledge of the biology and genetics has been advanced by such studies. No attempt will be made to review all the extensive data available on protein variation in parasitic protozoa.

Essentially, the study of electrophoretic protein variation is an indirect means of examining gene diversity. Most of the variation observed results from amino acid alterations within the polypeptides under study which in turn reflect nucleotide alterations within the structural genes coding for the polypeptides. In recent years, two new technologies, namely recombinant DNA and hybridoma techniques, have been developed. These techniques can also be applied to the study of genetic variation in parasitic protozoa and used to examine the same questions as those that have been addressed by the use of protein variation techniques. It is important to stress that, in this context, these techniques are essentially measuring the same parameter as that measured by protein variation, namely variation in the nucleotide sequence of different genes. When these newer techniques are used to examine speciation, population diversity etc., the same strategies as those used for similar studies using protein variation need to be adopted.

Much of the data available on protein variation in populations of parasitic protozoa come from a relatively small sample of this group and most of those studied in detail are pathogenic to man or his domestic animals. Thus, in this paper, only the main questions relating to this group will be discussed; briefly, these can be outlined as follows:

(1) Given that the parasitic protozoa studied replicate in both an insect vector and a mammalian host, what is a parasite population?

(2) Are these protozoa asexual or sexual and what is their ploidy?

(3) Can different populations, subspecies and species of morphologically similar protozoa be distinguished, how distinct are these groupings and how diverse are the parasites within a group?

(4) In a number of human parasitic protozoa a range of disease symptoms is observed and the 'same' parasite also infects a range of host species. Are the different diseases caused by different parasites and are the parasites causing disease in man different from those in wild or domestic animals?

All these questions have been examined to some degree by the study of protein variation and so such studies are not only aimed at providing an understanding of the population structure and genetics but also using this knowledge to examine applied questions with the ultimate aim of providing a broad understanding of the epidemiology of the parasite in relation to the diseases that it causes. Before considering how these questions have been examined, it is important first to consider how protein variation is measured, what it measures, what other techniques are available and what experimental strategies need to be adopted (in relation to the parasite material examined) to provide data with which to examine the questions outlined above.

THE MEASUREMENT OF GENETIC DIVERSITY

Most, if not all, the methods used to date to screen for protein variation are aimed at detecting charge differences, molecular weight differences or a combination of both parameters, between homologous proteins (Ferguson, 1980). Broadly, these techniques can be divided into two groups, those which involve the detection of specific protein molecules using a specific staining system or those which detect protein non-specifically such as Coomassie blue stain or autoradiography of radiolabelled proteins. The major advantage of the use of specific stains is that when electrophoretic variation is observed, it is reasonable to assume that one is comparing variants of the same protein, i.e. variation in the products of a single gene locus. In the case of non-specific protein stains one is able to detect diversity in a large number of proteins simultaneously; however, it is less clear cut which variant proteins are homologous and represent products of the same gene (unless genetic analysis can be undertaken). These points are illustrated in Fig. 1; in the upper panel, extracts of two stocks have been electrophoresed in a starch gel which was subsequently stained for malate dehydrogenase activity and it is clear that the two stocks exhibit variants of the same enzyme. In the lower panel, there is an autoradiograph of a 2D gel electrophoretic separation of radiolabelled proteins extracted from two strains of *Plasmodium falciparum*; a considerable number of polypeptides are observed and the majority have the same mobility (in both dimensions); however, those marked by arrows are of different mobility in the two stocks. It is difficult to be certain that, for example, polypeptide a in stock A is a variant of polypeptide b in stock B other than on the rationale that the variation in homologous proteins is likely to be small. that the variation in homologous proteins is likely to be small.

Figure 1 summarizes the two main methods for detecting protein variation between stocks. In the case of enzyme electrophoresis, a range of supporting media have been used (starch, polyacrylamide, agarose and cellulose acetate) and also separation based on the iso-electric point of the molecule under study (iso-electric focusing). Each method has both advantages and disadvantages at the practical level, but all are essentially measuring alterations in charge on the protein molecules. In the cases where detailed analysis has been undertaken, it has been shown that the majority of charge alterations arise by changes in the amino acid sequence although in some instances such changes in charge can be brought about by secondary modifications of the proteins such as amidation, glycosylation or oxidation (Harris & Hopkinson, 1976). Thus, by detecting electrophoretic differences in the same polypeptide in different stocks or strains of an organism, one is, albeit rather insensitively, detecting alterations in the amino acid sequence. As the amino acid sequence is determined by the nucleotide sequence of the gene for the polypeptide, variation in the nucleotide sequence of the gene is being detected. Due to the redundancy of the genetic code (i.e. a number of different codons determine the same amino acid) many nucleotide changes will go undetected; furthermore, as electrophoretic methods will only detect charge changes in proteins, many amino acid (and thereby nucleotide substitutions) changes will go undetected if no charge

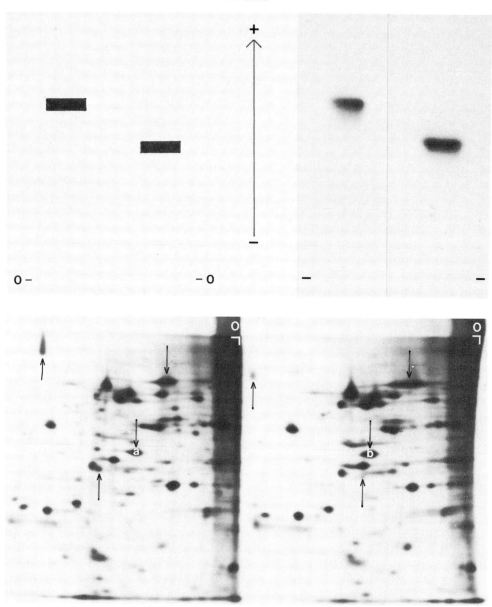

Figure 1. The upper panel is a photograph of a starch gel (after electrophoresis of extracts of two stocks of *T. brucei* spp.) stained for malate dehydrogenase activity. The lower panel is an autoradiograph of a 2D gel electrophoretic separation of biosynthetically labelled proteins of *Plasmodium falciparum* as described by Tait (1981). The homologous variant proteins are indicated by arrows and variants a and b of one protein are indicated.

change in the protein occurs e.g. if one neutral amino acid is substituted for another neutral amino acid. Thus, protein electrophoretic methods are a relatively insensitive means of detecting genetic diversity; estimates based on theoretical considerations suggest that some 30% of amino acid substitutions will be detected (Lewontin, 1974). These estimates do not include the fact that 'silent' substitutions are not detected either and if these are considered as well, the sensitivity of detecting variation in the nucleotide sequence of the gene under study is even lower than those estimates. These considerations raise two important points, firstly what alternative and more sensitive methods are available for detecting genetic diversity? Secondly, given the insensitivity of protein electrophoresis to detect genetic diversity, extreme caution must be exerted in concluding that two stocks or even groups of organisms are identical based on protein electrophoretic criteria.

Two, relatively new methodologies, offer the possibility of circumventing the lack of sensitivity of protein electrophoresis, namely, the use of recombinant DNA probes in conjunction with restriction enzyme digestion and the use of monoclonal antibodies detecting specific antigens. As the subject of this paper concerns protein variation, these techniques and the results obtained with them will not be considered in detail. The advantage of using DNA probes is two-fold; firstly, both expressed and non-expressed sequences of the genome can be examined and secondly, given that enough restriction enzymes are used, most nucleotide changes can be detected. Although this approach is beginning to be used to examine variation within and between groups of stocks (e.g. Pays *et al.*, 1983), no large body of data is available. Monoclonal antibodies, by detecting a particular small three dimensional region of a protein (considering only those recognizing proteins) are also theoretically more sensitive to changes in the amino acid sequence of the protein, although, as they are detecting gene products any 'silent' nucleotide changes will not be detected. In principle, monoclonal antibodies should detect a greater percentage of amino acid substitutions, however, as they only 'see' a small region (approximately 8–10 amino acids) of the protein a large number is required to examine the whole molecule. However, given that during their production a screening system is devised based on the detection of variation between stocks, only those detecting variation can be selected.

One of the major disadvantages inherent in using either enzyme electrophoresis or restriction enzyme analysis with gene probes is that the parasites under study must be grown to provide enough material for analysis. This requirement means not only that suitable methods of culture or growth have to be available but also that relatively large amounts of parasite material are required. One of the major advantages of the use of monoclonal antibodies is that, once a set of monoclonals recognizing polymorphism in a series of antigens has been isolated, it can be used to screen parasites at the single cell level using immunofluorescent techniques. This property, potentially, allows this method to be applied directly to samples from infected animals or man. In considering the relative merits of different techniques for measuring genetic diversity, the discussion is largely based on theoretical considerations as few or no studies have been made at an experimental level to compare these techniques using the same set of parasites, genes, proteins and antigens. Perhaps such a study would be warranted, in order to measure the relative sensitivities of these techniques.

EXPERIMENTAL QUESTIONS AND STRATEGIES

A large number of studies have been undertaken examining protein electrophoretic variation between stocks, subspecies and species of parasitic protozoa. The numbers of stocks of a species or subspecies examined and the relationship of the stocks in terms of date and place of isolation vary widely, such that it is often difficult to build up a comprehensive and logical picture of the variation observed. Generalized conclusions have been drawn relating either to similarity or difference based on the examination of a few stocks from different subspecies which happen to be available for study. It is therefore important to delineate the strategies required (in relation to the parasite material) in order to answer the main questions posed in the Introduction.

The simplest way to illustrate these strategies is to consider a generalized hypothetical parasitic protozoan that incorporates a number of the basic features encountered and to outline the strategies that can be adopted to answer or examine the questions posed. Having done this, it is then possible to examine, by reference to specific examples, how these questions have been examined experimentally. The hypothetical, generalized, parasitic protozoan has the following features.

(1) a morphologically identical parasite infects man, domestic animals and wild game.

(2) the parasite is transmitted by a number of different species of an insect vector and undergoes various developmental stages within the insect.

(3) the parasite only causes disease in man in certain areas and two distinct types of disease are found which can be distinguished clinically.

(4) the parasite is found in animals in a wide area covering two continents, and the limited areas of human infection are also widely dispersed.

This description covers some of the main features of a number of pathogenic parasitic protozoa and allows the main questions to be examined by using protein electrophoresis as a means of measuring genetic diversity. These questions can be briefly summarized as follows: is the parasite asexual or sexual, haploid, diploid or polyploid? Can man infective parasites be differentiated from those infecting animals and are different clinical symptoms caused by different parasites? Are discrete non-interbreeding (in the case of sexual parasites) populations found across a wide area or is there one large interbreeding population? How diverse are the parasites within a single host or vector? Although a number of other questions could be included, these cover those which, if answered, would give a rather complete picture of the biology, genetics, speciation and epidemiology of the parasite in relation to its hosts and vectors as well as the diseases caused. In addition, if such studies are extended to other closely related species of parasite, the evolutionary relationships between such species can be examined.

Given the outline description of the hypothetical generalized parasitic protozoan and the questions that can be examined by measuring genetic diversity using protein electrophoresis, what overall strategies can be adopted to examine these questions? Aside from any considerations of the technical advantages and disadvantages of protein electrophoresis, a crucial consideration in order to gain meaningful data, is the nature of the parasite material examined.

A scheme of the sort of material required to examine the questions outlined is shown diagrammatically in Fig. 2. A series of isolates are made from infected individual organisms (human, animal and insect) in four geographically distant areas; a single clone of each parasite established from each isolate and 10–20 isolates made from each host type. Using such a strategy, a series of cloned parasites is established with which it is possible to measure the diversity within a host or vector within one area and the diversity between areas by screening extracts of purified parasites for variation in 10–20 protein coding loci. For example, by comparing parasites in Area A isolated from man with those from the same area from animals,

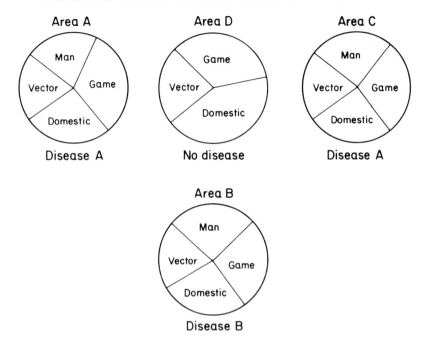

Figure 2. A diagrammatic representation of a collecting strategy for a hypothetical protozoan parasite. The circles indicate small geographical areas (A,B,C,D) in which isolates are made from the various hosts and vectors (sectors of each circle). In Areas A and C, human infection is observed with very similar clinical symptoms, in area B human infection is also observed but the clinical symptoms are distinct from those cases in areas A and C, and in area D no human disease is observed.

it is possible to ask whether they belong to the same or a different group of parasites. Similarly, by comparing human isolates from Area A and C (causing disease A) with those from Area B (causing disease B), it is possible to estimate the variation due to geographical isolation between parasites causing the same disease and to compare this with the parasites causing disease B and therefore examine whether diseases A and B are caused by distinct parasites or by the same parasite. By making all possible comparisons, it is then possible to examine the nature and degree of within and between group variation in relation to host, vector, disease and geographical location. In addition (see below for details), the question of the ploidy and existence of genetic exchange can be examined with such data; furthermore, the investigation of these properties is essential for the interpretation and analysis of the data obtained.

In practice, it is often extremely difficult to meet these requirements and so, in many cases, a compromise has to be made between the ideal and the practicable which can lead to difficulties in drawing definite conclusions. The aim of outlining this scheme and the questions is three-fold; firstly, to try to define the sort of information that can be obtained from the study of protein variation in populations; secondly, to stress the importance of a logical strategy in relation to the parasite material examined and, thirdly, to point out that such an approach is required independent of the means (protein electrophoresis, monoclonal antibodies, or DNA probes) of measuring genetic diversity. In the following sections, the points raised are examined by considering specific examples of the investigation of genetic diversity using protein variation.

GENETICS AND PLOIDY

Most of the work involved in analysing or detecting the existence of genetic mechanisms in parasitic protozoa has relied heavily on the use of enzyme electrophoretic variants as markers. As the topic of the genetics and ploidy of *T. cruzi* (Miles, 1983), the *Kinetoplastida* (Tait, 1983) and parasitic protozoa in general (Walliker, 1983a) has been extensively reviewed recently, only the main features and recent developments will be briefly discussed here. The relevance of ploidy and existence or not of a sexual cycle to the analysis of protein variation in parasite populations (or groups) is of importance for a number of reasons. The interpretation of enzyme electrophoretic patterns (and also 2D protein variation) will vary depending on whether the organism is haploid or diploid. If the patterns shown in Fig. 3 are obtained after electrophoresis of extracts of two stocks, then one would interpret the double banded pattern as a heterozygote generated by variation at a single locus in a diploid, whereas in a haploid, such a pattern would imply that two loci coded for the enzyme, one of which was variant (see Fig. 3). The diversity of enzyme electrophoretic patterns in different stocks is considerably different in an asexual organism compared with that found in a sexual organism. In simple

Figure 3. Starch gel electrophoresis of extracts of two stocks *T. brucei* spp. stained for alkaline phosphatase. In stock A a single band of activity is observed while in stock B two bands of equal activity are observed, one of which is identical in mobility to the single banded pattern.

terms, asexual organisms tend to show low levels of variation between individual stocks and a clonal population structure is found. This has been observed in *T. cruzi* (Tibayrenc *et al.*, 1984; Miles *et al.*, 1984), *E. coli* (Ochman & Selander, 1984) and the sea anemone, *H. luciae* (Schick & Lamb, 1977). In contrast, sexual organisms tend to show high levels of interstock variation, although the actual level of diversity varies. This situation is observed in *T. brucei* spp. (Gibson *et al.*, 1980; Tait, 1980; Tait, 1983), *Plasmodium* (Carter, 1973) and a wide range of higher organisms (Ferguson, 1980). These considerations are of considerable importance if comparisons are being made between parasites from, for example, different geographical areas or hosts. This is perhaps best illustrated by considering the use of the term zymodeme; this term is appropriate for asexual organisms; because of the low level of variation and clonal population structure, few zymodemes are found and therefore an adequate description of the population can be made. In the case of a sexual organism, the high levels of variation result in the description of very large numbers of zymodemes. For example, work with human enzyme electrophoretic variation using some 100 different enzymes (Harris & Hopkinson, 1976) results in each individual belonging to a different zymodeme, thus the description is not of great value in describing populations in this context. Overall, it is therefore of considerable importance to know whether a sexual cycle exists and whether the organism is haploid, diploid or polyploid, aside from the rationale that such knowledge is very basic to understanding the biology of the organisms under study.

Current knowledge of the genetics and ploidy of the parasitic protozoa is very limited and only a few species have been studied at all from a genetic standpoint. Three basic approaches to this question have been taken; firstly, the observation of gametes and their fusion to form zygotes. Secondly, the mixing of genetically marked stocks and subsequent demonstration of recombination and, thirdly, evidence based on the nature and frequency of enzyme variation in natural populations. The current state of our knowledge is summarized in Table 1 for those organisms where evidence exists.

In the case of rodent malaria species and some species of *Coccidia*, genetic exchange has been directly demonstrated by mixing stocks which are variant at a number of loci (Walliker, Carter & Morgan, 1973; Walliker, Carter & Sanderson, 1975; Rollinson, Joyner & Norton, 1979; Pfefferkorn & Pfefferkorn, 1980); furthermore, the use of enzyme variants in these studies and their subsequent segregation in

Table 1. Evidence for genetic exchange and the ploidy of parasitic protozoa

Organism	Gametes and fusion	Ploidy	Recombination by mixture	Recombination enzyme variation
Plasmodium	√	haploid	√	√
Coccidia	√	haploid	√	ND
Theileria	√	?	ND	ND
Babesia	√	?	ND	ND
Trypanosoma:				
a. *T. cruzi*	—	diploid	—	—
b. *T. brucei* spp.	—	diploid	√	√

ND, Not determined; —, evidence against.

crosses has established that these parasites are haploid throughout their life cycle except in the zygote (diploid). Recent unpublished work (Betschart *et al.*, 1984) has shown that meiosis and subsequent hybridization occurred in stocks of *T. brucei* spp. when they were mixed and transmitted through tsetse flies. These studies also confirmed that *T. brucei* spp. are diploid at least for the loci examined in this work. Thus, in these three groups, it is clear that a sexual cycle exists and that gene exchange occurs. Although genetic exchange has not been demonstrated in non-rodent malaria species, *Theileria* or *Babesia*, the observation of gametes and their fusion to form zygotes suggests, by analogy with the rodent malaria species and *Coccidia*, that it does take place.

Extensive enzyme electrophoretic surveys have been made of stocks of various species of *Leishmania* (Rassam, Al-Mudhaffer & Chance, 1979; Miles *et al.*, 1981b; Lainson *et al.*, 1982), *Trypanosoma cruzi* (Miles *et al.*, 1980, 1984; Miles, 1983; Tibayrenc *et al.*, 1984), *Trypanosoma brucei* spp. (Gibson *et al.*, 1980; Tait, 1980; Mehlitz *et al.*, 1982; Tait *et al.*, 1984, 1985) and *Trypanosoma congolense* (Young & Godfrey, 1983). On the basis of the frequency and type of variant observed in comparison with those predicted by models of sexual and asexual reproduction, it is possible to provide evidence for or against a sexual cycle (Tait, 1983). When the data from *T. cruzi* are examined in this way, no evidence for a sexual system is found although these organisms appear to be diploid (Tibayrenc *et al.*, 1981, 1984; Miles *et al.*, 1984). In contrast, similar data provide evidence for a sexual cycle (and diploidy) in *T. brucei* spp. (Gibson *et al.*, 1980; Tait, 1980) and more recently a similar, but novel, analysis based on the predicted degree and nature of the variation of sexual and asexual organisms has confirmed *T. cruzi* and New World *Leishmania* spp. as asexual but *T. brucei* spp., *T. congolense* and Old World *Leishmania* spp. as sexual (Cibulskis, pers. comm.).

On the basis of the data obtained to date, the parasitic protozoa can be divided into three groups as regards their mode of reproduction; those most probably having an obligatory sexual cycle (*Plasmodium, Coccidia, Theileria* and *Babesia*), those having a non-obligatory sexual cycle (*T. brucei* spp., *T. congolense*, and Old World *Leishmania* spp.) and those which are asexual (*T. cruzi* and New World *Leishmania* spp.). However, in many cases, further evidence is required to establish these findings beyond doubt.

POPULATIONS, SUBSPECIES AND SPECIES

Two of the questions which have been examined using protein electrophoresis as a means of measuring genetic diversity are, firstly, do non-interbreeding populations occur in different areas of a country or continent and, secondly, can different subspecies or species be defined in cases where morphological differentiation is difficult? To some extent, these questions overlap with those aimed at asking whether different hosts or vectors are infected by different parasite genotypes. In this section, examples will be used to illustrate the results obtained in studies where these questions have been examined without reference (specifically) to the host, disease or vector.

Before examining the first question, namely does gene flow occur between groups of parasites across a wide geographical area or are discrete genetically isolated populations observed, it is important to define the criteria by which it is possible to distinguish between these possibilities. It is self evident that only parasites which undergo a sexual cycle can be considered in this context. The criteria used to define two populations as non-interbreeding are somewhat subjective. These are largely based on the observation of different allele frequencies in the populations sampled, on the occurrence of alleles specific to a particular area, or on the absence of individuals possessing both the most frequent alleles (in the separate geographical areas) at two or more loci. If population A has a high frequency of allele a at locus 1 and allele b at locus 2, while population B has a high frequency of allele z at locus 1 and allele y at locus 2, then individuals of genotype z,b (in a haploid) or za, yb (in a diploid) will be very rare or absent if no interbreeding of the populations takes place. If enough isolates are available, other means of distinguishing breeding from non-breeding populations are available; for example, if each population were found to be in Hardy–Weinberg equilibrium, and were interbreeding, then pooling data from both populations and treating them as one would result in good agreement with Hardy–Weinberg proportions (in the absence of selection). As the number of isolates screened is often small in the case of parasitic protozoa, the rather more subjective criteria outlined above are those most used. The best means of illustrating these points and the various approaches is to consider two examples, firstly from enzyme variation studies in *Plasmodium* and secondly from similar studies in *Trypanosoma*.

A series of cloned isolates from the natural host (*Thannomys rutilans*) of rodent malaria were screened for electrophoretic variation of four enzymes (Carter and Walliker, 1975; Walliker, 1983a) and a sample of the results obtained is summarized in Table 2. The numbers refer to different electrophoretic variants of each enzyme and it can be seen that two groups from the Central African Republic could be distinguished; the first possessing GPI-4, PGD-2 or -3, LDH-2, -3, -4 or -5, GDH-5 and the second GPI-5 or -9, PGD-5, LDH-7 and GDH-6. Two main conclusions can be drawn from these results; firstly, in isolates A–G, all but one combination of variants at the PGD and LDH loci occurred suggesting that random mating (and recombination) was occurring in this population. Secondly, examining isolates

Table 2. Enzyme variation in a series of 9 isolates of *Plasmodium* from rodent malaria from the Central African Republic (Walliker, 1983a)

Isolate	GPI	Enzyme variant PGD	LDH	GDH
A	4	2	2	5
B	4	2	3	5
C	4	2	4	5
D	4	2	5	5
E	4	3	2	5
F	4	3	4	5
G	4	3	5	5
H	9	5	7	6
I	5	5	7	6

Each number represents a particular electrophoretic mobility after starch gel electrophoresis, different numbers reflecting different electrophoretic mobility. GPI, glucose phosphate isomerase; PGD, 6-phosphogluconate dehydrogenase; LDH, lactate dehydrogenase; GDH, glutamate dehydrogenase.

H and I (and a number of other isolates of the same phenotype), it can be seen that they differed (in enzyme electrophoretic mobility) at all four loci and there was no evidence for cross-fertilization between the groups A–G and H,I as no isolates were found with combinations of variants from each group. This strongly supports the conclusion that no interbreeding was occurring between the groups. On the basis of such data, the two groups were designated as separate species. Studies on isolates of *P. yoelii*, *P. chabaudi* and *P. vinckei* made from different geographical areas have established that a number of the electrophoretic types in each species are common to all regions while others appear to be specific to one area (Walliker, 1983b). For example, the variants observed for three enzymes in isolates of *P. yoelii* from the Central African Republic and Nigeria are shown in Table 3. The variant GDH-4 is common to both areas while ADA-2 is specific to the Central African Republic and ADA-1 to Nigeria. Similar considerations apply to the variants of the enzyme GPI (Table 3). Thus, there appear to be genetically distinct groups

Table 3. Enzyme variation in isolates of *P. yoelii* from different geographical regions

Country	Enzyme variants		
	GPI	GDH	ADA
Central	1	4	2
African	2	4	2
Republic	10	4	2
Nigeria	2	4	1

Electrophoretic variants are designated by different numbers as described in the footnote to Table 2. GPI, glucose phosphate isomerase; GDH, glutamate dehydrogenase; ADA, adenosine deaminase.

within each species which are geographically separated; on this basis, these groups have been designated as subspecies (Walliker, 1983a). Too few isolates from each area have been studied to establish whether these distinct groups within a species form one large interbreeding group or whether they form distinct non-interbreeding groups; laboratory studies have shown that mating can occur between subspecies of *P. yoelii* (Knowles, Sanderson & Walliker, 1981) and of *P. chabaudi* (Lainson, 1982), thus showing that genetic exchange between geographically isolated groups is possible. It is still an open question whether this occurs in the 'wild', although the existence of apparently region specific variants argues against this. An essentially similar analysis has been undertaken with *P. falciparum* using enzyme electrophoretic variation and a considerably greater number of isolates (see Walliker, 1983a,b for reviews). In contrast to the rodent malaria, comparison between isolates from Thailand (Thaitong, Sueblinwong & Beale, 1981) and The Gambia (Carter & McGregor, 1973) shows virtually no differences, suggesting, either that these particular markers are less variable in *P. falciparum* and therefore do not show the existence of genetically isolated populations, or that *P. falciparum* constitutes a single large interbreeding population. Application of 2D-gel electrophoresis as a means of measuring genetic variation in *P. falciparum* (Tait, 1981; Walker & Tait, unpublished) has provided some evidence, albeit incomplete, that area specific variants do occur and that *P. falciparum* is divided into discrete non-interbreeding populations.

A rather similar analysis has been undertaken with enzyme variation in *T. brucei* spp. (Gibson *et al.*, 1980; Mehlitz *et al.*, 1982; Tait *et al.*, 1984, 1985) although considerable differences exist both in terms of the methods of analysis, the fact that these parasites are diploid and in the extent of the data available. To take a specific example, enzyme electrophoretic variation at 20 loci has been screened for in a series of cloned animal isolates from Nigeria and in a series of cloned tsetse isolates from Kiboko, Kenya of *T. b. brucei* (Tait *et al.*, 1984, 1985). Ignoring, for the moment, the fact that one set of isolates are from the mammalian host and the other from the vector, the data can be compared to examine whether area specific variants occur and whether these two groups are genetically isolated. Using the sample of data shown in Table 4, it is clear that area specific variants occur e.g. TDH-2 for Kiboko and ALAT-2 and -3 for Nigeria (Table 4); however, an allele *frequency* difference is observed rather than complete (area specific) fixation of one variant or the other. The absence of TDH-2 from Nigeria and its high frequency in Kiboko coupled with the reverse situation for ALAT-2, argue strongly that no gene flow occurs between these populations although strong evidence exists for gene flow within each population (Tait, unpublished).

Because the main differences between these populations occur in the frequency of particular variants, it is reasonable to conclude that they belong to the same subspecies. Furthermore, estimates of the average difference between these populations (considering all loci), using the genetic distance measure D, of Nei (1972) yields values of this statistic of the same order of magnitude as those obtained

Table 4. Frequency of enzyme variants in geographically separated populations of *T. b. brucei*

| Enzyme | Variants | Observed numbers | |
		Kenya	Nigeria
TDH	1	4	9
	1–2	8	0
	2	5	0
ALAT	1	17	0
	1–2	0	2
	2	0	5
	2–3	0	1
	3	0	1

The table shows electrophoretic variants of threonine dehydrogenase (TDH) and Alanine aspartate amino-transferase (ALAT) in a series of cloned stocks of *T. b. brucei* isolated from Kiboko, Kenya and from Nigeria. The variants are designated as described by Tait (1980), namely each different number represents a different electrophoretic mobility of the enzyme under study, while numbers linked by a dash indicated hybrid patterns. The observed numbers refer to the number of stocks found to have a particular enzyme electrophoretic pattern.

by similar comparisons of geographically and genetically isolated populations of the same subspecies of other organisms (Ayala *et al.*, 1974; Zimmerman *et al.*, 1978). Similar findings using a somewhat different approach, namely numerical taxonomy, have been made by other authors (Gibson *et al.*, 1980). In these studies, it has been concluded that, within the same subspecies, there is a distinction between East and West African stocks.

Similar enzyme electrophoretic comparisons have been made between *T. b. gambiense* and *T. b. brucei* (Gibson *et al.*, 1980; Mehlitz *et al.*, 1982; Tait *et al.*, 1984). In contrast to the findings with comparisons between geographically isolated populations of the same subspecies, these comparisons show very marked differences in variant frequencies and in the case of one enzyme (PepC) a subspecies specific variant. However, many of the variants are shared between the subspecies; calculation of the genetic distance between *T. b. gambiense* and either of the *T. b. brucei* populations gives values which are of a similar order to those obtained for similar comparisons of subspecies in other organisms and, in addition, 2–3 fold greater than the values obtained between the geographically separated populations of *T. b. brucei*. These findings strongly support the view that *T. b. gambiense* is a distinguishable subspecies of *T. brucei*.

The degree of difference observed between subspecies of *T. brucei* is in marked contrast to that found in the studies of *T. cruzi* (Miles *et al.*, 1977; Miles *et al.*, 1980; Miles *et al.*, 1984). Either by intuitive analysis, examining variants shared or distinct or by measures of genetic distance (Tibayrenc & Miles, 1983; Miles *et al.*, 1984), three very clear and extremely distinct groups or zymodemes of *T. cruzi* are found. The three zymodemes, although having some enzyme electrophoretic types in common, have a large number of enzyme electrophoretic differences. Measurement of the genetic distance of Nei (1972) between the three main Brazilian zymodemes gave values between 1 and 2 orders of magnitude greater than those between *T. b. gambiense* and *T. b. brucei*. Thus, on a relative scale these zymodemes are genetically very distinct; comparisons of *T. cruzi* strains from other geographical areas of S. America confirms the division into three very distinct groups and shows that there is considerable genetic divergence within a group (values of D equivalent to those between subspecies).

The studies discussed here illustrate the application of enzyme electrophoresis to distinguishing between groups of morphologically very similar organisms and to examining the population structure of parasitic protozoa. Despite the inherent difficulties in collecting and growing enough material for analysis, it is clear that such studies have made a major contribution to our understanding of the genetic diversity, population structure and speciation of some of the parasitic protozoa.

DISEASE, HOST AND PARASITE GENOTYPE

The study of protein variation and the measurement of genetic diversity has, in addition to the examination of subspeciation in parasitic protozoa, been used to examine whether different disease symptoms caused by morphologically identical parasites are the result of infection by different parasites and to examine, with parasites which infect a number of mammalian hosts, whether the same group of parasites is found in all hosts. To illustrate some of the results in this field, two examples are considered, firstly *T. b. rhodesiense* and its relationship to *T. b. gambiense* and *T. b. brucei* and, secondly, the relationships between the hosts, vectors and disease caused by different zymodemes of *T. cruzi*. The latter will only be considered briefly due to the enormous complexity of this question, in relation to *T. cruzi*.

The main findings concerning comparisons between *T. b. gambiense*, *T. b. rhodesiense* and *T. b. brucei* and the relationships between different outbreaks of acute, *T. b. rhodesiense* sleeping sickness are derived from the data of Gibson *et al.* (1980), Gibson & Gashumba (1983), Dukes *et al.* (1983) and Tait *et al.* (1985). Comparison of different isolates from man in the same area have shown that the level of interstock variation is low and these stocks appear to represent only a few genotypes. This is in marked contrast to the interstock variation found in isolates from tsetse (Tait, 1980) and non-human hosts (Gibson *et al.*, 1980; Tait *et al.*, 1985). However, the same variants are found both in humans and animals and no 'rhodesiense specific' markers have been identified. Furthermore, comparisons of the genetic distance between *T. b. rhodesiense* (Nyanza) and both of the *T. b. brucei* populations mentioned in the previous section show that *T. b. rhodesiense* is no more distinct from either group of non-human isolates than the two groups of *T. b. brucei* are from each other, although *T. b. rhodesiense* is distinct and a separate subspecies from *T. b. gambiense* (Tait *et al.*, 1984). Comparisons between geographically separated *T. b. rhodesiense* isolates from Zambia and Kenya show (Gibson *et al.*, 1980) that there are minor differences between populations. Thus, it seems clear that *T. b. rhodesiense* constitutes a highly homogeneous group of stocks which are indistinguishable from *T. b. brucei* except by their ability to infect man. Electrophoretic variation in the enzyme alkaline phosphatase has been studied in a single *T. b. rhodesiense* population (Tait *et al.*, 1985) and was found to be heterozygous in all the stocks examined. This observation suggests that either the breeding structure of *T. b. rhodesiense* is different from *T. b. brucei* or that selection (presumably by ability to infect man) is occurring at some closely linked loci. Further analysis is required to establish whether this observation is a general property of *T. b. rhodesiense* and to investigate its genetic basis.

Studies of isolates from animals in West Africa and comparison (by enzyme electrophoresis) of these with isolates from man has established that *T. b. gambiense* occurs in domestic and wild animals (Gibson *et al.*, 1978; Gibson *et al.*, 1980; Scott *et al.*, 1983; Tait *et al.*, 1984). Thus, a reservoir of human infection exists within domestic and game animals, although the significance of such an animal reservoir as a source of human infection remains to be investigated. Studies on enzyme variation (Mehlitz *et al.*, 1982) and restriction enzyme site polymorphism in antigen genes (Pays *et al.*, 1983) of a large number of human isolates from West Africa has shown that such isolates can be divided into two groups; the first group is distinguishable from *T. b. brucei* and *T. b. rhodesiense* by such molecular and biochemical markers, while the second group is indistinguishable from *T. b. rhodesiense/T. b. brucei*. The first group is probably what is classically referred to as *T. b. gambiense* while the identification of the second group suggests that 'rhodesiense-like' trypanosomes occur in West Africa. Further studies are required to confirm these observations more firmly and further '*gambiense* specific' markers would considerably aid such studies.

Overall, the studies on *T. brucei* spp. clearly illustrate the value of protein electrophoretic variation as a means of investigating the existence of animal reservoir hosts, the relationship between parasite genotype and clinical disease and the epidemiology of the human disease. Similar studies have been undertaken to characterize *T. cruzi* by enzyme electrophoresis and to analyse the results in relation to geographical variation, the human disease caused, the species of vector and the species of mammalian host (Miles *et al.*, 1977, 1981a,b, 1984; Barrett *et al.*, 1980; Miles, 1983; Tibayrenc & Desjeux, 1983). Space does not allow the discussion of this work in any detail; in order to illustrate how protein variation can be used to define and understand the relationship between disease, host and parasite genotype some of the findings are discussed below.

The earlier work of Miles and co-workers (Miles *et al.*, 1978) showed that isolates from S.E. Brazil could be divided into three very distinct groups (zymodemes) with a low level of intragroup variation. Surveys of isolates from both man, domestic animals, wild animals and insect vectors, established that one zymodeme (Z2) was found extensively in both chronic and acute Chagas' disease, whereas the two other zymodemes (Z1 and Z3) were rarely found in man and only in acute cases of the disease. Studies of sylvatic animal isolates (and their associated vectors) established that Z3 predominantly occurred in arborial mammals while Z1 was found in various species of burrowing animals. Both zymodemes can infect a wide range of mammalian species and species of the triatome vector and so there is some considerable degree of overlap between these groups in relation to the mammalian species infected. In contrast, the major human zymodeme (Z2) appeared to have no sylvatic source but exclusively infects man and his domestic animals. Further studies of human isolates (Barrett *et al.*, 1980) in the same area of Brazil further confirmed Z1 and Z3 as sources of acute human infection and supported the view that these cases were caused by sylvatic *T. cruzi* stocks 'invading' domestic households.

Since these earlier studies were made, further characterization of a large number of isolates from Bolivia, Chile, and the Amazon Basin in Brazil have been made. A considerable proportion of this work has been directed at defining the relationships between the original Brazilian zymodemes and those found in geographically separate areas (Tibayrenc & Miles, 1983). These studies have shown that there is considerable genetic divergence between different geographical areas but that there are groupings in these other areas related to the original zymodemes. In the studies on isolates from the Amazon basin (Miles *et al.*, 1981a), only zymodemes 1 and 3 were detected, the majority of isolates being from sylvatic animals although cases of acute human disease caused by both zymodemes were found. No evidence for Z2 was found in 123 stocks of *T. cruzi* screened, suggesting that Z2 does not infect sylvatic animals and is confined, excluding imported human cases, to humans and domestic animals in the South. However, zymodemes related to Z2 are found in both Bolivia and Chile (to the West).

Although a wealth of further data are available from these studies, particularly in relation to the vector species and epidemiology of *T. cruzi*, the findings discussed illustrate clearly how the study of protein variation has begun to define the genotypes infective to man, the diversity within a group and the existence and relationships between the domestic and sylvatic cycles of this protozoan.

CONCLUSIONS AND PROSPECTS

In this paper, only a small fraction of the available data on protein variation in parasitic protozoa has been discussed, however, the aim has been to illustrate how such studies, using a few specific examples, have advanced our knowledge of the genetics, speciation, relationship between human infection and parasite genotype, population structure and genetic diversity of these parasites. I think it is abundantly clear that these studies have made important contributions to our knowledge and, more importantly, have shown that biochemical and molecular methods can be used to gain insight into the basic biology and epidemiology of parasitic protozoa in situations where morphological and other criteria are of little use.

One of the major disadvantages of the application of protein electrophoresis to the study of the questions examined in this paper is the requirement for considerable amounts of relatively pure preparations of parasite material and thereby the need for growing the parasites within the laboratory. This means that the number of isolates that can be examined is relatively small making generalized conclusions difficult. Any new methodology which could circumvent this disadvantage would have immense value if it could allow the detection of genetic variation without the need for growth or purification. The isolation of monoclonal antibodies to a range of parasitic protozoa (McMahon-Pratt & David, 1981; McBride, Walliker & Morgan, 1983; Miles, 1983) allows the detection of variation at the single cell level and therefore circumvents the disadvantages of protein electrophoresis. However, a clear relationship between the variation observed with such monoclonals and genetic diversity needs to be established prior to their use, and in particular that the variation in the antigens examined is not due to variation in gene expression rather than structural gene variation. Although, the use of these techniques circumvents some of the disadvantages of protein electrophoresis, it does not circumvent (at least wholly) the lack of sensitivity inherent in examining variation in gene products rather than the genes themselves. The use of DNA probes combined with restriction enzyme digestion of genomic DNA offers greater and more direct detection of genetic diversity; however, growth of the parasites is required to undertake such studies.

In conclusion, although these new techniques are being applied to examine the questions outlined here and offer many advantages over protein electrophoresis, these techniques are not without limitations and do not necessarily offer a panacea. Part of this paper is aimed at trying to develop logical strategies in relation to the parasite material examined so that various relevant questions can be asked. These considerations are applicable independent of the method of detecting gene diversity and therefore it is hoped will be of some general relevance outside protein electrophoresis.

ACKNOWLEDGEMENTS

I would like to express my gratitude to the Wellcome Trust for continued support.

REFERENCES

AL-TAQI, M. & EVANS, D. A., 1978. Characterisation of *Leishmania* spp. from Kuwait by isoenzyme electrophoresis. *Transactions of the Royal Society of Tropical Medicine and Hygiene, 72:* 56–65.
AYALA, F. J., TRACY, M. L., HEDGECOCK, D. & RICHMOND, R. C., 1974. Genetic differentiation during the speciation process in *Drosophila. Evolution, 28:* 576–592.

BARRETT, T. V., HOFF, R. H., MOTT, K. E., MILES, M. A., GODFREY, D. G., TEIXEIRA, R., ALMEIDA DE SOUZA, J. A. & SHERLOCK, I. A., 1980. Epidemiological aspects of three *Trypanosoma cruzi* zymodemes in Bahia State, Brazil. *Transactions of the Royal Society of Tropical Medicine and Hygiene, 74:* 84–90.

BETSCHART, B., MARTI, S., JENNI, L., TAIT, A., WELLS, J. M. & LEPAGE, R., 1984. Unpublished.

CARTER, R., 1973. Enzyme variation in *Plasmodium berghei* and *Plasmodium vinckei*. *Parasitology, 66:*, 297–307.

CARTER, R. and McGREGOR, I. A., 1973. Enzyme variation in *Plasmodium falciparum* in the Gambia. *Transactions of the Royal Society of Tropical Medicine and Hygiene, 67:* 830–837.

CARTER, R. & WALLIKER, D., 1975. New observations on the malaria parasites of rodents of the Central African Republic — *Plasmodium vinckei* subsp. Nov and *Plasmodium chabaudi* Landau, 1965. *Annals of Tropical Medical and Parasitology, 69:* 187–196.

DUKES, P., SCOTT, C. M., RICKMANN, L. R. & WUPARA, F., 1983. Sleeping sickness in the Luangwa Valley of Zambia. A preliminary Report of the 1982 outbreak in Kayasya Village. *Bulletin de le Société Pathologie Experimentale, 76:* 605–613.

FERGUSON, A., 1980. *Biochemical Systematics and Evolution*. Glasgow: Blackie.

GIBSON, W. C. & GASHUMBA, J. K., 1983. Isoenzyme characterization of some *Trypanozoon* stocks from a recent trypanosomiasis epidemic in Uganda. *Transactions of the Royal Society of Tropical Medicine and Hygiene, 77:* 114–118.

GIBSON, W. C., MEHLITZ, D., LANHAM, S. M. & GODFREY, D. G., 1978. Identification of *Trypanosoma brucei gambiense* in Liberian pigs and dogs by isoenzymes and by resistance to human plasma. *Tropenmedizin und Parasitologie, 29:* 335–345.

GIBSON, W. C., MARSHALL, T. F. de C. & GODFREY, D. G., 1980. Numerical analysis of enzyme polymorphism. A new approach to the epidemiology and taxonomy of trypanosomes of the sub-genus Trypanozoon. *Advances in Parasitology, 18:* 175–245.

HARRIS, H. & HOPKINSON, D. A., 1976. *Handbook of Enzyme Electrophoresis in Human Genetics*. Amsterdam: North Holland.

KNOWLES, G., SANDERSON, A. & WALLIKER, D., 1981. *Plasmodium yoelii*: genetic analysis of crosses between two rodent malaria subspecies. *Experimental Parasitology, 52:* 243–247.

KREUTZER, R. D., SEMKO, M. E., HENDRICKS, L. D. & WRIGHT, N., 1983. Identification of *Leishmania* spp. by multiple isoenzyme analysis. *American Journal of Tropical Medicine and Hygiene, 32:* 703–715.

LAINSON, F. A., 1982. Genetic crosses between rodent malaria sub-species. *Parasitology, 84:* xxxii–xxxiii.

LAINSON, R., SHAW, J. J., MILES, M. A. & POVOA, M., 1982. Leishmaniasis in Brazil: XVII Enzymic characterisation of a Leishmania from the armadillo, *Dasypus novenicinctus*, from Pora state. *Transactions of the Royal Society of Tropical Medicine and Hygiene, 76:* 810–811.

LEWONTIN, R., 1974. *The Genetic Basis of Evolutionary Change*. New York: Columbia Press.

McBRIDE, J. S., WALLIKER, D. & MORGAN, G., 1983. Antigenic diversity in the human malaria parasite *Plasmodium falciparum*. *Science, 217:* 254–257.

McMAHON-PRATT, D. & DAVID, J. R., 1981. Monoclonal antibodies that distinguish between New World species of *Leishmania*. *Nature, 291:* 581–583.

MEHLITZ, D., ZILMANN, U., SCOTT, C. M. & GODFREY, D. G., 1982. Epidemiological studies on the animal reservoir of *Gambiense* sleeping sickness. Part III. Characterization of Trypanozoon stocks by iso-enzymes and sensitivity to human serum. *Tropenmedizin und Parasitologie, 33:* 113–118.

MILES, M. A., 1983. The epidemiology of South American Trypanosomiasis-biochemical and immunological approaches and their relevance to control. *Transactions of the Royal Society of Tropical Medicine and Hygiene, 77:* 5–23.

MILES, M., TOYE, P. J., OSWALD, S. C. & GODFREY, D. G., 1977. The identification of isoenzyme patterns of two distinct strain groups of *Trypanosoma cruzi* circulating independently in a rural area Brazil. *Transactions of the Royal Society of Tropical Medicine and Hygiene, 71:* 217–225.

MILES, M. A., SOUZA, A., POVOA, M. & SHAW, P. J., 1978. Isozymic heterogeneity in the first autochthonous patients with Chagas's disease in Amazonia Brazil. *Nature, 272:* 819–821.

MILES, M. A., LANHAM, S. M., SOUZA, A. Ade & POVA, M., 1980. Further enzyme characters of *Trypanosoma cruzi* and their evaluation for strain identification. *Transactions of the Royal Society of Tropical Medicine and Hygiene, 74:* 221–237.

MILES, M. A., POVOA, M. M., DE SOUZA, A. A., LAINSON, R., SHAW, J. J. & KETTERIDGE, D. S., 1981a. Chagas's disease in the Amazon Basin: II. The distribution of *Trypanosoma cruzi* zymodemes 1 and 3 in Para State, North Brazil. *Transactions of the Royal Society of Tropical Medicine and Hygiene, 75:* 667–674.

MILES, M. A., LAINSON, R., SHAW, J. J., POVOA, M. & DE SOUZA, A. A., 1981b. Leishmaniasis in Brazil: XV. Biochemical distinction of *Leishmania mexicana amazonensis*, *Leishmania braziliensis braziliensis* and *Leishmania braziliensis guyanensis* — aetiological agents of cutaneous Leishmaniasis in the Amazon Basin of Brazil. *Transactions of the Royal Society of Tropical Medicine and Hygiene, 75:* 524–529.

MILES, M. A., APT, W., WIDMER, G., POVOA, M. M. & SCHOFIELD, C. J., 1984. Isozyme heterogeneity and numerical taxonomy of *T. cruzi* stocks from Chile. *Transactions of the Royal Society of Tropical Medicine and Hygiene, 78:* 526–535.

NEI, M., 1972. Genetic distances between populations. *American Naturalist, 106:* 283–292.

OCHMAN, H. & SELANDER, R. K., 1984. Evidence for clonal population structure in *Escherichia coli*. *Proceedings of the National Academy of Sciences, U.S.A., 81:* 198–201.

PAYS, E., DEKERCK, P., VAN ASSEL, S., STEINERT, M., LERAY, D. & VAN MEIRVENNE, N., 1983. Comparative analysis of a *T. b. gambiense* antigen gene family and its potential use in epidemiology of sleeping sickness. *Molecular and Biochemical Parasitology, 7:* 63–74.

PFEFFERKORN, L. C. & PFEFFERKORN, E. R., 1980. *Toxiplasma gondii*: Genetic recombination and drug resistance. *Experimental Parasitology, 50:* 305–316.

RASSAM, M. B., AL-MUDHAFFER, S. A. & CHANCE, M. L., 1979. Isozyme characterization of *Leishmania* species from Iraq. *Annals of Tropical Medical Parasitology, 73:* 527–534.

ROLLINSON, D., JOYNER, L. P. & NORTON, C. C., 1979. *Eimeria maxima*: the use of enzyme markers to detect the genetic transfer of drug resistance between lines. *Parasitology, 78:* 361–367.

SCHICK, J. M. & LAMB, A. N., 1977. Asexual reproduction and genetic population structure in the colonising sea anemone *Halipanella luciae*. *Biological Bulletin, 153:* 604–617.

SHIRLEY, M. W. & ROLLINSON, D., 1979. Coccidia: The recognition and characterisation of populations of *Eimeria*. *Symposia of the British Society for Parasitology, 17:* 7–30.

SCOTT, C. M., FREZIL, J-L., TOUDIC, A. & GODFREY, D. G., 1983. The sheep as a potential reservoir of human trypanosomiasis in the Republic of the Congo. *Transactions of the Royal Society of Tropical Medicine and Hygiene, 77:* 397–401.

TAIT, A., 1980. Evidence for mating and diploidy in trypanosomes. *Nature, 287:* 536–537.

TAIT, A., 1981. Analysis of protein variation in *Plasmodium falciparum* by two-dimensional electrophoresis. *Molecular and Biochemical Parasitology, 2:* 205–218.

TAIT, A., 1983. Sexual processes in the kinetoplastida. *Parasitology, 86:* 29–57.

TAIT, A., BABIKER, E. A. & LERAY, D., 1984. Enzyme variation in *Trypanozoma bruceii* spp. I. Evidence for the sub-speciation of *T. b. gambiense*. *Parasitology, 89:* 311–332.

TAIT, A., BARRY, J. D., WINK, R., SANDERSON, A. & CROW, J. S., 1985. Enzyme variation in *T. brucei* spp: II Evidence for *T. b. rhodesiense* being a set of variants of *T. b. brucei*. *Parasitology, 90:* 89–100.

THAITONG, S., SUEBLINWONG, T. & BEALE, G. H., 1981. Enzyme typing of some isolates of *Plasmodium falciparum* from Thailand. *Transactions of the Royal Society of Tropical Medicine and Hygiene, 75:* 268–270.

TIBAYRENC, M. & DESJEUX, P., 1983. The presence in Bolivia of two distinct zymodemes of *Trypanosoma cruzi*, circulating sympatically in a domestic transmission cycle. *Transactions of the Royal Society of Tropical Medicine and Hygiene, 77:* 73–75.

TIBAYRENC, M. & MILES, M. A., 1983. A genetic comparison between Brazilian and Bolivian zymodemes of *Trypanosoma cruzi*. *Transactions of the Royal Society of Tropical Medicine and Hygiene, 77:* 76–83.

TIBAYRENC, M., CARION, M. L., SOLIGNAC, M. & CARLIER, V., 1981. Arguments genetique contre l'existence d'une sexualité actuelle chez *Trypanosoma cruzi*. *Comptes-rendus de l'Academie des Sciences, Paris, 293:* 207–209.

TIBAYRENC, M., ECHALAR, L., DUJARDIN, J. P., POCH, O. & DESJEUX, P., 1984. The microdistribution of isoenzymic strains of *T. cruzi* in Southern Bolivia, new isoenzyme profiles and further arguments against Mendelian sexuality. *Transactions of the Royal Society of Tropical Medicine and Hygiene, 78:* 519–525.

WALLIKER, D., 1983a. *The contribution of genetics to the study of parasitic protozoa*. Letchworth: Research Studies Press Ltd.

WALLIKER, D., 1983b. Enzyme variation in malaria parasite populations. In G. S. Oxford & D. Rollinson (Eds), *Protein Polymorphism: Adaptive and Taxonomic Significance*. Systematics Association Special Volume No. 24: 27–35. London and New York: Academic Press.

WALLIKER, D., CARTER, R. & MORGAN, S., 1973. Genetic recombination in *Plasmodium berghei*. *Parasitology, 66:* 309–320.

WALLIKER, D., CARTER, R. & SANDERSON, A., 1975. Genetic studies on *Plasmodium chabaudi*: recombination between enzyme markers. *Parasitology, 70:* 19–24.

YOUNG, C. J. & GODFREY, D. G., 1983. Enzyme polymorphism and the distribution of *T. congolense* isolates. *Annals of Tropical Medicine and Parasitology, 77:* 467–481.

ZIMMERMANN, E. G., KILPATRICK, C. W. & HART, B. J., 1978. The genetics of speciation in the rodent genus *Peromyscus*. *Evolution, 32:* 565–579.

Genetic resistance to *Plasmodium falciparum*: studies in the field and in cultures *in vitro*

L. LUZZATTO, E. A. USANGA AND G. MODIANO*

Department of Haematology, Royal Postgraduate Medical School, Ducane Road, London W12 0HS, and
*Istituto di Genetica, Citta Universitaria, 00185, Roma

Species of the genus *Plasmodium* are protozoal parasites with a complex life cycle. Different species infect a variety of vertebrate hosts including reptiles, birds and mammals. There is considerable evidence that *Plasmodium falciparum*, the most lethal of the human parasites, has played a significant role in human evolution by selecting host resistance genes which are now polymorphic in many human populations living in malaria-endemic areas. In this paper, we discuss two examples. (1) The Tharu population of the Terai valley of Southern Nepal have had a historical reputation for a capacity to survive in that heavily malarious area which was not inhabitable by other population groups. Subsequent to malaria control measures having been instituted, we have gathered epidemiologic evidence that residual cases of malaria are six times less frequent in Tharu people when compared to sympatric non-Tharus. We also have preliminary *in vitro* evidence that relative resistance against *P. falciparum* may be due to a lower invasion rate of host red blood cells. (2) Females heterozygous for glucose 6-phosphate dehydrogenase (G6PD) deficiency are known to have relatively lower *P. falciparum* parasitaemias than either normal or G6PD-deficient hemizygous males. We now show that *P. falciparum* can adapt *in vitro* to G6PD-deficient red cells. This explains both the successful parasite cycle in G6PD-deficient individuals and the impaired growth in heterozygotes, who are genetic mosaics as a result of X-chromosome inactivation.

KEY WORDS:—Malaria—glucose 6-phosphate dehydrogenase—*Plasmodium falciparum*—host-parasite interaction—red cell genetics—balanced polymorphism—X-chromosome.

CONTENTS

INTRODUCTION

Numerous examples of host–parasite interactions in a variety of biological systems are presented in this volume. For those who are interested in *human* biology, and every practising physician should be, the burning question is of course how far

Ecology and Genetics of Host–Parasite Interactions
ISBN: 0 12 593 690 7

the concepts involved are relevant to human populations today. Fortunately, through the foresight and insight of some pioneers of human genetics and evolution, it is already clear that the answer is that they are highly relevant. Indeed, selection of particular genotypes by the malaria parasite has become a textbook item by now (Cavalli-Sforza & Bodmer, 1971). However, for all our enthusiasm about population genetics and population dynamics related to balanced polymorphism, we have really only begun to glimpse at the underlying mechanisms, as opposed to having merely a description of these systems. This paper summarizes our attempts to analyse the host–parasite interaction in at least one polymorphic system, and reports on what is possibly a new finding in the genetics of malaria resistance, which may be characteristic of a unique population perhaps through the action of a unique gene.

The world distribution of malaria has changed little in recent years. Some major successes in malaria control were scored in certain parts of the world both before and after World War II, but, subsequently, a variety of social, political and economic as well as biological constraints have drastically limited further progress in this battle (Wernsdorfer, 1983).

In spite of the high rate of malaria transmission, and the very high mortality and morbidity toll that this entails, all these malaria areas are populated, and some of them very heavily so. This indicates that some sort of balance between the host and the parasite does exist. An illustration of how this comes about can be given by the age-dependence of malaria parasitaemia in an hyperendemic area (Fig. 1). It can be seen that parasitaemia falls sharply during the first 5 years of life, suggesting that some form of acquired resistance develops. We now know that, contrary to previous beliefs, immune mechanisms play a very important and complex role in the development of this resistance. We can also infer that genetic factors, at least in hyperendemic areas, would be of importance primarily during this phase of life. Basically, a genetic resistance factor will be selected for if it can enable the individual to survive until acquired immunity has had a chance to develop.

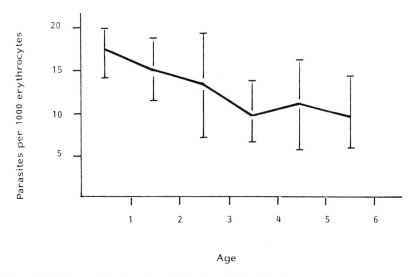

Figure 1. Malaria as a function of age in Nigerian children. Median parasite densities. Vertical bars indicate 95% confidence limits (from Bienzle *et al.*, 1981).

Table 1. Genetics of host and susceptibility to malaria parasites

Form of parasite	Site of resistance	Possible mechanism of relative resistance which may be subject to genetic variation	Evidence of genetic variation in resistance
Sporozoites	Blood	Destruction by antibodies	None
	Liver	Impeded penetration of hepatocytes	None
Cryptomerozoites and cryptoschizonts	Liver	Impeded reproduction or survival in hepatocytes	None
Merozoites	Blood plasma	Destruction by antibodies	Likely
Trophozoites	Erythrocytes	Impeded penetration	Possible
and schizonts	Erythrocytes	Impeded reproduction or survival within red cells	
	Blood plasma	Destruction by antibodies	Likely
	R.E. system	Increased ability to remove parasitized red cells	Likely
Various forms	Immuno-competent cells	Cellular mediated immunity (macrophage activation?)	Possible

In principle, resistance against the malaria parasite could depend on genetic variations in a variety of cells and tissues (Table 1). However, so far, what we know is limited to erythrocyte genes (reviewed by Luzzatto, 1979). This is not surprising, since the main pathology associated with human malaria, which eventually kills the patient, is due to the rapidly expanding parasite population produced by the schizogonic cycle which goes on in red cells. The well-known protective effect of the haemoglobin S gene in AS heterozygotes characteristically occurs in the age group of 2–5 years (Gilles, 1964). Subsequently, there is little difference in parasitaemia between AA and AS individuals. Those who survive have developed acquired immunity. Interestingly, there is evidence that in areas with less severe malaria, the AS heterozygote advantage may actually be prolonged into adult life (Fleming, 1981).

A system which may be regarded as at least equally important in malaria resistance is that of glucose 6-phosphate dehydrogenase (G6PD). This enzyme plays a key role in the metabolism of red cells and other cells, and current biochemical evidence indicates that this role is primarily with respect to protection from oxidative damage. Most cells are exposed to peroxide and other activated oxygen radicals and the main mechanism for detoxifying peroxides is through glutathione peroxidase. This enzyme depends on supply of GSH, the regeneration of which relies on glutathione reductase, and this in turn depends on a steady supply of NADPH, which is largely provided by G6PD. In man, G6PD is characterized by a tremendous amount of genetic variability, with at least 300 different variants already known; and by a great deal of polymorphism, since at least 30 of the allelic genes underlying such variants do have polymorphic frequencies (up to 30%) in a variety of human populations (Luzzatto & Battistuzzi, 1984). Some years ago, Bienzle *et al.* (1972) showed by field work in Nigeria that the G6PD genotype was important in determining the severity of *Plasmodium falciparum* parasitaemia. This system, however, differs from the haemoglobin S system in that G6PD is an X-linked gene and the relative protection against malaria turned out to be a prerogative of heterozygous females. These are genetic mosaics, as a result of X-chromosome inactivation; in heterozygotes, there was a marked difference in the parasite rate of the G6PD-normal and of the G6PD-deficient red cells, with the latter having much lower numbers of parasites (Luzzatto, Usanga & Reddy,

208   L. LUZZATO *ET AL.*

1969). Thus, hemizygous males with only G6PD-deficient red cells were not protected, whereas heterozygous females with a mixed cell population were. This paradox will be dealt with later.

MALARIA IN THE THARU POPULATION OF NEPAL

In contrast to the well characterized situation of stable hyperendemic malaria in S.W. Nigeria, which probably has changed little over centuries or perhaps millennia, a very different situation obtains in the Kingdom of Nepal in central Asia (Fig. 2). From the geographic point of view, this country is divided into the mountainous areas in the North, the Himalaya ranges, and the plains in a vast Southern territory which is known as the Terai. This area was bedevilled by very severe malaria: so much so, that it was traditionally regarded by most people as practically uninhabitable. It was accepted that only one particular population, called the Tharu, regarded by classical anthropology as of Mongolian stock, could survive in this inhospitable land. There is documented evidence that military leaders and anthropologists had difficulties in exploring this area because of rampant malaria, and attempts to settle other people in the territory were abandoned because of the high rate of malaria mortality. Since the early 1960s, the Nepalese Malaria Eradication Organization (NMEO), with assistance from the World Health Organization and the London School of Hygiene and Tropical Medicine, has embarked on a campaign for malaria control which has been largely successful (see Table 2), especially thanks to complete elimination of the vector, *Anopheles minimus* (White, 1982). Indeed, since the late 1970s, the situation has been one of 'residual cases' only, and this consists now more of imported than of indigenous

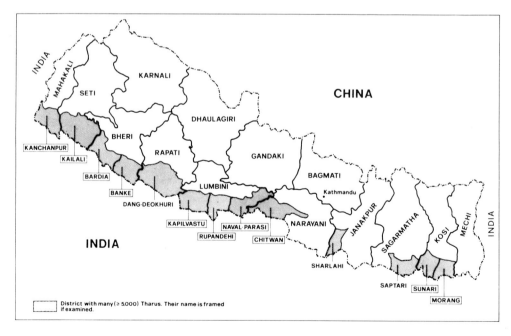

Figure 2. Map of Nepal showing the area inhabited by the Tharus.

Table 2. Malaria control in the Terai*

Year	Parasite rate in children %
Pre-1956	69
1959–60	38
1975	$\simeq 0.5$

*Data in Tables 2–4 have been compiled from the records of the Nepal Malaria Eradication Organization through the kindness of Dr S. Shrestha (see Terrenato et al., 1985).

Table 3. Sample data on malaria epidemiology in the Terai*

Year	Cases/100 000	
	P. vivax	P. falciparum
1975	164	56
1976	135	40
1977	152	30
1978	160	17
1979	146	18
1980	147	10

*See Table 2.

cases. *Plasmodium vivax* malaria prevalence has reached a plateau at the low level of approximately 150 cases per 100 000 per year, whereas the number of cases of *P. falciparum* is still declining (Table 3).

As a result of this largely successful campaign, the Terai has become, for the first time, an attractive agricultural land not only for the Tharu but also for non-Tharu. Today, these people live side-by-side in this area and, in many villages, a mixed population is found.

This unique epidemiological situation made it possible to test directly whether the previously claimed innate resistance of Tharus against malaria was an anthropological myth or a reality. We were very fortunate in obtaining the collaboration of Dr Shrestha of the NMEO, who made available to us the very extensive records of that programme. Table 4 shows that in five districts with a

Table 4. Incidence of malaria in sample areas in the Terai*

Area	Cases/100 000	
	Non-Tharu	Tharu
Kanchanpur	610	101
Kailali	360	10
Rupandehi	250	47
Chitwan	99	45
Sunari	115	7

*See Table 2.

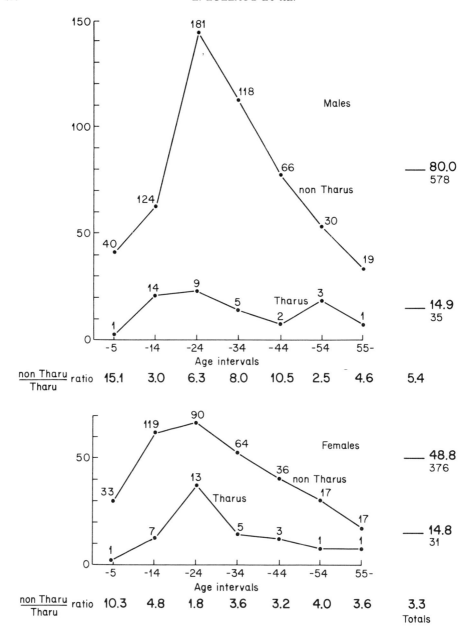

Figure 3. Age dependence of incidence of indigenous cases of *P. vivax* malaria. Under each panel the age specific non-Tharu/Tharu ratios are given. Figures on graphs indicate the absolute numbers of malaria cases.

mixed population, the frequency of residual cases in Tharus was lower by an average factor of about 6 compared with non-Tharus. It is pertinent to note that this is an hypoendemic area. Thus, the possibility that this difference might be due to the Tharus becoming more rapidly or more effectively immunized as a result of repeated attacks, becomes unlikely. Indeed, we have recently shown that the difference holds true even in the very young age groups, i.e. in children born after most of the control programme had already taken place (Fig. 3).

(a)

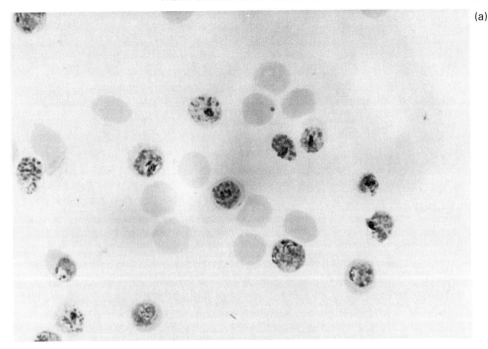

(b)

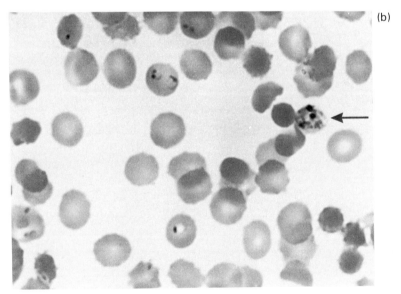

Figure 4. Photomicrograph of *P. falciparum* in culture in G6PD(+) and G6PD(–) red cells. *Top:* schizonts in G6PD(+) red cells showing normal morphology with the characteristic pigments. *Bottom:* parasites in G6PD(–) red cells showing morphologically abnormal schizont (arrowed). Merozoites invasion of G6PD(–) red cells and their subsequent development to trophozoites appears normal in G6PD(–) red cells. The major schizogonic lesion in these cells is at the trophozoite→schizont stage.

The availability of an *in vitro* system for the culture of *P. falciparum* made it possible to test whether difference in malaria susceptibility between Tharus and non-Tharus could be revealed at the level of the red cells. Samples were collected in the field and cultures set up within 48 h of collection. Figure 4 shows that there was no

absolute resistance of red cells to invasion by *P. falciparum*. Indeed, successful
infection *in vitro* was obtained in all cases. The second important point was technical:
there seemed to be absolutely no problem with the collection and transportation
of the samples since the average invasion rate obtained for non-Tharu controls
was identical to that of local (London) controls. On the other hand, the distribution
of parasite invasion rate in the Tharu red cells was significantly shifted towards
lower levels. Interestingly, when the further development of trophozoites and
schizonts from the young rings was followed up, no difference at all was apparent
in these aspects of the schizogonic cycle. Thus, the difference between red cells
seems to be specifically at the stage of invasion, suggesting a possible difference
in the membrane or in some process associated with parasite penetration. This
indicated clearly where to look in further attempts to pinpoint the site of genetic
difference.

MECHANISM OF PROTECTION IN G6PD HETEROZYGOTES

The availability of *in vitro* cultures gives us also an opportunity to go back to
the paradox outlined earlier regarding G6PD. Attempts to infect G6PD-deficient
red cells *in vitro* were again successful. Indeed, quite contrary to what has just been
reported for the Tharu people, invasion of G6PD(–) red cells at the ring stage
was normal: however, the morphology of trophozoites and schizonts was abnormal
(Fig. 4). When the cultures were followed up and the yield of parasites after a whole
cycle in G6PD-deficient cells assessed, there was an inhibition of growth of just
over 50% (Table 5). It is noteworthy that, in spite of this relatively low yield of
parasites, the cycle could be completed within these cells. (In the terminology of
classical genetics, the G6PD(–) mutation is leaky for parasite-resistance.) We
therefore asked the question as to what would be the fate of those parasites that
have survived further transfer to G6PD(–) cells. In fact, we were able to obtain
continuous cultures of *P. falciparum* in G6PD-deficient cells, and this made it possible
to compare the efficiency of parasite development in G6PD-deficient cells starting
from G6PD-normal cells and from G6PD-deficient cells (Table 6). The difference
observed indicates that after a number of cycles, parasites have developed the ability
to grow as successfully in these G6PD(–) cells as they do in normal cells.
Descriptively, this may be regarded as an adaptive phenomenon and we shall refer
to these parasites as adapted to G6PD-deficient red cells.

What could be the mechanism of adaptation? It is possible that adaptation is
related to G6PD itself. There has been some controversy as to whether *P. falciparum*

Table 5. Impaired growth of *P.
falciparum* in G6PD deficient red cells*

Parasites at 48 h	% of control
A –	Med.
46	41
38	53
42	48
41	45

*E. A. Usanga & L. Luzzatto (unpublished).

Table 6. Growth of *P. falciparum in vitro* depends on G6PD status of donor and recipient erythrocytes*

Type of transfer	Efficiency of transfer		
	Rings/1000 red cells at 24 h	Schizonts/1000 red cells at 50 h	Total parasites/1000 red cells at 75 h
G6PD(+)→G6PD(+)	24	8.9	85
G6PD(+)→G6PD(−)	26	4.5	53
G6PD(−)→G6PD(−)	25	9.8	87

*From Luzzatto *et al.* (1983)

produces its own G6PD (see Hempelmann & Wilson, 1981). If it does, it must be very little, especially since the related enzyme, 6-phosphogluconate dehydrogenase, has been demonstrated in the same parasite quite easily by both cytochemical and electrophoretic techniques (Carter & Walliker, 1977).

A specific model might be as follows. When *P. falciparum* is in a G6PD-normal red cell, it somehow can make use of the host cell enzyme and it produces none or very little of its own. When it is transferred to G6PD-deficient red cells, the scarcity of this enzyme is detrimental to parasite growth, and many parasites fail to develop and die. At the same time, this environment perhaps acts as a signal for the derepression of the parasite's own gene for G6PD. Thus, a parasite-coded enzyme begins to be made, but the lag in this derepression phenomenon explains the need of several cycles for complete adaptation. This model predicts (Fig. 5) that a parasite-coded G6PD would be found in parasitized G6PD(−) red cells but not in parasitized G6PD(+) red cells. Indeed, in extracts of G6PD-deficient A − red cells, we have been able to demonstrate the presence of two bands of G6PD activity. One migrates like the host red cell enzyme and the other migrates with a slower mobility which happens to coincide with that of the normal red cell enzyme B. Thus, we have evidence that the adaptation phenomenon, as demonstrated by continuous *in vitro* culture, is associated with the production of a novel type of G6PD.

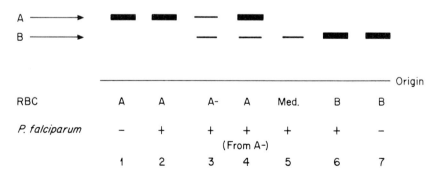

Figure 5. G6PD electrophoretic pattern of lysates of G6PD(+) and G6PD(−) red cells parasitized by *P. falciparum*. Lysates of parasitized G6PD-normal red cells migrate like their corresponding host cell lysates (lanes 1 and 2, and lanes 6 and 7). Although lysate of parasitized G6PD Mediterranean variant migrates like that of the host (lane 5), the host cell lysate had undetectable activity on electrophoresis. Lysate of parasitized G6PD A − red cells shows two G6PD activity bands; one in the same position as the host band, and a slow band in the B position (lane 3). The slow band in parasitized G6PD A − is still detectable when parasites are transferred from A − cells to G6PD A red cells (lane 4). This parasite-specific band disappears after one schizogonic cycle in the new A host cell.

This enzyme remains to be characterized and this task will be very difficult because of the very small amounts involved. What we have already shown is that no such enzyme band is seen when the parasites are grown in G6PD A normal red cells.

CONCLUSION

Complex interactions between two organisms are the landmark of symbiosis and of parasitism, and they are bound to be especially intimate in the case of intracellular parasitism. No matter how remote the phylogenetic relationships between the two organisms may be, it is suggestive that at some stage and to a certain extent the two have co-evolved. Among human parasites, *Plasmodium falciparum* has been extremely successful in its evolutionary adaptation to the host. For instance, *P. vivax* relies for erythrocyte penetration on the Duffy 'receptor', which may be genetically absent without any harm to the host cell. By contrast, *P. falciparum* seems to require for penetration only membrane components that are not dispensable and, consequently, red cells that are totally refractory to infection have not yet been discovered. On the other hand, the host has also evolved and widened the pressure of the parasite, and genetically determined quantitative variations in susceptibility to *P. falciparum* are highly prevalent in many populations. Such genetic variation may affect the penetration, or the growth, or the ultimate disposal of the parasite. While these resistance factors have been historically crucial for survival in malarious areas, they help us today to analyze the biology of *Plasmodium*, and they may also suggest ways to control the parasite cycle in the interest of public health.

REFERENCES

BIENZLE, U., AYENI, O., LUCAS, A. O. & LUZZATTO, L., 1972. Glucose-6-phosphate dehydrogenase and malaria. Greater resistance of females heterozygous for enzyme deficiency and of males with non-deficient variant. *Lancet, i:* 107–110.

BIENZLE, U., GUGGENMOOS-HOLZMANN, I. & LUZZATTO, L., 1981. *Plasmodium falciparum* malaria and human red cells. I. A genetic and clinical study in children. *International Journal of Epidemiology, 10:* 9–15.

CARTER, R. & WALLIKER, D., 1977. Biochemical markers for strain differentiation in malarial parasites. *Bulletin of the World Health Organization, 55:* 339–345.

CAVALLI-SFORZA, L. L. & BODMER, W. F., 1971. *The Genetics of Human Populations*, San Francisco: W. H. Freeman and Company.

GILLES, H. M., 1964. *Akufo: An Environmental Study of a Nigerian Village Community*. Ibadan: Ibadan University Press.

FLEMING, A. F., 1981. Haematological manifestations of malaria and other parasitic diseases. *Clinics in Haematology, 10:* 983–1011.

HEMPELMANN, E. & WILSON, R. J. M., 1981. Detection of glucose-6-phosphate dehydrogenase in malarial parasites. *Molecular Biochemistry and Parasitology, 2:* 197–204.

LUZZATTO, L., 1979. Genetics of red cells and susceptibility to malaria. *Blood, 54:* 961–976.

LUZZATTO, L. & BATTISTUZZI, G., 1984. Glucose-6-phosphate dehydrogenase. Chapter 4, *Advances in Human Genetics, 14:* 217–329.

LUZZATTO, L., USANGA, E. A. & REDDY, S., 1969. Glucose-6-phosphate dehydrogenase deficient red cells: resistance to infection by malarial parasites. *Science, 164:* 839–842.

LUZZATTO, L., SODEINDE, O. & MARTINI, G., 1983. Genetic variation in the host and adaptive phenomena in *Plasmodium falciparum* infection. In *Malaria and the Red Cell*: 159-173. Ciba Foundation Symposium 94, London: Pitman.

TERRENATO, L., SHRESTHA, S., PARAJULI, M., LUZZATTO, L., MODIANO, G., MORPURGO, G. & ARESE, P., 1985. Decreased malaria morbidity in the Tharu people compared to sympatric populations in Nepal. *Bulletin of the World Health Organization* (submitted for publication).

WERNSDORFER, W. H., 1983. Paludisme pharmacorésistant: situation d'urgence. *Chronique de l'Organisation Mondiale de la Santé, 37:* 12–15.

WHITE, G. B., 1982. Malaria vector ecology and genetics. *British Medical Bulletin, 38:* 207–212.

The gene-for-gene hypothesis: parable or paradigm

JOHN BARRETT

Department of Genetics,
University of Cambridge,
Downing Street, Cambridge CB2 3EH, U.K.

This paper discusses the extent to which gene-for-gene relationships are typical of plant host–parasite interactions and examines the argument that such relationships may be a consequence of the plant breeding process and the cultivation of resistant varieties.

KEY WORDS: — Gene-for-gene hypothesis — plant pathogens — plant breeding — disease resistance

CONTENTS

Parable:
"Fictitious narrative used to typify moral or spiritual relations" (*Concise Oxford Dictionary*)

Paradigm:
". . . accepted examples of actual scientific practice . . . (which) . . . provide models from which spring particular coherent traditions of scientific research." (Thomas S. Kuhn: *The Structure of Scientific Revolutions*)

INTRODUCTION

Flor's description of complementary genetic systems in flax (*Linum usititattissimum*) and its fungal parasite *Melampsora lini* is possibly one of the most important events in the development of ideas about plant host–parasite interactions and the epidemiology of disease in crops. The gene-for-gene hypothesis has become familiar to many biologists outside plant pathology as interest in co-evolutionary processes has grown over the last few years. This paper attempts to review, briefly, the

Ecology and Genetics of Host-Parasite Interactions
ISBN: 0 12 593 690 7

evidence for gene-for-gene interactions, and their role in the evolution of plant host–parasite systems.

In a series of papers, Flor (1956, for review) reported the results of experiments in which he crossed cultivars which were either resistant or susceptible to different strains of the flax rust fungus and simultaneously crossed the rust strains which were either virulent or avirulent on each of the flax cultivars. Table 1 shows the results of one such experiment. The cultivar Ottawa was susceptible to race 21 but resistant to race 22; Bombay was resistant to race 21 but susceptible to race 22. By turning the data around, it can be seen that race 21 was avirulent on Bombay but virulent on Ottawa and race 22 was virulent on Bombay but avirulent on Ottawa.

Table 1

| Race | Host crosses | | | | | | |
	Ottawa	Bombay	F1	F2			
21	S	R	R	R	S	R	S
22	R	S	R	R	R	S	S
				110	32	43	9

| Variety | Parasite crosses | | | | | | |
| | Race | | F1 | F2 | | | |
	21	22					
Ottawa	V	A	A	A	V	A	V
Bombay	A	V	A	A	A	V	V
				78	27	23	5

In crosses between Ottawa and Bombay, it was found that the F1 was resistant to both race 21 and 22. In the F2, the contrasting characters observed in the parental lines segregated 9/16 resistant to both races of the rust, 3/16 resistant to race 21 but susceptible to race 22, 3/16 susceptible to race 21 but resistant to race 22 and 1/16 susceptible to both races. In crosses between races 21 and 22, the F1 was unable to attack either variety. The F2 segregated 9/16 avirulent on either variety, 3/16 virulent on Ottawa but avirulent on Bombay, 3/16 virulent on Bombay but avirulent on Ottawa and 1/16 with virulence for both cultivars. From these and many similar results, he was able to conclude that:

(1) Resistance to a rust race was inherited at a single locus with resistance dominant to susceptibility.

(2) Virulence was inherited at a single locus with avirulence dominant to virulence.

Combining these two conclusions, he argued that the two genetic systems were complementary and summarized his results as the 'gene-for-gene' hypothesis: 'for each gene conditioning rust reaction in the host there is a specific gene conditioning pathogenicity in the parasite' (Flor, 1956).

Since then, the gene-for-gene hypothesis has become a cornerstone in the study of host–parasite interactions in plant pathology. As a result of Flor's pioneering work, many other systems showing 'race-specific' resistance have been investigated and gene-for-gene interaction sought; for example, Moseman's work on the barley-powdery mildew system (Moseman, 1959). The most recent list of gene-for-gene interactions has been given by Vanderplank (1982), although the list is derived primarily from Day (1974) (Table 2). (In a recent paper, Michelmore *et al.* (1984) have described a gene-for-gene interaction in the *Bremia latucae/Latuca sativa* (lettuce) system).

Table 2. List of gene-for-gene interactions (after Day, 1974 and Vanderplank, 1982)

Rusts:	Linum — *Melampsora lini*
	Zea — *Puccinia sorghi*
	Triticum — *Puccinia graminis tritici*
	Triticum — *Puccinia striiformis*
	Triticum — *Puccinia recondita*
	Avena — *Puccinia graminis avenae*
	Helianthus — *Puccinia helianthi*
	Coffea — *Hemileia vastatrix*
Smuts:	Triticum — *Ustilago tritici*
	Avena — *Ustilago avenae*
	Hordeum — *Ustilago hordei*
Bunts:	Triticum — *Tilletia caries*
	Triticum — *Tilletia contraversa*
	Triticum — *Tilletia foetida*
Mildews:	Hordeum — *Erysiphe graminis hordei*
	Triticum — *Erysiphe graminis tritici*
Other fungi:	Malus — *Venturia inaequalis*
	Solanum — *Phytophthora infestans*
	Lycopersicon — *Cladosporium fulvum*
	Solanum — *Synchrytrium endobioticum*
Nematodes:	Solanum — *Heterodera rostochiensis*
Insects:	Triticum — *Mayetolia destructor*
Bacteria:	Gossypium — *Xanthomonas malvacearum*
	Leguminosae — *Rhizobium*
Viruses:	Lycopersicon — TMV
	Lycopersicon — spotted wilt
	Solanum — potato virus X

HOW MANY HOST–PARASITE SYSTEMS UNEQUIVOCALLY SHOW GENE-FOR-GENE INTERACTIONS?

Even a cursory examination of Table 2 will reveal that all of the systems listed involve a cultivated host species. In the 28 which Vanderplank lists, there are only 12 host species and nine of the interactions included are between wheat and various of its parasites. In some cases, the demonstration of a clear-cut difference between resistant and susceptible host lines, and a corresponding all-or-nothing ability of some pathogen strains to infect has been interpreted as a demonstration of a gene-for-gene interaction, even in the absence of genetic evidence from one or other of the organisms. For example, *Hemileia vastatrix* has no known sexual stage and no genetic studies have been carried out on it and yet it is included in the list. Note also that *Rhizobium* is included in the list; despite an apparent specificity of strains for different host species and cultivars, and intensive work on the molecular biology of the symbiosis, no complementary genetic systems have yet been demonstrated (Beringer, 1983). Indeed, in Day's original list, nine of the systems are listed as only possibilities, but Vanderplank does not differentiate between those demonstrated and those suggested.

One of the problems in composing any list is that it draws attention to the contents of the list, not to items which are not included in it. To put this in perspective, it is only necessary to consider the number of pathogenic organisms which can produce disease in or on a single plant species. For example, a practical guide to cereal diseases in the U.K. lists 21 fungal pathogens of economic importance on barley alone (Gair, Jenkins & Lester, 1972). Some of these diseases show specificity for varieties, e.g. *Erysiphe graminis*, some show species specificity, e.g. *Septoria nodorum*, and some show no detectable specificity, e.g. *Claviceps purpurea*. Plant host–parasite systems show the whole range of possible interactions one could hope to dream up and at one end of the spectrum are the gene-for-gene interactions. In concentrating attention on this small group, it is too easy to forget that there are many interactions which do not behave in this way.

The wild relatives of some crop species, e.g. *Hordeum spontaneum*, *Avena sterilis*, have been investigated for variation in resistance using isolates of a pathogen known to be pathogenic for different resistance genes in the cultivated species. Conversely, variation in pathogenicity in wild parasites has been investigated by testing isolates on cultivars known to carry different resistance genes (e.g. Wahl, 1970; Wahl *et al.*, 1978; Dinoor, 1977). From the phenotypes observed in such tests inferences have been made about the presence or absence of resistance or virulence genes but it would appear that no-one has yet reported a rigorous genetic analysis of a wild host–parasite system. On the other hand, the obvious commercial importance of crop species has meant that there has been a concentration of effort on cultivated species, making it more likely that genetic phenomena would be uncovered in cultivated species.

DO PLANT GENE-FOR-GENE INTERACTIONS
SHOW A STRICT ONE-FOR-ONE RELATIONSHIP?

When Flor proposed the gene-for-gene hypothesis, it was on the basis of two alleles at a single locus in both host and parasite, with resistance dominant to susceptibility and virulence recessive to avirulence and it is in this form that it is generally presented, i.e. the interactions will be built up from a series of diallelic complementary loci.

Perhaps the most extensive genetic analysis of any plant host–parasite system has been that carried out by Mayo, Shepherd and their colleagues on the flax–flax rust system pioneered by Flor. In their most recent publications (e.g. Lawrence, Mayo & Shepherd, 1981a; Lawrence, Shepherd & Mayo, 1981b) they report that a total of 29 resistance genes has been identified and that these fall into five recombination groups. In the rust, they have evidence for 24 genes controlling pathogenicity which matches resistance genes. They have tested 19 of these virulence genes and find that they fall into four recombination groups (Table 3), which, while showing consistency with the resistance gene groupings, are not identical to them. They have not reported any recombination between pathogenic characters inherited

Table 3. Present status of flax/flax rust system (Source: Lawrence *et al.*, 1981a,b)

29 Resistance genes identified in 5 'allelic' groups				
K	L	M	N	P
1	13	7	3	5

24 Matching pathogenic phenotypes identified of which
19 have been tested for segregation:
      14 show avirulence dominant to virulence
       5 show interaction with a second locus such that only genotypes iiAa and iiAA express pathogenicity.
      Genes controlling pathogenicity fall into 4 groups

in the same group because progeny sizes tend to be small, less than 200, and detection of close linkage will be difficult. Similarly, the *Mla* locus in cultivated barley has multiple 'alleles' for resistance to powdery mildew. But there is evidence that powdery mildew can combine virulence for different cultivars carrying different *Mla* resistance alleles. This suggests that virulence for each *Mla* allele is inherited independently. Whilst more complex systems such as these do not violate the spirit of the gene-for-gene hypothesis, the intriguing question of what is meant by a 'gene' in this context is raised.

Notwithstanding this problem, the gene-for-gene hypothesis implies that that however inherited, resistance genes will be matched on a one-for-one basis by single factors controlling pathogenicity in the parasite. In recent reviews, Person, Christ & Pope (in press) and Christ (1984) have surveyed the literature of the inheritance of resistance and pathogenicity. They cite five systems in which resistance is controlled by two loci, but it is not clear how many loci are involved in the pathogen (Table 4); all of these systems are included in Day's list (Table 2). On the other hand, they refer to six systems in which pathogenicity for resistance controlled by a single locus is matched by two loci in the pathogen. Lest it be forgotten that both resistance and pathogenicity can be inherited as quantitative characters, Person *et al.* list examples of both. It should be also noted that the genetic analysis of obligate plant parasites is difficult and quantitative genetic analysis doubly so. Consequently, the number of rigorous quantitative genetic investigations is very limited and this of itself adds to the impression that host–parasite interactions are controlled by simple genetic systems.

There has been a steadily accumulating literature over the last few years of interactions between loci and the effects of genetic background on the expression of resistance and pathogenicity characters. In the barley-powdery mildew system, which shows a classic gene-for-gene interaction, pathogen phenotypes can easily be isolated which are pathogenic on varieties carrying resistance genes singly or in combination. Within a group of varieties nominally carrying the same resistance gene(s), specialization of different mildew isolates to each variety can be discerned. Indeed, Wolfe, Barrett & Jenkins (1981) have been able to demonstrate that the magnitude of this effect is sufficient to reduce levels of disease in mixed stands of barley varieties with the same resistance gene(s) in exactly the same way that a mixture of varieties with different resistance genes can reduce disease. Chin & Wolfe (in press) have demonstrated that where mildew isolates can attack two varieties with different resistance genes, the mildew isolates can still show specificity for the variety from which they were originally isolated. Data such as these show that specificity can occur at a genetic level other than that controlled by major resistance or virulence genes.

Table 4

Recessive resistance

Triticum — *Puccinia striiformis*
Triticum — *Puccinia graminis tritici*
Triticum — *Puccinia recondita*
Avena — *Puccinia graminis avenae*
Zea — *Puccinia sorghi*
Hordeum — *Ustilago hordei*

Dominant pathogenicity

Puccinia graminis tritici — Triticum
Puccinia graminis avenae — Avena
Puccinia coronata — Avena
Melampsora lini — Linum
Uromyces phaseoli — Phaseolus
Ustilago hordei — Hordeum

Control by two genes

Resistance
Hordeum — *Ustilago nuda*
Triticum — *Puccinia graminis tritici*
Triticum — *Puccinia recondita*
Avena — *Puccinia graminis avenae*
Avena — *Puccinia coronata*

Pathogenicity
Puccinia graminis tritici — Triticum
Puccinia recondita — Triticum
Puccinia graminis avenae — Avena
Melampsora lini — Linum
Uromyces phaseoli — Phaseolus
Ustilago hordei — Hordeum

Systems in which polygenic inheritance has been shown

Resistance
Triticum — *Puccinia striiformis*
Triticum — *Puccinia graminis tritici*
Triticum — *Puccinia recondita*
Avena — *Puccinia coronata*
Hordeum — *Puccinia hordei*
Solanum — *Phyophthora infestans*
Zea — *Cochliobolus carbonum*
Brassica — *Leptosphaeria maculans*

Pathogenicity
Ustilago hordei — Hordeum
Ustilago maydis — Zea
Ceratocystis ulmi — Ulmus
Gaeumannomyces graminis tritici — Triticum

ARE DOMINANCE RELATIONSHIPS ALWAYS AS DESCRIBED BY FLOR?

It has become part of the conventional wisdom of the study of plant host–parasite systems, that resistance and avirulence are dominant. Indeed, complex arguments about the nature of the biochemical and molecular basis of host–parasite interactions have been built up on this assumption (e.g. Ellingboe, 1982; Vanderplank, 1978). That this 'rule' should have become so widely accepted is all the more surprising when the literature is consulted. In one of the earliest papers on the inheritance of disease resistance, Biffen (1905) reported recessive resistance to yellow rust in wheat. Person *et al.* (in press) list six host–parasite systems in which recessive resistance has been reported. Luig and Rajaram (1971) have reported the results of tests on segregating wheat lines and showed that the expression of resistance in heterozygotes (i.e. dominance) depended on the genetic background of the wheat line and the environmental conditions under which the tests were carried out. The fact remains, however, that, in general, resistance does tend to be dominant but there are reasons to believe that it is probably more due to the activities of plant breeders than any intrinsic properties of the character itself.

The investigation of dominance relations in plant pathogens is based on an extremely small number of examples from the small number of cases in which gene-for-gene interactions have been demonstrated. The prokaryotes can be eliminated and the Ascomycetes (e.g. *Erysiphe graminis*, *Venturia inaequalis*) are haploid in the infective stage. The only examples in which the dominance relations of pathogenicity can, and have been, investigated are confined almost exclusively to the Basidiomycetes, the rusts and smuts. In 1946, Flor reported the observation of dominant pathogenicity in the flax rust fungus and Person *et al.* list examples of dominant pathogenicity in the cereal rusts, *Puccinia graminis tritici*, *P. graminis avenae*, *P. coronata*, flax rust, bean rust and loose smut of barley. In their analysis of segregation of pathogenicity in flax rust, Lawrence *et al.* (1981a) have detected a 'suppressor' locus which effectively reverses the dominance of avirulence. It must be admitted, however, that in the majority of cases reported, virulence tends to be recessive.

THE ORIGIN OF GENE-FOR-GENE INTERACTIONS

It should be clear from previous sections that the investigation of gene-for-gene interactions has been confined to cultivated species and, furthermore, that there is a suspicion that their existence may be a consequence of the process of plant breeding and crop husbandry (Day, 1974). This section will examine this contention.

When a plant breeder is seeking disease resistance, his ideal is the most extreme expression of the character possible, with simple inheritance, so that segregating generations can be easily classified. Immediately, then, the breeder will select from the material available to him resistance characters which are simply inherited, preferably at a single locus. Resistance with more complex inheritance will be discarded unless no other variation is available. The next step will probably be to backcross the resistance source to agronomically superior lines which are susceptible to disease. This necessarily means that resistance genes will be selected as heterozygotes during the backcross programme and a dominant character obviously makes progeny testing easier. In addition, the breeder will probably be selecting, either consciously or unconsciously, individuals from the backcross progeny with the best expression of resistance. The backcrossed line could then be used as a parent in a breeding programme and, since disease resistance is one of the principal characters to be selected, the breeder will select for enhanced expression in the segregating generations. Although this is a somewhat simplified account of plant breeding, it does show that the breeding process itself will tend to favour dominant resistance and that it will tend to put resistance genes into genetic backgrounds which enhance expression and consequently increase dominance. In assessing progeny for resistance, individual plants will tend to be classified as either 'resistant' or 'susceptible'. Thus, heterozygotes which express any acceptable level of resistance will be classified as resistant and dominant, even though they may not be as resistant as the homozygote. A breeding programme for disease resistance selects for resistance to the prevailing pathogen population, which necessarily implies that corresponding pathogenicity, if it exists, is rare. When released commercially, a new resistant cultivar rapidly increases in popularity partly because of its resistance. An increasing area of cultivation exposes it to a larger pathogen population than it had been exposed to during breeding and this makes the selection of rare variants more likely. To overcome the resistance, it would appear that a large phenotypic change is required and although in theory this could just as easily be achieved by a polygenic trait as by a single locus change (cf. insecticide resistance, Wood, 1981), it appears that some species produce such variants more easily by a single point change and these are selected. But this is a slightly too simple view. There are a number of biological factors, which increase the probability of this mechanism for producing pathogenic mutations which apply to most of the species in which gene-for-gene interactions have been demonstrated. The pathogen is exposed to the host predominantly during an asexual or vegetative stage of its life cycle and so the sexual process which is important in generating diversity by recombination and transgressive segregation is absent during a significant proportion of the selective process; for example, powdery mildew goes through 10–20 asexual generations but only one sexual cycle per annum. In other words, the primary selection by the host is between pathogen clones. In some economically important pathogens, the sexual cycle is completely absent in some areas, e.g. *Puccinia graminis* and *P. recondita* in the Great Plains and *Puccinia graminis* in Australia. In other species, the sexual stage is not an obligate part of the life cycle, e.g. *Erysiphe graminis* in N.W. Europe. For other species, especially seed-borne diseases, the sexual cycle is the culmination of a systemic, often asymptomatic, disease e.g. *Ustilago maydis*. There is accumulating evidence that in predominantly asexual species, populations are made up of a restricted number of clones (e.g. Roelfs & Groth, 1980; Selander & Levin, 1980) and consequently the range of quantitative variation must be limited. This suggests that under the conditions of intense selection, restricted genetic variability and predominantly asexual reproduction, single gene changes are more likely. Indeed, Luig & Watson (1970) have reported isolating over 50 different phenotypes in a single *Puccinia graminis* clone in Australia.

In a clonally reproducing diploid species, deleterious mutants with partially dominant or recessive effects on fitness, in the absence of the selective host, have such high heterozygote mutation-selection equilibrium frequencies, that the detection of dominant pathogenicity is almost certain during the screening of candidate 'resistant' lines (Barrett, in press). Thus, resistant lines matched by dominant pathogenicity will tend to be selected against by the breeder. For dominant pathogenicity to be rare enough in the unselected population in the absence of the selective host, the mutation must have almost completely dominant effects on fitness.

The classical theory of the evolution of dominance in random mating populations requires the generation of a high frequency of heterozygotes during the substitution of an allele, but, in pathogens of cultivated plants, substitution takes place instantaneously because the 'wild-type' is lethal on a resistant variety. Consequently high frequencies of heterozygotes will not be generated. Therefore, unless pathogenicity was dominant *de novo*, there is little opportunity for pathogenicity to acquire dominance as it spreads through the population. This would be true even for a random mating sexual population, e.g. hessian fly, but as we have seen in the plant pathogens we are dealing with, the species are either clonal or effectively clonal during most of the selection process. Consequently, the opportunities for the reshuffling of modifier genes and the genetic background which is a prerequisite for the evolution of dominance will either be absent or very restricted.

During the initial stages of the evolutionary response of a pathogen to a resistant variety, a number of different alleles at a single locus or mutants at a number of loci may be able to overcome the resistance with varying degrees of effectiveness, but by the time the 'breakdown' of the resistance of the variety has been recognized and a genetic investigator takes his sample(s), the population on the host is likely to be dominated by a single genotype and the investigator will be led to the conclusion that a gene-for-gene interaction exists. It appears that no investigation has yet been carried out to determine whether phenotypically similar pathogen isolates are genotypically identical, nor has the possibility that different loci in different pathogen populations control the same pathogenic phenotype been explored.

Although I would be the first to admit that this argument is speculative, I believe that there are features about the process of plant breeding and agriculture which will favour the spread of simple genetic responses to resistant varieties, if the pathogen is capable of producing them. Because of these unique features, it is difficult to extrapolate from agro-ecosystems and predict what will take place in wild eco-systems. For example: In a wild system, a novel resistant genotype can only spread and have its expression modified by natural selection and, at every stage, there will be an effect on the pathogen population and feedback from it. On the other hand, in an agricultural system, resistance is selected and enhanced away from any influence of the pathogen population and then it is introduced to the pathogen population, which has never experienced it before, at a frequency which would have taken natural selection many generations to achieve. Indeed, the use of resistant varieties in agriculture is more akin to imposing an environmental abiotic stress on the pathogen population than a continuous co-evolutionary process. As a consequence of this, it is difficult to see how co-evolutionary and molecular models built upon the base of gene-for-gene interactions can reasonably be considered to be descriptions of processes in natural ecosystems.

Gene-for-gene interactions are an extreme form of specificity. There are other levels of specificity which can be used to illustrate the possible problems in extrapolating from agricultural systems to natural ecosystems. Many pathogens on crop species show specificity for particular host species and different biotypes adapted to different host species can exist within a single pathogen species. For example, *Erysiphe graminis* has biotypes adapted to barley, oats and wheat. The specificity is so complete that it can be used as a taxonomic criterion, so *E. graminis* f. sp. *hordei* is a biotype (*forma speciales*) adapted to barley, *E. graminis* f. sp. *tritici* to wheat and so on. Within an agricultural area, classification into *formae speciales* is usually unequivocal. However, if *Erysiphe graminis* is sampled from a wild ecosystem, the host specificity is no longer present to the same extent and a single isolate may be able to attack a wide range of different host species (Table 5). A more detailed examination of the reports from which these data have been

Table 5. Examples of host ranges of plant pathogens in
wild ecosystems

Erysiphe graminis (Wahl *et al.*, 1978)

Source	Species	Genera	Tribes	N
Hordeum murinum	17	13	4	44
Phalaris paradoxa	33	20	7	40
Alopecurus myosuroides	53	30	6	74

Puccinia coronata (Eshed & Dinoor, 1981)
(106 species tested from 43 genera)

Source	Genera	Tribes
Agrostidae	37	7
Festucidae	33	7

extracted reveals that there is no taxonomic consistency between the species which can be attacked.

The prime objective of crop husbandry is to protect crop plants from environmental stresses which reduce yield and, for most crops in highly developed agricultural systems, the only uncontrolled stresses are weather and disease. This necessarily means that disease is perceived as a significant factor in reducing the productivity of crop plants. On the other hand, disease in a natural community is just one of the problems plants have to contend with and it may not be the most significant factor in reducing the reproductive success of the host plant. In a wild eco-system, the evolutionary importance of novel host genotypes to the pathogen population is quite different to the problems faced by a pathogen of a cultivated species when confronted with a newly introduced resistant variety. Since host variation for the pathogen and pathogen variation for the host species are but a part of their respective problems, it would be necessary to postulate the existence of a gene for every environmental stress if the gene-for-gene hypothesis was extended, *reductio ad absurdum*.

CONCLUSIONS

For whatever reasons, its logic, symmetry or simplicity, the gene-for-gene hypothesis has a strong intellectual appeal. What I hope to have argued in this paper is that even in the agro-ecosystems in which it was developed, it is a simplification and to try and draw wide-ranging conclusions about biologically more complex natural ecosystems based on the gene-for-gene hypothesis could be misleading.

In no other area of evolutionary biology have single gene effects been so influential in shaping the development of ideas. Not even in the classic examples of population genetics which have their roots in single gene effects, e.g. industrial melanism, mimicry, insecticide resistance, has there been any problem in assimilating evidence of different modes of inheritance into the thinking. Yet, despite the evidence that gene-for-gene systems are but a small subset of a range of possible interactions between host and parasite, the concept maintains a stranglehold on thinking about co-evolutionary processes in plants and their pathogens.

REFERENCES

BARRETT, J. A. The dynamics of genes in pathogen populations. In M. S. Wolfe & C. E. Caten (Eds), *Populations of Plant Pathogens: Their Dynamics and Genetics.* Oxford: Blackwell Scientific Publications (in press).

BERINGER, J. E., 1983. The Rhizobium–Plant interaction. In A. Puhler (Ed.), *Molecular Genetics of the Bacteria–Plant Interaction*: 9–13. Berlin: Springer-Verlag.

BIFFEN, R. H., 1905. Mendel's laws of inheritance and wheat breeding. *Journal of the Agriculture Society, 1:* 4–48.

CHIN, K. M. & WOLFE, M. S. Evolution of *Erysiphe graminis* in mixed stands of *Hordeum vulgare* (in press).

CHRIST, B. J., 1984. *Effects of selection on populations of* Ustilago hordei. Ph.D. Thesis, University of British Columbia.

DAY, P. R., 1974. *Genetics of Host–Parasite Interactions*: 238. San Francisco: W. H. Freeman & Co.

DINOOR, A., 1977. Oat crown rust resistance in Israel. *Annals of the New York Academy of Sciences, 287:* 357–366.

ELLINGBOE, A. H., 1982. Host resistance and host–parasite interactions: a perspective. In M. S. Mount and G. H. Lacey (Eds), *Phytopathogenic Prokaryotes Vol. 2*: 103–117. New York and London: Academic Press.

ESHED, N. & DINOOR, A., 1981. Genetics of pathogenicity in *Puccinia coronata*: the host range among grasses. *Phytopathology, 71:* 156–163.

FLOR, H. H., 1946. Genetics of pathogenicity in *Melampsora lini. Journal of Agricultural Research, 73:* 335–357.

FLOR, H. H., 1956. The complementary genic systems in flax and flax rust. *Advances in Genetics, 8:* 29–54.

GAIR, R., JENKINS, J. E. E. & LESTER, E., 1972. *Cereal Pests and Diseases*: 184 pp. Ipswich: Farming Press Ltd.

LAWRENCE, G. J., MAYO, G. M. E. & SHEPHERD, K. W., 1981a. Interactions between genes controlling pathogenicity in the flax rust fungus. *Phytopathology, 71:* 12–19.

LAWRENCE, G. J., SHEPHERD, K. W. & MAYO, G. M. E., 1981b. Fine structure of genes controlling pathogenicity in flax rust *Melampsora lini. Heredity, 46:* 297–313.

LUIG, N. H. & RAJARAM, S., 1971. The effect of temperature and genetic background on host gene expression and interaction to *Puccinia graminis tritici. Phytopathology, 62:* 1171–1174.

LUIG, N. H. & WATSON, I. A., 1970. The effect of complex genetic resistance in wheat on the variability of *Puccinia graminis* f. sp. *tritici. Proceedings of the Linnean Society of New South Wales, 95:* 22–45.

MICHELMORE, R. W., NORWOOD, J. M., INGRAM, D. S., CRUTE, I. R. & NICHOLSON, P., 1984. The inheritance of virulence in *Bremia latucae* to match resistance factors 3, 4, 5, 6, 7, 8, 9, 10 and 11 in lettuce (*Latuca sativa*). *Plant Pathology, 33:* 301–315.

MOSEMAN, J. G., 1959. Host–pathogen interaction of the genes for resistance in *Hordeum vulgare* and for pathogenicity in *Erysiphe graminis* f. sp. *hordei. Phytopathology, 49:* 469–472.

PERSON, C. O., CHRIST, B. J. & POPE, D. D. The Genetic determination of variation in pathogenicity. In M. S. Wolfe & C. E. Caten (Eds), *Populations of Plant Pathogens: Their Dynamics and Genetics.* Oxford: Blackwell Scientific Publications. (in press).

ROELFS, A. P. & GROTH, J. V., 1980. A comparison of virulence phenotypes in wheat stem rust populations reproducing sexually and asexually. *Phytopathology, 70:* 855–862.

SELANDER, R. K. & LEVIN, B. R., 1980. Genetic diversity and structure in *Escherichia coli* populations. *Science, 210:* 545–547.

VANDERPLANK, J. E., 1978. *Genetic and Molecular Basis of Plant Pathogenesis.* 167 pp. Berlin: Springer-Verlag.

VANDERPLANK, J. E., 1982. *Host–pathogen Interactions in Plant Disease*: 207 pp. New York and London: Academic Press.

WAHL, I., 1970. Prevalence of geographic distribution of resistance to crown rust in *Avena sterilis. Phytopathology, 60:* 746–749.

WAHL, I., ESHED, N., SEGAL, A. & SOBEL, Z., 1978. Significance of wild relatives of small grains and other wild grasses in cereal powdery mildews. In D. M. Spencer (Ed.), *The Powdery Mildews*: 83–100. London and New York: Academic Press.

WOLFE, M. S., BARRETT, J. A. & JENKINS, J. E. E., 1981. The use of cultivar mixtures for disease control. In F. J. Jenkyn & R. T. Plumb (Eds), *Strategies for the Control of Cereal Disease*: 73–80. Oxford: Blackwell Scientific Publications.

WOOD, R. J., 1981. Insecticide resistance: genes and mechanisms. In J. A. Bishop & L. M. Cook (Eds), *Genetic Consequences of Man Made Change*: 53–96. London and New York: Academic Press.

Bacteria and phage: a model system for the study of the ecology and co-evolution of hosts and parasites

BRUCE R. LEVIN AND RICHARD E. LENSKI*

Department of Zoology,
University of Massachusetts,
Amherst, Massachusetts 01003 U.S.A.

The results are reviewed of theoretical and experimental investigations of the population biology of bacteria and bacteriophage, emphasizing those aspects of general interest in the study of host–parasite ecology and evolution.

1) *Existence Conditions:* the conditions are considered under which phage can invade bacterial populations and will stably co-exist with these hosts. Particular emphasis is given to the effects of phage resistant bacterial clones on these communities, and hypotheses are presented to account for the observation that experimental populations of bacteria and virulent phage are more stable than anticipated from theory.

2) *Co-evolution:* The nature and effects of selection on the interacting populations of bacteria and phage are examined. Evidence is presented that the resulting co-evolution is a constrained process, rather than the indefinite gene-for-gene arms race previously postulated.

3) *Latency:* Temperate bacteriophage are analogous to the latent viruses of eukaryotes. We critically discuss three classes of hypotheses for the ecological conditions and selective pressures responsible for the evolution and maintenance of temperate (as opposed to virulent) modes of phage reproduction.

4) *Immunity:* Bacterial restriction-modification systems are similar to the immune systems of higher organisms. The hypothesis is considered that restriction-modification systems evolved and are maintained for defence against phage infection and we speculate on the effects of this type of immune system on the population dynamics of bacteria and phage.

5) *Coda:* This review is concluded with a brief consideration of the use of phage for the biological control of bacteria.

KEY WORDS: — Bacteria — phage — ecology — co-evolution — population biology — restriction-modification immunity — lysogeny.

CONTENTS

*Address after July 1, 1985: Department of Ecology and Evolutionary Biology, University of California, Irvine, California 92717 U.S.A.

Ecology and Genetics of Host–Parasite Interactions
ISBN: 0 12 593 690 7

INTRODUCTION

Studies of the population biology of host–parasite associations generally address one or more of the following issues: existence conditions; co-evolution; latency; and physiological immunity. Under what conditions will the parasite population become established and maintain a stable association with its host? What is the nature of co-evolution in the host and parasite populations and what are the consequences of this co-evolution for the long-term persistence of their association? Under what conditions will latent phases evolve and be maintained in the parasite population and what are the effects of latency on the long-term persistence of the host–parasite association? Under what conditions will physiological immunity evolve and be maintained in host populations and what are the effects of the immune system on the population dynamics of the host–parasite association?

In an effort to answer these questions, one considers either *real* or *model* systems. The distinction between real and model is, by and large, one of motivation. Real systems are generally chosen for practical reasons, especially concern with a specific clinically or agriculturally significant host–parasite association. Model systems are chosen primarily for simplicity and manipulative convenience, and secondarily because they are a tenable analogue of some real system. In this paper, we review studies addressing these questions on the population biology of host–parasite associations with a model system of bacteria and bacterial viruses.

While bacteria and bacterial viruses, or phage, are commonly thought of as reagent-like tools of molecular biology rather than objects of ecological and evolutionary study, the relationship between these organisms is certainly that of host and parasite. Phage can reproduce only inside a bacterial cell, and this infection is usually deleterious (often lethal) to the bacterium. Several features make the bacteria-phage system a convenient model for exploring the ecological and evolutionary dynamics of host–parasite interactions. Bacteria and phage are readily cultured and sampled in the laboratory. In well-agitated liquid culture, their dynamics are governed by mass action, an assumption implicit in almost all mathematical models of interacting populations. Their high densities and short generations make it possible to perform evolutionary experiments in the course of a few weeks. And because bacteria and phage have served as model organisms in microbial genetics and molecular biology, there is an abundance of well-characterized strains and well-developed procedures for their culture and sampling. There is also a wealth of 'background' information on the physiology of phage infection and on growth and the genetic and molecular bases of the interaction between these viruses and their hosts.

Whether or not answers to the questions posed in the introduction can be generalized from this (or any other) simple model system to more complex host–parasite associations is moot. What we wish to stress is that the bacteria–phage system is one in which these questions can be addressed in a rigorous, experimental fashion. Before reviewing efforts to answer these questions, we briefly summarize some of the basic features of the bacteria–phage interaction.

Phage are generally divided into two classes, *virulent* and *temperate*. For both classes, the infection of a bacterium begins with the adsorption of the phage to specific sites on the bacterial surface, followed by the injection of the phage's genetic material into the bacterium. For virulent phage, there follows a period during which the phage genome is replicated and encapsulated intracellularly, culminating in the lysis (bursting) of the cell and the release of tens or hundreds of progeny phage (Ellis & Delbruck, 1939). Temperate phage may also replicate by this *lytic* process, or the DNA of the infecting phage may be integrated into the bacterial genome, a phenomenon known as *lysogeny* (Lwoff, 1953). The temperate phage genome (now called a *prophage*) is replicated alongside the bacterial genome and is inherited by each of the daughter cells (now called *lysogens*). Occasionally, the prophage may be lost (*segregation*) or stimulated to enter the lytic cycle (*induction*). [Lysogeny is thus analogous to the association between latent eukaryotic viruses and somatic cells.] The distinction between temperate and virulent phage is made solely on functional (and not phylogenetic) grounds; with one or a few mutations, temperate phage can lose their ability to form lysogens (Lwoff, 1953; Ptashne, 1971).

Bacteria have an arsenal of defences against phage infection. These are of two basic types, resistance and immunity. In the case of *resistance*, the bacterium is refractory to the phage, while in the case of *immunity*, phage adsorb to the cell and inject their genetic material, but their replication is aborted. Resistance is typically acquired by mutation of a single chromosomal gene (Luria & Delbruck, 1943), while immunity is often acquired by the carriage of a plasmid or prophage that codes for this property. Prophage render lysogens immune to reinfection by free temperate (but not virulent) phage of the same or closely related species. Immunity to phage infection may also be achieved through a restriction–modification system (Arber & Linn, 1969) coded for by plasmid, chromosome or prophage-borne genes. With this type of immune system, injected phage DNA is recognized as foreign, and through the action of enzymes known as restriction endonucleases is destroyed by cutting at specific nucleotide sequences. As in the case of our own immune system, this bacterial system has a mechanism for recognition of self. This is accomplished through modification enzymes which methylate bases at specific nucleotide sequences and thereby physically protect that DNA from cutting by the associated restriction enzyme. However, there is a small probability that an infecting phage's DNA is 'accidentally' modified; if so, all progeny phage are also modified and able to infect the bacteria carrying that restriction–modification system with full efficiency.

Not surprisingly, phage may possess counter-defences against the defences of their bacterial hosts. Phage populations can sport *host-range* mutants that are capable of infecting not only 'wild-type' (sensitive) bacteria, but also mutant bacteria resistant to wild-type phage (Luria, 1945). Certain phage possess characteristics which render them protected from the restriction endonucleases of bacteria (Kruger & Bickle, 1983). Some phage have the potential for mutualistic associations with bacteria. Many temperate phage encode gene products that are of direct benefit to their host bacterium (in addition to the repressors responsible for immunity to reinfection) and phage can serve as vectors for host gene recombination (*transduction*).

Stent (1963) provides an excellent (albeit somewhat dated) review of the basic biology of phage.

THE CONDITIONS FOR THE EXISTENCE OF PHAGE

Theory and observations

Existence conditions can be partitioned into two components, establishment (successful invasion) and maintenance (stable co-existence). The conditions for establishment are straightforward; a phage population can successfully invade a bacterial population as long as its rate of growth exceeds its rate of loss (due to mortality or other causes). For virulent phage introduced into chemostat populations of bacteria, establishment can occur as long as the product of the adsorption rate parameter, burst size, and bacterial population density exceeds the dilution rate of the chemostat (Levin, Stewart & Chao, 1977). The establishment conditions for temperate phage in continuous culture are somewhat broader than those for virulent. If lysogens have a competitive advantage over non-lysogens, temperate phage can become established even when this lytic invasion condition does not obtain (Stewart & Levin, 1984). If, however, lysogens are at a competitive disadvantage, the invasion conditions for temperate phage are very similar to those for virulent phage.

While successful invasion is a necessary condition for stable maintenance, it is not a sufficient condition. Models of the population biology of virulent phage in continuous culture admit to solutions specifying stable equilibria, stable oscillations, and oscillations leading to extinction of bacteria and/or phage (Levin et al., 1977). This formal theory also predicts that if phage-resistant bacteria have a disadvantage when competing with sensitive bacteria in phage-free culture, their presence will not upset stable associations that do exist (Campbell, 1961; Levin et al., 1977). Due to the production of lysogens, which are immune to reinfection, invasions by temperate phage are unlikely to yield the oscillations of increasing amplitude which may destabilize the virulent phage and bacterial community. As a result, the conditions for the stable persistence of these 'benign' phage are anticipated to be substantially broader than those for virulent phage (Stewart & Levin, 1984).

There have been a number of experimental studies of the population dynamics of *Escherichia coli* and virulent phage in chemostats (Paynter & Bungay, 1969; Horne, 1970; Levin et al., 1977; Chao, Levin & Stewart, 1977; Lenski, 1984b; Lenski & Levin, 1985). These investigations have considered a number of different strains of *E. coli* and different species of phage. In all, apparently stable associations between the phage and bacterial populations were observed, although Lenski and Levin (1985) reported occasional extinctions of *E. coli* B and virulent phage T4. These stable associations obtained for both phage-limited and resource-limited communities. In the former situation, the dominant population of phage was able to infect all bacteria present, the bacterial density at equilibrium was orders of magnitude lower than that in phage-free culture, and there was an abundance of unused resource. In the latter situation, the dominant bacterial population was resistant to all of the coexisting phage, the equilibrium cell density was similar to that of a phage-free community, and excess resource was not available. These experimental phage-bacterial communities persisted for substantial periods; Horne (1970) reported the maintenance of *E. coli* B and phage T3 communities for more than a year. We are aware of only two published studies of the population dynamics of temperate phage in chemostats and, in both, apparently stable associations were observed (Noack, 1969; Paynter & Bungay, 1970).

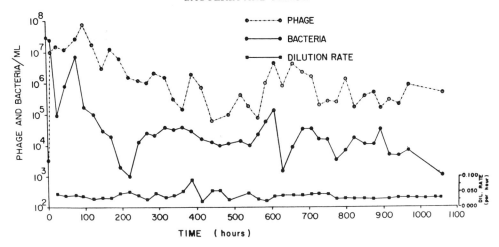

Figure 1. Phage-limited chemostat community comprised of virulent phage T7 and the bacterium *E. coli* B. Reprinted from Chao *et al.* (1977) with the permission of *Ecology*.

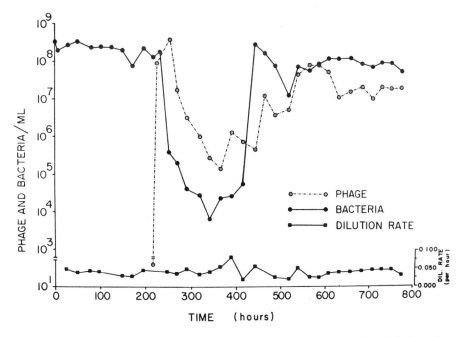

Figure 2. Resource-limited chemostat community comprised of virulent phage T7 and the bacterium *E. coli* B. Reprinted from Chao *et al.* (1977) with the permission of *Ecology*.

In Figures 1 and 2, we present the results of chemostat experiments with virulent phage T7 and *E. coli* B in phage- and resource-limited states, respectively (Chao *et al.*, 1977). The phage population in the later stages of both of these communities consisted of (at least) two genotypes, the original wild-type phage and a host-range mutant. The bacterial population in Fig. 1 contained (at least) two genotypes, the original sensitive clone and a mutant clone resistant to the wild-type phage. A third bacterial clone that was resistant to both the wild-type and host-range phages evolved in the community depicted in Fig. 2.

It would, of course, be nice to say that the mathematical models of the phage/bacteria system represent accurate analogues of the interaction between *E. coli* and its virulent phage in continuous culture. Unfortunately, the returns on this assessment are somewhat mixed. The predicted and observed results agree in two important ways: 1) in studies with phages T2 and T4 and *E. coli* B, the absolute densities of phage and bacteria in phage-limited chemostats were close to those anticipated from the model (Levin *et al.*, 1977; Lenski and Levin, 1985); and 2) in all cases where the phage were maintained in a resource-limited bacterial community, the phage-resistant clone had a marked disadvantage when competing with the sensitive clone in phage-free culture (Levin *et al.*, 1977; Chao *et al.*, 1977; Lenski and Levin, 1985). However, the observed behaviour of virulent phage and bacteria in chemostats differs from that predicted by the models in one very significant way; the experimental communities are considerably more stable than anticipated (Levin *et al.*, 1977).

Not only do stable communities of virulent phage and *E. coli* obtain in continuous culture, they also occur in serially transferred batch culture. Under these conditions, the phage are not subject to continuous 'mortality' through washout. Thus, the phage population is anticipated to have adequate time and reach sufficient densities to 'seek out' and adsorb to all sensitive cells that are present (see also Rodin and Ratner, 1983b). Nevertheless, in a recent study with *E. coli* K-12 and the phages T2, T4, T5, T6, T7 and λvir in liquid and surface serial transfer culture, long-term persistence was noted in the vast majority of populations examined: Table 1 (Levin, Lenski & Evans, unpublished). As can be seen, the likelihood of persistence of these communities depended on both habitat and phage species.

Table 1. Extinction of phage in serial transfer culture

Phage	Liquid			Surface		
	No. of Cultures	No. of Transfers	No. of Extinctions*	No. of Cultures	No. of Transfers	No. of Extinctions*
T2	3	15	0	49	20	0
T4	3	15	1[†]	50	11	0
T5	3	15	3	50	11	49
T6	3	15	0	49	20	0
T7	3	15	0	49	12	18
λ^{Vir}	3	25	1	49	12	0

*In cultures where phage were present at the end of the experiment, the phage density exceeded 10^6 per ml or per colony for the liquid and surface serial transfer cultures, respectively.
[†]In all three liquid populations, T4 producing small plaques evolved. In one T4 culture, phage apparently went extinct, although this was difficult to demonstrate unequivocally, because the plaques had become too small.

Also noteworthy in Table 1, there are rather striking species differences in extinction rate in surface culture. There were high rates of extinction for T5 and T7, but no extinctions for T2, T4, T6, and λvir. Phages T5 and T7 produce large plaques on lawns of sensitive cells, and infections with these phage tend to spread through colonies. When growing bacterial colonies run into T5 or T7, the vast majority of sensitive cells are killed; the colony is translucent, rather than opaque like uninfected colonies. Phages T2, T4 and T6 and λvir, however, produce small plaques, and when sensitive colonies grow into phage of these types, the infections tend to be more localized; the cells in the colony that first encounter the phage die, but the infection does not spread much beyond its original focus. As a consequence, bacterial colonies infected with these small-plaque phage are opaque but have wedge-shaped cuts in them.

At this time, there have not been sufficient studies to evaluate how well the population dynamics of temperate phage fit those anticipated from models of these interactions. However, the study of Noack (1969) suggests that simple models can be used to predict the equilibrium concentration of free phage in chemostats. While not sufficient as a test of the fit of formal theory, the results of some preliminary studies done with *E. coli* K-12 and temperate phages λ, $\phi80$ and P1 (CM^{-lc} clr 100) in liquid and surface serial transfer culture certainly suggest that temperate phage/bacterial associations are generally stable. Save for the mutant P1 (CM^{-lc} clr 100) at high temperatures (where induction occurs at an unusual high rate), extinctions were not observed in any of three liquid and 48 or more surface populations for each of these temperate phage (Levin, Lenski & Evans, unpublished).

Mechanisms for the stable persistence of virulent phage

In our view, the most interesting unanswered question concerning existence conditions is — What are the mechanisms accounting for the greater than anticipated stability of *E. coli*–virulent phage communities in chemostats and serially transferred batch culture? At this juncture, we can offer only an element of faith, a general hypothesis, and a specific embellishment of that hypothesis. The element of faith is that there is a single dominant factor that accounts for the stability of the associations between all virulent phage and their host bacteria. The general hypothesis is that there are refugia for sensitive cells in our experiments. The embellished form of this hypothesis is that in liquid culture, this refuge is physiological rather than spatial. We postulate that there is physiological variation in sensitivity to phage infection such that in a population of genetically sensitive bacteria, there is nonetheless a minority of cells that are transitorily insensitive to phage infection.

While we do not consider this physiological refuge hypothesis to be tested, there are three lines of evidence in support of it. The first is theoretical; it can work. By incorporating a transitorily resistant bacterial population (derived by 'migration' from the sensitive population and migrating back into that population) into the model of Levin *et al.* (1977), the stabilty of the association between virulent phage and bacteria is considerably augmented. The oscillations in amplitude are damped, and the phage population and the sensitive cell population that supports it continue to persist. This can obtain even when the model is for a serially transferred batch culture (the worst-case for persistence). The second line of evidence is the apparent absence of spatial refugia in liquid. These populations are well-agitated, and none of the wall populations of these communities are transferred. The final line of evidence comes from studies of the physiological regulation of the production of the phage receptor sites and their incorporation into the bacterial cell wall. The phage λ receptor protein is not restored to its full complement during every cycle of binary fission, but rather goes several to many cell cycles (with the density of receptors diluted by half during each cycle) before the receptors are restored (Ryter, Shuman & Schwartz, 1975). Because the extent of physiological variation among cells in phage-sensitivity is dependent on the carbon source in which they are growing (Howes, 1965; Ryter *et al.*, 1975), we believe this hypothesis is directly testable.

While physiological refugia may also play a role in the stabilization of surface communities, we suspect that spatial refugia are also important in this structured habitat. For the T-even phage and λvir, the geometry of infection and cell growth on surfaces almost certainly contributes to the persistence of the community. It is even possible that cells infected with these phage fail to physically burst when embedded in a colony. Indeed, so little is known about phage infection in surface culture that virtually any plausible hypothesis has to be entertained.

CO-EVOLUTION

There are two basic paradigms concerning the supposed nature of co-evolution of parasites and their hosts. According to the antagonistic paradigm, selection favours hosts and parasites which exhibit novel defences and counterdefences (Van Valen, 1973; Dawkins & Krebs, 1979), while according to the mutualistic paradigm, selection favours hosts and parasites which exhibit increased tolerance and reduced virulence (Burnet & White, 1972). Whether host–parasite co-evolution is antagonistic or mutualistic is likely to be highly dependent on the mode of parasite transmission (May & Anderson, 1983). If successful reproduction by the parasite is in any way dependent on the host's survival (or vice versa), then selection may favour mutualistic adaptations such as reduced parasite virulence. If parasite reproduction is not dependent on the host's survival (and vice versa), then selection will favour antagonistic adaptations such as increased exploitation by the parasite.

Because reproduction by virulent phage necessarily entails the death of its host bacterium, their co-evolution is anticipated to be exclusively antagonistic (Levin & Lenski, 1983), at least in spatially unstructured (mass action) habitats (see also Wilson, 1980). If all else is equal, selection acting on the phage would be to increase their rate of adsorption to sensitive cells, while selection acting on the bacteria would be to reduce this rate of adsorption. Bacteria that are resistant to phage adsorption typically arise by a single mutation, and these resistant mutants will generally be favoured as long as the phage are present. As a result, selection in the phage population would favour host–range phage mutants (also commonly generated by single gene changes) that are capable of adsorption and growth on these resistant bacteria. The evolution of these host-range phage then sets the stage for selection favouring a second-order resistant bacterial mutant, and following that a second-order host-range phage, and so on. Thus, bacteria and virulent phage seem an ideal system for observing an unending gene-for-gene (Flor, 1956; Barrett, 1983) arms race between host and parasite. In fact, Stent (1963:181) states that "The co-existence of bacteria and bacterial viruses is thus sustained by a delicate mutational equilibrium that saves both protagonists from total extinction", a scenario that has now been modelled by Rodin & Ratner (1983a,b).

However, the results of studies on both the molecular genetics and the population dynamics of bacteria and their phage parasites are inconsistent with this unending arms race hypothesis (Lenski, 1984a; Lenski and Levin, 1985). Resistance and host-range mutations tend to engender a reduction in competitive ability (relative to wild-type clones) in the absence of selection specifically favouring these mutants (Chao *et al.*, 1977; Lenski & Levin, 1985). These trade-offs are not surprising on physiological grounds. The phage adsorption sites on the bacterial surface exist, of course, for specific cellular functions which have only secondarily been parasitized by phage (Schwartz, 1980); mutations in the genes coding for these structures may affect the ability of the bacteria to exploit its environment. As discussed in the preceding section on existence conditions, such trade-offs between resistance and competitive ability permit phage to persist even though they may be completely unable to infect the resistant strain.

In fact, even with intense selection, there seem to be limits to the number of host-range states that can be generated for the phage (Hofnung, Jezierska & Braun-Breton, 1976; Lenski & Levin, 1985). While one cannot say that further host-range mutants of these phage do not exist, the estimated rate of spontaneous mutation must be generally less than 10^{-11} (Lenski & Levin, 1985); i.e. mutation rates lower than those associated with point mutations, and not readily estimable. This asymmetry in the co-evolutionary potential of bacteria and virulent phage apparently exists because mutations conferring resistance may occur by either the alteration or the loss of certain gene functions, while only host-range mutations that counter the former can occur (Hofnung et al., 1976; Schwartz, 1980; Lenski, 1984a; Lenski & Levin, 1985). If these results are at all general (and of course we believe they are), then one would anticipate that bacteria have a co-evolutionary edge over virulent phage. This interpretation is supported by experimental studies of E. coli and several different virulent phage in chemostats (Horne, 1970; Chao et al., 1977; Lenski & Levin, 1985). The most evolved communities are almost invariably resource-limited, rather than phage-limited, and have bacteria that are resistant to all co-occurring phage as the dominant clones. (Communities containing virulent phage T2 come closest to violating this rule. First-order resistance to this phage usually requires two separate mutations (Lenski, 1984b), and there are at least two orders of host-range phage mutations (Lenski & Levin, 1985). Even so, one can select a resistant bacterial clone for which one cannot isolate a corresponding host-range mutant (Lenski & Levin, 1985), although it may take a long time for all of this to occur in chemostats (Paynter & Bungay, 1969; Levin et al., 1977).)

Selection on temperate phage and their hosts can also operate in this antagonistic fashion. However, as a consequence of lysogeny, their co-evolution can also be mutualistic (Levin & Lenski, 1983). Selection acting on the lysogen population operates on both parasite- and host-determined characters. Thus, a prophage-coded character that augments the fitness of the lysogenic cell would be favoured by selection, and the resulting co-evolution could certainly be characterized as mutualistic. As noted in the introduction, there are, in fact, a variety of adaptive bacteria phenotypes that are encoded by prophage-borne genes and that are likely to be products of mutualistic co-evolution: 1) reinfection immunity; 2) antibiotic resistance (Williams Smith, 1972); 3) toxin production/pathogenicity (Freeman, 1951; Uchida, Gill & Pappenheimer, 1971); and 4) restriction-modification (Arber & Linn, 1969). In addition, for some unknown reason, lysogens for the phages λ, P1, ϕ80 and μ have competitive advantages over non-lysogens even when no specific phage-determined phenotype is selected (Edlin, Lin & Bitner, 1977; Lin, Bitner & Edlin, 1977; Dykhuizen, Campbell & Rolfe, 1978). Finally, temperate phage can serve as vectors for the transfer of chromosomal genes (i.e., transduction), although this may not be an evolved function, but rather an accidental consequence of phage replication (Levin & Lenski, 1983).

THE EVOLUTION AND MAINTENANCE OF LYSOGENY

The establishment and maintenance of a lysogenic association between a phage and its host is a relatively complex process. For the phage λ, the 'decision' to lyse or lysogenize a bacterium involves a number of operators, promoters and structural genes, the functions of which seem to be uniquely for this process (Ptashne, 1971; Ptashne et al., 1980). Analogously complex and specific machinery for lysogeny exists in other, apparently independently evolved, temperate phage (Sternberg & Austin, 1981). It therefore seems reasonable to assume that lysogeny is a highly evolved character (Campbell, 1961; Joklik, 1974), and there must be a set of ecological conditions under which a lysogenic mode of phage replication is favoured over a purely lytic one. For an individual phage infecting a bacterium, this 'benign' mode of replication is likely to occur at a very much lower rate than lytic replication, because prophage reproduction is limited to the comparatively modest bacterial growth rate. Even so, the difference in growth rates for populations of temperate and virulent phage is likely to be small, all else being equal, as the probability of lysogeny is generally small even for temperate phage. However, unless the carriage of a prophage actually augments the host bacterium's fitness, virulent phage would have a selective advantage and replace the temperate phage, at least under equilibrium conditions, owing to their higher rate of replication and their ability to infect lysogens (Stewart & Levin, 1984).

A number of hypotheses have been put forth addressing the 'why be temperate' question. These hypotheses are non-exclusive, largely untested, and fall into three basic classes.

One class requires the action of some form of interdemic (group) selection. One form of this hypothesis can be extracted from the writing of Dove (1971) and Echols (1972), and rests on the premise that temperate phage are less likely to drive their hosts (and consequently themselves) to extinction than virulent phage. Thus, temperate phage could have a global advantage even though experiencing a disadvantage within any deme. An alternative group selection hypothesis has been offered by Campbell (1961), who suggested that a group-level advantage for temperate phage may occur as the result of temperate phage acting as vectors for host recombination.

There may be a temptation to discount these group selection hypotheses because of the relatively stringent conditions for this type of selection to operate (see Levin & Kilmer, 1974; Wilson, 1980). However, we hesitate to discard these hypotheses solely on grounds of parsimony, especially since there has yet to be a formal consideration of the *a priori* conditions for this process to operate in bacterial and viral populations and so little is known about the demic structure of natural communities of these organisms. On the other hand, there are some empirical observations which cast doubt on the validity of the premises of the specific group selection hypotheses presented above. As noted in the preceding consideration of existence conditions, the association between some virulent phage and their hosts can be quite stable. Thus, it may well be that the rates of population extinction for virulent and temperate phage are not too different. In the case of temperate λ, no extinctions were observed for any of three liquid and 48 surface serial transfer populations. For a virulent mutant of λ, one extinction was observed in three liquid populations and none in 49 surface populations. These liquid populations were maintained for 25 transfers (with a transfer fraction of 0.01) and the surface populations for 10–12 transfers (Levin, Lenski & Evans, unpublished data). The densities of virulent and temperate (free and integrated) phage were comparable, except for the single extinction noted above. Moreover, virulent as well as temperate phage can serve as vectors for host recombination (Wilson *et al.*, 1979), so that any such advantage for temperate phage over virulent phage would be quantitative rather than qualitative. For *E. coli* at least, the rate of recombinational gene replacement is similar to that of mutation (Ørskov & Ørskov, 1961; Selander & Levin, 1980; Levin, 1981; Caugant *et al.*, 1981). Thus, if the group advantage by recombination is contingent upon a high rate of host gene shuffling, then it is unlikely to be obtained for temperate coliphage.

While existing evidence does not bode well for these group selection hypotheses, the amount of this evidence is quite modest. Furthermore, group selection hypotheses need not be restricted to the differential extinction and host recombination mechanisms described above (see Wilson, 1980). Thus, at this time, it seems most prudent to consider group-level arguments viable, if not excessively appealing.

The second class of hypotheses assumes that the carriage of the prophage augments the fitness of the host bacterium. This fitness advantage can be direct, for example, prophage-determined antibiotic resistance. With a fitness advantage for lysogens over non-lysogens, temperate phage would either co-exist with or have a net advantage over virulent phage (Stewart and Levin, 1984). As noted in the preceding section on co-evolution, there is a variety of well-characterized prophage-determined phenotypes which are likely to augment cell fitness, at least in certain environments. There are also the observations of seemingly general, but uncharacterized, fitness advantages for lysogens over non-lysogens (Edlin *et al.*, 1977; Lin *et al.*, 1977; Dykhuizen *et al.*, 1978). Thus, it seems reasonable to assume that selection favouring prophage-determined phenotypes contributes to the maintenance of some extant temperate phage. However, this mechanism seems unlikely to have led to the evolution of temperate phage from virulent phage ancestors, because it requires the expression of the beneficial phage gene in a living (not fatally infected) bacterium. Stated another way, the phage would have to be temperate to become temperate (Levin & Lenski, 1983). On the other hand, it seems reasonable to assume that phage are derived from bacterial genetic material and it is therefore possible that some primordial bacterial viruses were temperate rather than virulent.

An alternative to this direct lysogen advantage mechanism has been postulated by Levin & Lenski (1983) and Stewart & Levin (1984). According to this hypothesis, an advantage to a lysogenic clone can derive solely through the allelopathic effects of free phage, and there is no need for the expression of beneficial prophage-borne genes. This indirect lysogen advantage requires a physically structured habitat, where lysogens and sensitive non-lysogens compete as colonies rather than as individual cells (as in mass culture). As a consequence of induction and diffusion of free phage, sensitive cells in the vicinity of lysogenic colonies are killed (or, at a much lower rate, converted into lysogens). Because of this, the lysogenic colonies are able to sequester limiting resources and thus obtain a competitive advantage. This structured habitat/allelopathy mechanism has been demonstrated to generate a competitive advantage for colicinogenic bacteria (Chao & Levin, 1981). While it has yet to be tested for temperate phage, we find it an appealing hypothesis.

The third class of 'why be temperate' hypotheses can be described as 'diapause' mechanisms (a term suggested by Conrad Istock). In essence, these hypotheses rest on the premise that lysogeny provides a refuge for the phage genome in hostile environments. For example, if populations of bacteria and phage periodically encounter situations where free phage are killed but lysogens survive, then temperate phage could have a selective advantage over virulent phage.

An alternative form of the diapause hypothesis has been suggested by Campbell (1961) and Levin & Lenski (1983), and treated more formally by Stewart & Levin (1984). When the density of bacterial hosts is very low, the rate of lytic replication may be insufficient to offset phage mortality. In contrast, lysogenic replication does not require the phage to 'find' new host cells; prophage can increase at the modest bacterial growth rate even when hosts are rare (provided, of course, that there are sufficient resources for bacterial growth). Thus, at low bacterial densities, temperate phage could have an advantage over virulent phage, all else equal. There is a caveat to this low host density hypothesis, however, as shown by Stewart & Levin (1984). If bacterial densities are constant and sufficiently low to give temperate phage an advantage over otherwise identical virulent phage, then neither the virulent nor temperate phage would be able to successfully invade the bacterial population. On the other hand, if bacterial densities are allowed to fluctuate, there do exist conditions where temperate phage can become established and outcompete virulent phage, owing to their lower rate of decline when hosts are rare (Stewart & Levin, 1984). Thus, the low host density hypothesis rests on the assumption of non-equilibrium dynamics, a likely condition in 'feast or famine' habitats such as the gut (Koch, 1971).

RESTRICTION-MODIFICATION IMMUNITY

While one may get the impression that restriction endonucleases are reagents that have been recently invented by molecular biologists, this is certainly not the case. These site-specific DNA-cutting enzymes are naturally occurring products of bacteria and are coded for by genes borne on bacterial chromosomes, plasmids or prophage. They are produced by a phylogenetically diverse group of bacteria and have a broad array of restriction sites, as a brief perusal of the catalogues of supplies for DNA manipulation readily illustrates.

The original discovery of restriction–modification and contemporary *in vivo* assays for these systems have relied on the phenotype of immunity to phage infection (Luria, 1953). As a consequence of host restriction, the probability of a productive adsorption by a phage (with unmodified DNA) can be several orders of magnitude lower than in the absence of restriction. It seems reasonable to hypothesize that restriction–modification systems evolved and are maintained as mechanisms for defence against phage infection. This interpretation is supported by the plethora of mechanisms which phage have apparently evolved to avoid host restriction (Kruger & Bickle, 1983).

As compelling as this hypothesis for the evolution and maintenance of restriction–modification immunity seems, it remains untested. Indeed, there are some observations which may not be fully consistent with it. The fact that so many phage have mechanisms to avoid restriction actually calls into question whether defence against phage infection is an adequate selective pressure for the maintenance of extant restriction–modification systems. Also calling into question this phage defence hypothesis are: 1) the apparent co-evolutionary advantage that bacteria derive from envelope resistance alone (as discussed in the preceding section on co-evolution); 2) the relatively high rate of erroneous modification of phage (on the order of 10^{-3}); and 3) the observation that restriction endonucleases can be isolated from organisms living in environments that would seem to be inhospitable to phage (McConnell *et al.*, 1978).

Whether or not restriction immunity evolved as a defence against phage, it clearly could have an important effect on the conditions for the establishment and stable persistence of phage sensitive to these enzymes. In the absence of restriction immunity, the conditions for invasion of phage are (more or less) independent of the number of phage. On the other hand, for restriction-sensitive phage to invade a population of bacteria producing restriction endonucleases, the number of phage would have to be sufficiently high to yield at least one successful infection and the resulting modified progeny. Thus, it seems reasonable to assume that restriction immunity would protect bacterial populations from phage invasion. Once restriction is overcome in a monoclonal bacterial population, however, the conditions for the persistence of the phage should be similar to those in the absence of this immunity. But this may not be the case if the bacterial population contains several clones producing different restriction endonucleases; this interesting possibility has not been formally modelled or experimentally tested. Could it be that frequency-dependent selection favouring rare restriction endonuclease types plays an important role in maintaining the considerable clonal diversity observed for *E. coli* (Selander & Levin, 1980; Caugant, Levin & Selander, 1981)?

CODA

In this review, we have emphasized bacteria and phage as a model system for exploring what we consider to be some of the most interesting aspects of the ecology and evolution of hosts and parasites. It would be naïve (as well as arrogant) to assert that *all* of the results obtained from the examination of the population biology of this prokaryotic system can be readily generalized to more complex eukaryotic hosts and parasites. However, we do believe that some of these results are extrapolatable to more complex host–parasite systems. It is also hoped that most of the questions raised here and the approaches being used to test hypotheses will, at least, be of interest to those working on the population biology of other host–parasite systems.

While this review is restricted to theoretical and laboratory studies, the hypotheses generated will be fully tested *only* when their predictions have been examined in natural populations of bacteria and phage. For example, the constraints on the co-evolution of bacteria and virulent phage that have been demonstrated in the laboratory predict that, although virulent phage may have an important role in determining the clonal composition of populations of coliform bacteria, they usually would have little effect on the overall density (Lenski & Levin, 1985). Although we are unaware of evidence that is inconsistent with these predictions, most studies of bacteria and phage in natural communities seem at best only indirectly relevant to this or other questions considered here (Dhillon *et al.*, 1970; Dhillon *et al.*, 1976; Furuse *et al.*, 1983). Thus, in spite of their limited aesthetic appeal, further 'field' studies of the population biology of coliform bacteria and their phage are clearly necessary.

While emphasis has been placed on bacteria and phage as a 'model' system, it is also a 'real' system, with potential clinical and agricultural significance. In fact, for the first two decades after the discovery of bacteriophage, the primary motivation for studying these viruses was their potential as agents for the 'biological control' of bacterial pathogens (see e.g. D'Herelle, 1922). During the 1930s, at least three pharmaceutical companies marketed phage in the United States (Peitzman, 1969). However, as the efficacy of antibiotics became apparent, research on phage therapy essentially stopped, and until very recently was regarded as a failure (Stent, 1963; Wilson & Miles, 1964; Peitzman, 1969).

Renewed interest in phage therapy in recent years probably derives from concerns about the increased problems of resistance by many bacteria to antibiotics (Anderson, 1968; Mitsuhashi, 1971; Falkow, 1975), and the realization that phage are self-replicating and naturally (rather than commercially) co-evolving anti-bacterial agents. Possible applications of phage for both clinical and agricultural purposes have received recent coverage in the popular scientific press (Miller, 1983; Dixon, 1984). To be sure, the studies reviewed here indicate that there are greater constraints on the 'co-evolutionary potential' of phage than there are on bacteria, and this may be one factor that contributed to the 'failure' of phage therapy in its first go-round. But co-evolutionary potential is not the whole story; in fact, quite recently Williams-Smith and Huggins (1982) used phage successfully to treat experimental bacterial infections in mice. This was accomplished through the clever choice of phage for which the target bacterium lost its pathogenicity as a direct consequence of the evolution of resistance. It remains to be seen whether phage can be isolated for other bacterial targets such that the bacteria lose their undesirable properties by becoming resistant to the phage (Lenski, 1984c). If this strategy can be generalized (or other strategies developed), then perhaps phage may become something like the 'magic bullet' envisioned by Sinclair Lewis' (1925) fictitious Dr Arrowsmith.

ACKNOWLEDGEMENTS

We wish to thank Debbie Boudreau and Joyce Britt for aid in preparing this manuscript. This work has been supported by grants from the National Institutes of Health GM19848 and GM33782 and a BRSG grant from the University of Massachusetts. Some computer time for processing these words was provided by the P & S Apple Foundation.

REFERENCES

ANDERSON, E. S., 1968. The ecology of transferable drug resistance in the Enterobacteria. *Annual Review of Microbiology, 22:* 131–180.
ARBER, W. & LINN, S., 1969. DNA modification and restriction. *Annual Review of Biochemistry, 38:* 467–500.
BARRETT, J. A., 1983. Plant–fungus symbioses. In D. J. Futuyma & M. Slatkin (Eds), *Coevolution:* 137–160. Sunderland, Mass: Sinauer.
BURNET, M. & WHITE, D. O., 1972. *Natural History of Infectious Disease.* Cambridge: Cambridge University Press.
CAMPBELL, A. M., 1961. Conditions for the existence of bacteriophage. *Evolution, 15:* 153–165.

CAUGANT, D. A., LEVIN, B. R. & SELANDER, R. K., 1981. Genetic diversity and temporal variation in the *E. coli* population of a human host. *Genetics, 98:* 467–490.

CHAO, L. & LEVIN, B. R., 1981. Structured habitats and the evolution of anticompetitor toxins in bacteria. *Proceedings of the National Academy of Science USA, 78:* 6324–6328.

CHAO, L., LEVIN, B. R. & STEWART, F. M., 1977. A complex community in a simple habitat: an experimental study with bacteria and phage. *Ecology, 58:* 369–378.

DAWKINS, R. & KREBS, J. R., 1979. Arms races between and within species. *Proceedings Royal Society of London Series B, 205:* 489–511.

D'HERELLE, F., 1922. *The Bacteriophage: Its Role in Immunity.* (Translated by G. H. Smith). Baltimore: Williams and Wilkins.

DHILLON, T. S., CHAN, Y. S., SUN, S. M. & CHAU, W. S., 1970. Distribution of coliphages in Hong Kong sewage. *Applied Microbiology, 20:* 187–191.

DHILLON, T. S., DHILLON, E. K. S., CHAU, H. C., LI, W. K. & TSANG, A. H. C., 1976. Studies on bacteriophage distribution: virulent and temperate bacteriophage content of mammalian feces. *Applied and Environmental Microbiology, 32:* 68–74.

DIXON, B., 1984. Attack of the phages. *Science 84 (June):* 66–69.

DOVE, W. F., 1971. Biological inferences. In A. D. Hershey (Ed.), *Bacteriophage Lambda* : 297–312. New York: Cold Spring Harbor Laboratory, Cold Spring Harbor.

DYKHUIZEN, D., CAMPBELL, J. H. & ROLFE, B. G., 1978. The influences of prophage on the growth rate of *E. coli. Microbios, 23:* 99–113.

ECHOLS, H., 1972. Developmental pathways for the temperate phage: lysis vs lysogeny. *Annual Review of Genetics, 6:* 157–190.

EDLIN, G., LIN, L. & BITNER, R., 1977. Reproductive fitness of P1, P2, and Mu lysogens of *Escherichia coli. Journal of Virology, 21:* 560–564.

ELLIS, E. L. & DELBRUCK, M., 1939. The growth of bacteriophage. *Journal of General Physiology, 22:* 365–384.

FALKOW, S., 1975. *Infectious Multiple Drug Resistance.* London: Pion.

FLOR, H. H., 1956. The complementary genic systems in flax and flax rust. *Advances in Genetics, 8:* 29–54.

FREEMAN, V. J., 1951. Studies on the virulence of bacteriophage infected strains of *Corynebacterium diphtheriae. Journal of Bacteriology, 61:* 675–688.

FURUSE, K., OSAWA, S., KAWASHIRO, J., TANAKA, R., OZAWA, A., SAWAMURA, S., YANAGAWA, Y., NAGAO, T. & WATANABE, I., 1983. Bacteriophage distribution in human faeces: continuous survey of healthy subjects and patients with internal and leukaemic diseases. *Journal of General Virology, 64:* 2039–2043.

HOFNUNG, M., JEZIERSKA, A. & BRAUN-BRETON, C., 1976. *lam B* mutations in *E. coli* K12: growth of Lambda host-range mutants and effect of nonsense suppressors. *Molecular and General Genetics, 145:* 207–213.

HORNE, M. T., 1970. Coevolution of *Escherichia coli* and bacteriophage in chemostat culture. *Science, 168:* 992–993.

HOWES, W. V., 1965. Effect of glucose on the capacity of *Escherichia coli* to be infected by virulent Lambda bacteriophage. *Journal of Bacteriology, 90:* 1188–1193.

JOKLIK, W. K., 1974. Evolution in viruses. Symposium of the Society for General Microbiology, 24: 293–320.

KOCH, A. L., 1971. The adaptive responses of *Escherichia coli* to a feast and famine existence. *Advances in Microbiology, 6:* 147–217.

KRUGER, D. H. & BICKLE, T. A., 1983. Bacteriophage survival: multiple mechanisms for avoiding deoxyribonucleic acid restriction systems of their hosts. *Microbiological Reviews, 47:* 345–360.

LENSKI, R. E., 1984a. Coevolution of bacteria and phage: are there endless cycles of bacterial defenses and phage counterdefenses? *Journal of Theoretical Biology, 108:* 319–325.

LENSKI, R. E., 1984b. Two-step resistance by *Escherichia coli* B to bacteriophage T2. *Genetics, 107:* 1–7.

LENSKI, R. E., 1984c. Releasing 'ice-minus' bacteria. *Nature, 307:* 8.

LENSKI, R. E. & LEVIN, B. R., 1985. Constraints on the coevolution of bacteria and virulent phage: a model, some experiments, and predictions for natural communities. *American Naturalist, 125:* 585–602.

LEVIN, B. R., 1981. Periodic selection, infectious gene exchange and the genetic structure of *E. coli* populations. *Genetics, 99:* 1–23.

LEVIN, B. R. & KILMER, W. L., 1974. Interdemic selection and the evolution of altruism: a computer simulation study. *Evolution, 28:* 527–545.

LEVIN, B. R. & LENSKI, R. E., 1983. Coevolution in bacteria and their viruses and plasmids. In D. J. Futuyma & M. Slatkin (Eds), *Coevolution* : 99–127. Sunderland, Mass: Sinauer.

LEVIN, B. R., STEWART, F. M. & CHAO, L., 1977. Resource-limited growth, competition, and predation: a model and experimental studies with bacteria and bacteriophage. *American Naturalist, 111:* 3–24.

LEWIS, S., 1925. *Arrowsmith.* New York: Harcourt, Brace and World.

LIN, L., BITNER, R. & EDLIN, G., 1977. Increased reproductive fitness of *Escherichia coli* Lambda lysogens. *Journal of Virology, 21:* 554–559.

LURIA, S. E., 1945. Genetics of bacterium–bacterial virus relationship. *Annals of the Missouri Botanical Gardens, 32:* 235–242.

LURIA, S. E., 1953. Host-induced modification of viruses. *Cold Spring Harbor Symposia in Quantitative Biology, 18:* 237–244.

LURIA, S. E. & DELBRUCK, M., 1943. Mutations of bacteria from virus sensitivity to virus resistance. *Genetics, 28:* 491–511.

LWOFF, A., 1953. Lysogeny. *Bacteriological Reviews, 17:* 269–337.

MAY, R. M. & ANDERSON, R. M., 1983. Parasite–host coevolution. In D. J. Futuyma & M. Slatkin (Eds), *Coevolution*: 186–206. Sunderland, Mass: Sinauer.

McCONNELL, D. J., SEARCY, D. G. & SUTCLIFFE, J. G., 1978. A restriction enzyme, Thal, from the thermophilic mycoplasma, *Thermoplasma acidophilium. Nucleic Acids Research, 5:* 1729–1739.

MILLER, J. A., 1983. Microbial antifreeze: gene splicing takes to the field. *Science News, 124:* 132.

MITSUHASHI, S., 1971. Epidemiology of bacterial drug resistance. In S. Mitsuhashi (Ed.), *Transferable Drug Resistance Factor R*: 1–23. Baltimore: University Park Press.

NOACK, D., 1969. A model on the production of temperate phages in continuous culture. In *Continuous Cultivation of Microorganisms*: 233–241. Prague: Academia.

ØRSKOV, F. & ØRSKOV, I., 1961. The fertility of *Escherichia coli* antigen test strains in crosses with K12. *Acta Pathologica et Microbiologica Scandinavica, 51:* 280–290.

PAYNTER, M. J. B. & BUNGAY, M. R., III, 1969. Dynamics of coliphage infections. In D. Perlman (Ed.), *Fermentation Advances*: 323–335. New York and London: Academic Press.

PAYNTER, M. J. B. & BUNGAY, M. R., III, 1970. Responses in continuous culture of lysogenic *Escherichia coli* following induction. *Biotechnology and Bioengineering, 12:* 347–351.

PEITZMAN, S. J., 1969. Felix d'Herelle and bacteriophage therapy. *Transactions and Studies of the College of Physicians of Philadelphia, 37:* 115–123.

PTASHNE, M., 1971. Repressor and its action. In A. D. Hershey (Ed.), *Bacteriophage Lambda*: 221–237. New York: Cold Spring Harbor Laboratory, Cold Spring Harbor.

PTASHNE, M., JEFFREY, A., JOHNSON, A. D., MAURER, R., MEYER, B. J., PABO, C. O., ROBERTS, T. M. & SAUER, R. T., 1980. How the Lambda repressor and *cro* work. *Cell, 19:* 1–11.

RODIN, S. N. & RATNER, V. A., 1983a. Some theoretical aspects of protein coevolution in the ecosystem 'phage-bacteria'. I. The problem. *Journal of Theoretical Biology, 100:* 185–195.

RODIN, S. N. & RATNER, V. A., 1983b. Some theoretical aspects of protein coevolution in the ecosystem 'phage-bacteria'. II. The deterministic model of microevolution. *Journal of Theoretical Biology, 100:* 197–210.

RYTER, A., SHUMAN, H. & SCHWARTZ, M., 1975. Integration of the receptor for bacteriophage Lambda in the outer membrane of *Escherichia coli*: coupling with cell division. *Journal of Bacteriology, 122:* 295–301.

SCHWARTZ, M., 1980. Interaction of phages with their receptor proteins. In L. L. Randall & L. Philipson (Eds), *Virus Receptors, Part 1. Bacterial Viruses*: 59–94. London: Chapman and Hall.

SELANDER, R. K. & LEVIN, B. R., 1980. Genetic diversity and structure in *Escherichia coli* populations. *Science, 210:* 545–547.

STENT, G. S., 1963. *Molecular Biology of Bacterial Viruses*. San Francisco: Freeman.

STERNBERG, N. & AUSTIN, S., 1981. The maintenance of the P1 plasmid prophage. *Plasmid, 5:* 20–31.

STEWART, F. M. & LEVIN, B. R., 1984. The population biology of bacterial viruses: why be temperate? *Theoretical Population Biology, 26:* 93–117.

UCHIDA, T., GILL, D. M. & PAPPENHEIMER, A. M., 1971. Mutation in the structural gene for diphtheria toxin carried by the temperate phage Beta. *Nature, 233:* 8–11.

VAN VALEN, L., 1973. A new evolutionary law. *Evolutionary Theory, 1:* 1–30.

WILLIAMS SMITH, H., 1972. Ampicillin resistance in *Escherichia coli* by phage infection. *Nature, 238:* 205–206.

WILLIAMS SMITH, H. & HUGGINS, M. B., 1982. Successful treatment of experimental *Escherichia coli* infections in mice using phage: its general superiority over antibiotics. *Journal of General Microbiology, 128:* 307–318.

WILSON, D. S., 1980. *Natural Selection of Populations and Communities*. Menlo Park, California: Benjamin Cummings.

WILSON, G. G., YOUNG, K. K. Y., EDLIN, G. J. & KONIGSBERG, W., 1979. High frequency generalized transduction by bacteriophage T4. *Nature, 280:* 80–82.

WILSON, G. S. & MILES, A. A., 1964. *Topley and Wilson's Principles of Bacteriology and Immunity, Volume II.* Baltimore: Williams and Wilkins.

Host–parasite associations: their population biology and population genetics

ROBERT M. MAY

Department of Biology,
Princeton University,
Princeton, New Jersey 08544, U.S.A.

Various theoretical and empirical aspects of the overall population dynamics and population genetics of host–parasite associations are reviewed (with parasite defined broadly to include viruses, bacteria, protozoans and fungi along with helminths and arthropods). The conditions under which parasites may provide density-dependent regulation of their host population, and the dynamical character of the regulated state (stable point, stable cycles, chaos) are discussed, both for host populations with discrete generations and for host populations with continuously overlapping generations. Combining genetics and epidemiology, I also discuss gene-for-gene associations between hosts and parasites; the main conclusions are that such interactions tend to generate and maintain polymorphism (again either stably, or cyclically, or even chaotically), and that whether or not parasites evolve toward 'harmlessness' depends on the relationships among parasite virulence and transmissibility and the cost of host resistance.

KEY WORDS: — Host–parasite associations — population biology — population genetics — modelling — epidemiology — microparasites — macroparasites

CONTENTS

Ecology and Genetics of Host–Parasite Interactions
ISBN: 0 12 593 690 7

INTRODUCTION

Most parasitological research deals with the biology of individual parasites, or with the interaction between an individual host and the population of parasites within that host. For an understanding of the overall transmission and maintenance — and ultimately the control or eradication — of parasitic infections, however, we must deal with the interactions between the total populations of hosts and of parasites. The present paper therefore offers a brief review of recent work on the population biology of host–parasite associations. The paper is more in the nature of a signposted guide than a synoptic and self-contained review; it aims to sketch the essential character of the various results, referring to the existing literature for the details.

Throughout, the term 'parasite' is taken to include viruses, bacteria, protozoans and fungi along with the conventionally defined helminth and arthropod parasites. Insofar as broad distinctions among parasites are made, they are based on evolutionary and dynamical grounds rather than on conventional taxonomic ones. The main such distinction is between microparasites and macroparasites (Anderson and May, 1979). Biologically, microparasites are defined as those with direct reproduction, usually at high rates, within the host; they typically are small, have generation times much shorter than the lifespan of the host, and induce acquired immunity (often lifelong) in recovered hosts. Although there are many exceptions, microparasitic infections are characteristically of a transient nature. Viral and bacterial infections (such as smallpox and pertussis) are typical examples. Macroparasites usually have no direct reproduction within the host, are larger than microparasites, and have longer generation times (which can approach an appreciable fraction of the host lifespan); in those cases where an immune response is elicited, it is usually dependent on the number of parasites present in the host and is not long-lasting. Macroparasitic infections are typically of a persistent nature, with hosts being continually reinfected. Most helminth and arthropod parasites belong in this class.

More specifically, the distinction between microparasites and macroparasites is based on their dynamics (Anderson and May, 1979). Microparasites are essentially those for which the host population can be roughly divided into a relatively small number of distinct epidemiological classes (susceptible, infected, recovered and immune); to a good approximation, hosts either are or are not infected. For macroparasites, on the other hand, it is necessary to take account of the detailed distribution of parasites among individuals in the host population; there is an important distinction between infection (harbouring one or more parasites) and disease (harbouring a load sufficient to be pathogenic). One reflection of this distinction lies in the definition of the basic reproductive rate of the parasite, R_0: for a microparasite, R_0 is simply the number of infected hosts produced on average by one infected host individual in a wholly susceptible population; for a macroparasite it is necessary to count parasites, and R_0 is the average number of reproductively mature female offspring produced throughout the lifetime of a female parasite in the absence of density-dependent constraints.

The annotated bibliography is organized as follows. First, I discuss recent studies that focus on the overall population dynamics of host–parasite associations, treating them essentially as special cases of prey–predator interactions. Of particular interest is whether the parasite may regulate the magnitude of its host population and, if so, whether the regulated state is steady, or with cyclic oscillations, or apparently chaotic fluctuations. The answers are sketched separately for microparasites and macroparasites, interacting with host populations with discrete generations (difference equations) or with continuously overlapping generations (differential equations). Second, consideration is given to the special case when the host population is effectively constant (regulated by factors other than the parasite), and there is discussion of the population dynamics of microparasitic and macroparasitic infections with particular emphasis on programs of immunization or chemotherapy. Third, recent work on the overall population genetics of host-parasite associations is summarized; to date, this work is confined to microparasitic infections. Fourth, I mention some of the complications that arise when dynamic and genetic considerations are combined to explore what happens when a genetically polymorphic host population is regulated by a genetically polymorphic parasite.

DYNAMICS OF HOST-PARASITE ASSOCIATIONS

The work reviewed under this heading is mainly devoted to elucidating the circumstances under which parasites may regulate the abundance or geographical distribution of their host populations. Although prey-predator dynamics in general, and the possible regulation of prey populations by predators in particular, receive extended treatment in most ecology textbooks, corresponding discussion of host-parasite interactions has been unaccountably absent until very recently. As seen below, the dynamical behaviour of particular host-parasite systems provides some striking examples of central themes in contemporary ecology (including chaos and the stabilizing effects of patchiness and aggregation). For general reviews of the available evidence about the effects of parasites on the ecology of their hosts, see May (1983), Hassell et al. (1982) and Holmes (1982).

Host population with discrete generations: microparasites

Many populations, such as univoltine insects in temperate regions, have discrete generations that do not overlap. For such populations, the census data may be taken to be the number of adults emerging in generation t, N_t. Suppose such a population is regulated by a lethal pathogen that spreads in epidemic fashion throughout each generation before reproductive maturity is attained; the survivors then go on to reproduce, each producing on average λ offspring that survive to emerge as adults at the start of the next generation. The number of adults in successive generations are then related by a first-order non-linear difference equation,

$$N_{t+1} = \lambda N_t [1 - I(N_t)]. \tag{1}$$

Here, $I(N_t)$ represents the fraction of the population infected by the epidemic in generation t; $1 - I$ is thus the fraction surviving to reproduce. This fraction I is given by a simple extension of the Kermack-McKendrick (1927) equation (May and Anderson, 1983), and obeys the relation

$$1 - I = \exp(-IN_t/N_T). \tag{2}$$

Here N_T is a 'threshold' density, determined by the transmissibility, β, and virulence, α, of the pathogen ($N_t = \alpha/\beta$). Notice that eqs (1) and (2) can be expressed in dimensionless form by defining X_t to be the ratio of N_t to N_T:

$$X_t \equiv N_t/N_T. \tag{3}$$

If N_t is below threshold magnitude ($N_t < N_T$; $X_t < 1$), the pathogen cannot spread, and essentially nobody is infected: $I = 0$. If N_t is above threshold ($N_t > N_T$; $X_t > 1$), the pathogen does spread, infecting a larger and larger fraction as N_t increases: eq (2) has a solution $I \neq 0$.

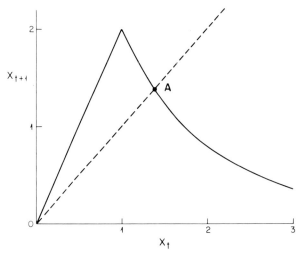

Figure 1. The solid line depicts the functional relationship or map determining the (dimensionless) population density in generation $t + 1$, X_{t+1}, in terms of that in generation t, X_t, for a population regulated by a pathogen; specifically, the map is for eq (1) with $\lambda = 2$. The spikey hump in the map derives from the discontinuous nature of the threshold phenomenon, whereby a deterministic epidemic spreads if and only if the host population exceeds a critical value. The dashed line corresponds to an unchanging population, $X_{t+1} = X_t$, so that the point A represents a possible equilibrium point. (From May, 1985.)

The 'map' relating the host population densities in successive generations is shown in Fig. 1, for the representative value $\lambda = 2$. The essential features of this figure hold for all values of λ: for N_t below threshold ($X_t < 1$) there is density independent growth at the rate λ; for N_t above threshold ($X_t > 1$) the pathogen inflicts pre-reproductive mortality that increases in severity as host density increases.

Clearly this lethal pathogen provides density dependent regulation of its host population, and it appears possible from Fig. 1 that the population may be regulated around the point $N_{t+1} = N_t = N^*$ which is labelled A in Fig. 1. The dynamics of this simple and natural model for a population regulated by disease are, however, astonishing. The system has no stable point nor any stable cycles for any value of $\lambda > 1$ (and for $\lambda < 1$ the population of course declines to extinction). Instead, the purely deterministic relation described by eqs (1) and (2) and Fig. 1 leads always to 'deterministic randomness'; the dynamical behaviour of the host population is always like the sample function of some random process.

Figures 2 and 3 illustrate this 'chaotic' dynamical behaviour. Figure 2 was obtained by plotting long runs of iterations of eq (1) for specific values of λ, and

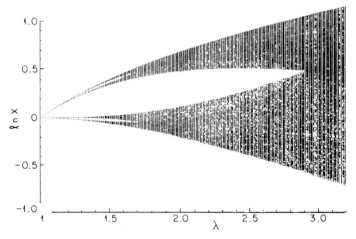

Figure 2. This figure is constructed by plotting the population values (on a logarithmic scale, $\ln X$) generated by iterating the difference equation (1) many times, for each of a sequence of λ-values. The diagram gives an impression of the probability distribution of population values generated by this purely deterministic difference equation; for a more full discussion, see May (1985).

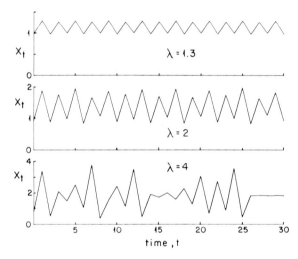

Figure 3. This figure shows the variation in the population, X, with time, t, as described by eq (1) for three values of λ. These three population trajectories further illustrate the character of the chaotic dynamical behaviour noted in Fig. 2 and discussed more generally in the text: (a) for $\lambda = 1.3$, the trajectory — although strictly aperiodic — is close to a 2-point cycle; (b) for $\lambda = 2$, the trajectory is obviously aperiodic, but still alternates up and down in successive generations; (c) for $\lambda = 4$, the trajectory is quite ragged.

it gives some idea of the probability distributions for host densities. For relatively small values of λ, the host population alternates between a band of relatively high values and a band of relatively low values; these bands are narrow for λ close to unity (and indeed there are four bands, which correspond to trajectories looking rather like a 4-point cycle, for λ less than about 1.68). For $\lambda > 2.91$ the two bands coalesce, and the population can take any value between upper and lower bounds. Figure 3 illustrates these properties by displaying three specific trajectories: for $\lambda = 1.3$ the trajectory — although in fact chaotic — is close to a 2-point cycle; for

$\lambda = 2$ the aperiodicity is marked, although the population density still clearly alternates up and down; and for $\lambda = 4$ the trajectory is quite irregular.

These results are derived and discussed in detail by May (1985). It is surprising that this simple and sensible model for a host–parasite interaction should not have been studied earlier. The system is, moreover, undoubtedly the simplest example of a purely chaotic deterministic system yet known, and it is remarkable that such pathological behaviour should arise from such natural biological assumptions.

More generally, it may be assumed that the pathogen is not invariably lethal, but rather that some infected hosts die (at a rate α) and others recover to an immune state (at a rate v). It may then be shown that the pathogen can regulate its host population if, and only if, it is sufficiently virulent:

$$\alpha > v(\lambda - 1). \tag{4}$$

The regulated state may be a stable point, or a stable cycle, if v is sufficiently large in relation to α (while still obeying eq (4); May, 1985).

At the opposite extreme from the above case of an epidemic infection is an endemic infection, in which all infected hosts simply recover to the susceptible state. This could be relevant to some insect populations, where acquired immunity is rare. Suppose all infected hosts recover ($\alpha = 0$), but do not reproduce while infected. The analogue of eqs (1) and (2) can then be seen simply to be

$$X_{t+1} = \lambda X_t, \ \ if \ X_t < 1, \tag{5a}$$

$$X_{t+1} = \lambda, \ \ if \ X_t > 1. \tag{5b}$$

This relation is illustrated in Fig. 4, where it is seen that an endemic infection of this kind will always regulate the host population to a stable equilibrium value.

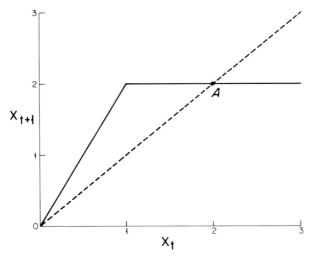

Figure 4. This map differs from that Fig. 1 in that it shows the relation between X_{t+1} and X_t for a host population regulated by an endemic infection: infected hosts recover directly back into the susceptible class; infected hosts are not killed by the infection, but they do not reproduce while infected. As in Fig. 1, the dashed line corresponds to an unchanging population, $X_{t+1} = X_t$. Here the equilibrium point A is globally stable.

More generally, we can let some infected hosts die, while others recover to the susceptible state. The results are relations intermediate between Figs 1 and 4, with dynamics ranging from stable equilibrium points to apparently chaotic trajectories.

Host population with discrete generations: macroparasites

Crofton (1971a,b) was the first to analyse models for hosts with discrete generations, whose densities are regulated by macroparasites. The basic model parallels that for microparasites: in each generation, host individuals acquire a burden of parasites as they advance to reproductive maturity; relatively heavily infected hosts die (and their parasites — whose generation time is synchronized with that of the hosts — die with them); relatively lightly infected hosts reproduce, to give on average λ offspring in the next generation (and their parasites also reproduce, each to give on average Λ free-living transmission stages, that will infect the next generation of hosts). Specifically, Crofton assumed hosts with fewer than a lethal level of L parasites would survive to reproduce, while those with more than L parasites would die. Guided by observed patterns of parasite distribution within host populations, Crofton (1971a) did not assume that parasites are acquired independently randomly by host individuals, but rather assumed the parasite distribution to be a negative binomial. That is, the parasite distribution was taken to be clumped, with most hosts having relatively light burdens, and a few having relatively heavy burdens; this accords with observed patterns where often 80–90% of helminths are found in 10% of the hosts. The degree of clumping is characterized by the parameter k of the negative binomial: for a negative binomial distribution

$$\frac{\text{variance}}{\text{mean}} = 1 + (\text{mean})/\text{k}. \tag{6}$$

Thus $k \to \infty$ gives the Poisson distribution, while $k \to 0$ gives a highly aggregated distribution (Crofton, 1971a; May, 1977a).

Crofton's numerical simulations (1971b) suggest that macroparasites can regulate their host populations in a steady way, provided parasite-induced mortality is severe enough and k small enough. For k too large (parasite distribution insufficiently clumped), Crofton found diverging oscillations of a kind familiar in many host–parasitoid models (Hassell, 1978). May (1977a) subsequently refined Crofton's model, replacing Crofton's step-function host survival (with its lethal level of L parasites) by a more continuously varying survival function (with the lethal level still roughly characterized by L parasites); May also made more realistic assumptions about the rate at which parasites are acquired by hosts. It can then be shown that the host population is regulated by the parasitic infection if, and only if (May, 1977a),

$$\lambda < [\Lambda \exp(-1/L)]^{k/(1+k)}. \tag{7}$$

That is, the basic reproductive rate of the parasite (discounted to a degree that depends on the amount of parasite clumping, k) must exceed that of the host for regulation to be possible. As found by Crofton, this equilibrium is a stable point provided k is small enough in relation to λ, and is always a stable point if $k < 1$. In some situations, the equilibrium may be such that the system recovers from small disturbances, but is unstable (undergoing diverging oscillations) to large perturbations (May, 1979).

Notice that clumping or overdispersion of parasites among host individuals is important for the stability of these systems. This re-echoes the major theme of much recent theoretical and empirical research on prey–predator systems in general: if the system is homogeneous (that is, if predators or parasites attack independently at random) it cannot persist, undergoing wild oscillations; but if there is sufficient heterogeneity (patchiness and differential aggregation, as in the Crofton model), there can be global persistence, produced by local differences. For a review of work relating to this theme, see Hassell and May (1984).

Host population with continuously overlapping generations: microparasites

At the opposite extreme from populations with discrete, non-overlapping generations, are those where generations overlap completely so that population growth is a continuous process. The basic model for the interaction between such a host population and a microparasitic infection takes the form of differential equations describing the rate of change of the numbers of susceptible, infected-and-infectious, and recovered-and-immune hosts, $X(t)$, $Y(t)$, $Z(t)$, respectively (Anderson & May, 1979):

$$dX/dt = a(X + Y + Z) - bX - \beta XY + \gamma Z, \qquad (8a)$$

$$dY/dt = \beta XY - (\alpha + b + v)Y, \qquad (8b)$$

$$dZ/dt = vY - (b + \gamma)Z. \qquad (8c)$$

Here, the host population is assumed to be 'homogeneously mixed', and new infections appear at a rate proportional both to the number of susceptibles and the number of infecteds, βXY; β is the 'transmission parameter'. The quantity a represents the per capita birth rate; b is the per capita death rate from causes other than the disease in question; α is the disease-induced death rate; v is the recovery rate; and γ is the rate of loss of immunity ($\gamma = 0$ if immunity is lifelong). This basic model differs from those of conventional epidemiological studies (e.g. Bailey, 1975) in that the host population is not taken to be constant, but rather increases exponentially at the rate $r = a - b$ in the absence of this infection.

Such a microparasite will regulate its host population to a stable equilibrium value provided

$$\alpha > r[1 + v/(b + \gamma)]. \qquad (9)$$

That is, the infection must be virulent enough (α large enough) to prevail over the host population's intrinsic growth rate ($r = a - b$) augmented by a factor that allows for the presence of acquired immunity. Although invertebrates are capable of mounting cellular or humoral responses to microparasitic infection, they rarely if ever manifest acquired immunity (that is, for invertebrates $\gamma \to \infty$); in this case, the infection will stably regulate its host population provided only that

$$\alpha > r. \qquad (10)$$

The above results are derived and a variety of possible refinements and applications discussed in Anderson and May (1979, 1981). Among the possible complications which may be included are: a latent, infected-but-not-yet-infectious, class (which makes regulation of the host population more difficult); vertical transmission, whereby some offspring of infected hosts are born infected (making regulation easier); diminished reproduction or even castration of infected hosts (again making regulation easier); and various complexities associated with indirect transmission via intermediate hosts (which can lead to sustained oscillations both in the incidence of infection and even in the magnitude of the host population). In particular, many viral or protozoan infections of forest insects have free-living transmission stages with long life spans, which can produce marked cyclic oscillations in the abundance of the host, with periods ranging from a few years to a few decades (Anderson & May, 1981; Regniere, 1984; Getz & Pickering, 1983).

Host population with continuously overlapping generations: macroparasites

The corresponding differential equations modelling the interaction between a host population with continuously overlapping generations and a macroparasitic infection were first constructed and studied by Anderson & May (1978).

A crucial aspect of host–macroparasite systems for which good data are available is the clumped or aggregated way the parasites are distributed among hosts. These observed distributions are usually described well by a negative binomial, with the parameter k characterizing the degree of aggregation as above (see eq (6)). Table 1 summarizes information about k for macroparasitic infections of humans and other animal hosts; essentially all these parasite distributions exhibit marked aggregation.

In constructing these host–macroparasite models, it is assumed that sufficiently high parasite burdens do indeed contribute to host deaths, with the mortality rate increasing either linearly or exponentially with increasing parasite numbers within a host. Such macroparasites are capable of regulating their host population, provided

$$\Lambda - (\mu + b + \alpha) > (a - b)(k + 1)/k. \tag{11}$$

Here, Λ is the rate of production of transmission stages (eggs, spores or cysts) per parasite; μ is the per capita parasite death rate; α is the proportionality constant such that αi is the parasite-induced mortality rate in a host harboring i parasites; a and b, as before, are the birth and disease-free death rates per host; and k is the clumping parameter in the negative binomial parasite distribution. The criterion (11) for hosts with continuously overlapping generations is broadly comparable to eq (7) for hosts with discrete generations: the left-hand side represents the parasite population growth rate (births, Λ, minus deaths from all causes — parasite death, natural host death, parasite-induced host death — $(\mu + b + \alpha)$), which must be able to outrun the host population growth rate $(a - b)$, corrected for parasite clumping. If eq (11) is satisfied, the parasite will always be capable of regulating its host population. On the other hand, if parasite-induced mortality effects are not substantial (α insufficiently large), this parasite-regulated host population level is likely to be so high that other density dependent regulatory effects intervene before it is reached. In short, regulation of a host population by macroparasites in general requires both that eq (11) be obeyed, and that α be large enough.

Macroparasites may regulate their host population to a stable equilibrium value,

Table 1. Values of the negative binomial clumping parameter k observed for distributions of parasites in human and other natural populations of hosts (excerpted from Anderson & May, 1978, 1982b)

	Parasite	Host	
Taxonomic group	Species	Species	Range of k values
Platyhelminthes	*Diclidophora denticulata*	*Gadus virens*	0.7
	Diplostomum gasterostei	*Gasterosteus aculeatus*	0.1–0.7
	Caryophyllaeus laticeps	*Abramis brama*	0.1–0.5
	Schistocephalus solidus	*Gasterosteus aculeatus*	0.7–2.4
Nematoda	*Chandlerella quiscoli*	*Culicoides crepuscularis*	0.5
	Toxocara canis	*Vulpes vulpes*	0.5
	Ascaridia galli	*Gallus gallus*	0.7
Acanthocephala	*Polymorphus minutus*	*Gammarus pulex*	0.6–3 1
	Echinorhynchus clavula	*Gasterosteus aculeatus*	0.07–0.5
Arthropoda	*Lepeophtheirus pectoralis*	*Pleuronectes platessa*	0.3–10.0
	Chondracanthopsis nodosus	*Sebastes marinus*	0.6
	Chondracanthopsis nodosus	*Sebastes mentella*	0.2
	Ixodes trianguliceps	*Apodemus sylvaticus*	0.04–0.4
	Liponysue bacoti	*Rattus rattus*	0.2
Nematoda	*Ascaris lumbricoides*	Humans, Iran	0.2–2.9
	Necator americanus	Humans, India	0.03–0.6
	Anclyostoma duodenale	Humans, Taiwan	0.05–0.4
Trematoda	*Schistosoma mansoni*	Humans, Brazil	0.03–0.5
Arthropoda	*Pediculus humanus capitis*	Humans, India	0.14

or in stably sustained cycles (Anderson & May, 1978; May & Anderson, 1978). Factors tending to produce a stable point are parasite aggregation (small x), parasite-induced host mortality that rises steeply with parasite load, and density dependent constraints on parasite numbers per host or on egg output per parasite. Factors tending to produce cyclic oscillations in host and parasite abundance are parasite-induced reduction in host reproduction, direct reproduction of parasites within hosts, and time delays in parasite reproduction and transmission.

Notice that macroparasites may be the sole agents providing density dependent regulation of the host population, even though very few hosts harbor a lethal load of parasites. It is a common misconception that the effects of a density dependent regulatory agent must be apparent in most host individuals; this simply is not so.

We can, indeed, give a simple yet general expression for the fraction of all host deaths that must be attributable to a particular microparasite or macroparasite, if that parasite is truly the regulator. Assuming only that the per capita host birth rate, a, and death rate from all other causes, b, are density independent constants (which, of course, is not usually so), we have (May, 1983)

$$\frac{\text{parasite-induced host deaths}}{\text{total host deaths}} = \frac{a - b}{a} . \qquad (12)$$

The result holds for both microparasites and macroparasites, independent of the mode of transmission and of the nature of immune processes. If a and b are not too disparate, so that $(a - b)/a$ is small, the parasite can be responsible for regulating the host population, even though few deaths will be laid at its door. Conversely, if $a \gg b$ (as is the case for many invertebrates), the infection needs to be responsible for most of the observed mortality before it can be a candidate for consideration as the regulatory agent.

PARASITE POPULATION DYNAMICS (HOST POPULATION CONSTANT)

There exists an enormous amount of data for parasitic infections of humans. Although not often making contact with these data, there also exists a considerable literature on mathematical models for microparasitic infections in human populations (e.g., Bailey, 1975; Dietz, 1975; Bartlett, 1960). Essentially all this theoretical work treats the human host population as constant, unaffected in magnitude by the presence of the infection. Human populations do, of course, change over time, but these changes take place slowly in relation to time scales of epidemiological interest; thus the appoximation of taking the human host population, N, to be a constant is sensible. This usually corresponds to putting $a = b$ and $\alpha = 0$ in the differential equation models of the second section (p. 250).

Microparasites

The basic equations are obtained by putting $a = b$ and $\alpha = 0$ in eq (8). The total population, $N = X + Y + Z$, is now some constant, determined by other factors. By considering eq (8b) for the increase in the number infected when a few infectious individuals are introduced into a population that is essentially wholly susceptible, one sees that an infection can establish itself only if N exceeds a threshold vlaue, $N > N_T$, with the definition (Kermack & McKendrick, 1927)

$$N_T = (b + v)/\beta. \tag{13}$$

Alternatively, one can note that the microparasite's basic reproductive rate, R_0 (as defined earlier p. 244), is here given by $R_0 = N/N_T$; obviously, we must have $R_0 > 1$ for the infection to persist within the population. In general, it is not possible to make any direct estimate of the transmission parameter β, and thus R_0 cannot usually be estimated from the above formulae. One can, however, estimate R_0 indirectly for this homogeneously mixed population, as follows. As the infection becomes established in the population, a decreasing fraction of the host population remains susceptible (with an increasing fraction having acquired immunity following infection). The microparasite's effective reproductive rate is thus diminished to $R = R_0 x$, where x is the fraction remaining susceptible. But, at equilibrium, $R = 1$; hence, R_0 and the equilibrium fraction susceptible, x^*, are related by

$$R_0 x^* = 1. \tag{14}$$

The quantity x^* can be estimated accurately from serological studies (or roughly as $x^* \sim L/A$, where L is average life expectancy and A is average age at infection). Finally, an extension of this simple argument shows that in order to eradicate the infection the proportion successfully immunized must exceed p_c, where

$$p_c = 1 - x^* = 1 - 1/R_0. \tag{15}$$

The above formulae are useful both in characterizing the basic reproductive rates of various childhood infections, and in providing a rough guide to the design of immunization programmes (Smith, 1970; Macdonald, 1952; Dietz, 1975; Anderson & May, 1982c; Fine & Clarkson, 1982; Warren et al., 1982; Fine et al., 1982). For more detailed analysis, and for tests of the models against public health data, it is necessary to add various realistic refinements, including full treatment of age specific susceptibility and infection rates (for a detailed review, see Anderson & May, 1983). Recent work adds further, more complicated, refinements which include: transmission parameters $\beta(a,a')$ which vary with the ages of the susceptible and infectious individuals who are in contact (Schenzle, 1984; Anderson & May, in press); spatial inhomogeneity, with hosts divided into groups of varying sizes ('cities and villages') and with intragroup transmission rates being systematically higher than intergroup ones (May & Anderson, 1984); genetic heterogeneity in the host population, with some individuals being intrinsically more susceptible to infection than others (Anderson & May, in press).

Relations like eq (15) and its more sophisticated later relatives derive from consideration of the final equilibrium eventually reached under a given immunization program. The dynamic path to this endpoint can be surprisingly complicated, with very pronounced oscillations in the incidence of infection sometimes being excited by particular kinds of immunization schedules (Knox, 1980; Anderson & May, 1983). Even before immunization, most childhood infections exhibited fairly marked cycles in the yearly incidence of infection (around 2 years for measles, 3 years for pertussis, 4–5 years for rubella); these cycles are beautiful examples of prey–predator cycles, with periods, T, given very accurately by the simple Lotka-Volterra expression which in this instance is

$$T \sim 2\pi(A\tau)^{\frac{1}{2}}. \tag{16}$$

Here, τ is the average duration of infectiousness (the characteristic predator time scale) and A is the average host age at infection (the characteristic host time scale). For detailed analysis of the available data in this light, see Anderson, Grenfell & May (1984).

Macroparasites

Mathematical models for the transmission and maintenance of macroparasitic infections in human populations (of constant size, N) have traditionally received less attention than those for microparasites. The classic early work is due to Macdonald (1965, 1973) on schistosomiasis. Neither Macdonald's work nor later elaborations (e.g. Nasell & Hirsch, 1973) made much contact with data pertaining to the dynamics of infection, but it was influential in producing concepts such as the possible 'breakpoint' (whereby the parasite population may decline to extinction if depressed below a certain level, essentially because mated adult pairs become unlikely).

Later work has suggested, however, that the parasite clumping patterns discussed above (and testified to by Table 1) may usually make breakpoint parasite densities too low to be of practical significance (May, 1977b; Bradley & May, 1978; Fine et al., 1982).

More interesting, to my mind, are recent studies which seek to relate the kind of host–macroparasite models developed in the second section (p. 251) to public health data on the prevalence and mean burdens of hookworm, *Ascaris* and other helminths in various human populations. These studies have some success in fitting observed patterns of age-specific prevalence and worm burden, or of reacquisition of worms following chemotherapy, with mathematical models employing relatively few biological parameters (such as the negative binomial k, the death rate μ of adult parasites, and the helminth basic reproductive rate, R_0); for details, see Anderson & May (1982b, 1985).

These theoretical studies can help in the design of chemotherapy programs, shedding light on such questions as the timing of successive episodes of chemotherapeutic intervention, or the relationship between effects of chemotherapy on mean worm burden (where large reductions may be possible) versus on prevalence (where low levels are difficult to attain). In particular, the models can be used to explore the advantages and disadvantages of selective treatment of the most heavily infected individuals in a community (Warren, 1981). Table 2 summarizes one such study, comparing the outcome of a program of randomly applied chemotherapy with one targeted to heavily infected hosts.

Table 2. The potential advantages of a programme of selective chemotherapy that focuses on heavily infected hosts*

	Fraction of host population to be treated		
Programme	0.40	0.20	0.10
Percentage reduction of mean parasite burden if treatment is at random	40	20	10
Percentage reduction of mean parasite burden under 'selective treatment' defined above	75	38	19

*Specifically, the programme concentrates — albeit with an element of uncertainty — on hosts with parasite burdens above or around the pristine average value; for details, see Anderson and May, 1982b. The parasites are assumed to be distributed among hosts according to a negative binomial with clumping parameter k = 0.5.

POPULATION GENETICS OF HOST–PARASITE ASSOCIATIONS

Genetics without epidemiology

Following early work by Mode (1958) and others, there now exists a large literature on the population genetics of 'gene-for-gene' interactions between hosts and pathogens. In these studies, there are specific associations between individual genotypes of hosts and corresponding genotypes of pathogens; such associations have been documented in detail for several pathogens of plants, especially crop plants. The genetic dynamics in these models is treated accurately, employing the conventional formalism of mathematical population genetics, but the fitnesses of the various host genotypes when attacked by specific pathogens are treated as constant. Thus, although host fitnesses ultimately depend on the relative gene frequencies in the parasite population, and likewise pathogen fitnesses depend on the relative gene frequencies in the host population, all the threshold and other non-linear effects associated with epidemiological processes are absent.

Such models are nevertheless interesting. They show that gene-for-gene associations between hosts and pathogens can easily maintain polymorphisms in the gene frequencies of both hosts and pathogen; these polymorphisms may be at some stable level, or they may oscillate in stable cycles. An excellent recent review of this area has been given by Levin (1983).

Genetics and epidemiology

Recent studies take the earlier gene-for-gene framework, but now calculate the various fitness functions from epidemiological analyses of the kind developed in the second and third sections earlier (pp. 245–255). The pioneering study here is by Gillespie (1975) who, however, only considered the statics and not the dynamics of his model. Studies of the full dynamics of such combined genetic and epidemiological models reveal interesting biological and mathematical features (May & Anderson, 1983; Beck, in press; Hamilton, 1980).

These models are notable, *inter alia*, as the first examples to my knowledge where a population genetic analysis has employed fitness functions whose frequency and density dependences are derived from an explicit ecological model (rather than being constructed in an *ad hoc* way). The essential character of the models can be appreciated by considering a haploid host with discrete, non-overlapping generations. We focus on a single locus with 2 alleles, A and a: genotype A is susceptible to pathogen genotype 1 (but resistant to pathogen genotype 2), and conversely host genotype a is susceptible to pathogen 2 (and resistant to pathogen 1). In the usual way, the gene frequency of A in generation $t + 1$, p_{t+1}, is related to that in generation t, p_t, by

$$p_{t+1} = p_t W_1 / \overline{W}_t. \tag{17}$$

The fitnesses of host genotypes A and a are labelled W_1 and W_2, respectively, and $\overline{W}_t$ is the mean fitness in generation t,

$$\overline{W}_t = p_t W_1 + (1 - p_t) W_2. \tag{18}$$

As in the simple models of the second section (p. 245), we assume that the pathogens spread epidemically through the populations of susceptible hosts, eventually infecting a fraction I_i of the hosts of genotype i $(i = 1,2)$; these infected hosts either die (at the disease-induced death rate α_i) or recover (at a rate v_i). The survivors then each produce on average λ_i offspring. It follows that the fitness of hosts of genotype i $(i = 1,2)$ is

$$W_i = \lambda_i [1 - s_i I_i]. \tag{19}$$

Here, s_i is the fraction of those infected who die, $s_i = \alpha_i/(\alpha_i + v_i)$, and I_i is given by the earlier eq (2) for each genotype.

For the time being, one can assume the pathogen serves only to determine the relative proportions of the various host genotypes, with some other ecological factor holding the total number of hosts to a constant density, K, in each generation. In this case, the number of hosts of genotype i, N_i, can be written $N_i = f_i K$ (with $f_1 = p$ and $f_2 = 1 - p$), and eq (2) takes the form

$$1 - I_i = \exp[-I_i R_i f_i]. \tag{20}$$

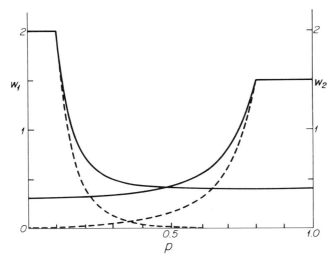

Figure 5. For a haploid host, this figure shows the fitnesses W_1 and W_2 of the genotypes A and a respectively, as functions of the gene frequency p. The fitnesses are given by eqs (19) and (20), with the parameter values $\lambda_1 = 2$, $\lambda_2 = 1.5$, $R_1 = 10$, $R_2 = 5$; the solid curves are for $s_1 = s_2 = 0.8$, and the dashed curves are for $s_1 = s_2 = 1$.

The reproductive rate R_i for pathogens of genotype i $(i = 1,2)$ is given as $R_i = K/N_{T,i}$, where $N_{T,i}$ is the threshold density for host genotype i.

Figure 5 illustrates the kind of frequency dependence exhibited by the fitness function of eqs (19) and (20) for this haploid host. When p is small (frequency of the allele A small; genotype A or 1 relatively rare), the density of the host genotype A is below the threshold for maintaining the parasite $(R_1 p < 1)$, and $W_1 = \lambda_1$. Once p is sufficiently large $(R_1 p > 1)$, the epidemic can 'take off', and thereafter the fitness W_1 falls as p increases. For values of the parasite reproductive rate, R_1, significantly in excess of unity, the fitness W_1 will tend to saturate to $W_1 \rightarrow \lambda_1 (1 - s_1)$ unless s_1 is very close to unity; for an invariably lethal infection $(v_1 = 0, s_1 = 1)$, W_1 will not saturate, but will decline exponentially as p increases. The fitness of the other host genotype (labelled a or 2) exhibits similar behaviour as p decreases from 1 to 0. Obviously, the details depend on the relative magnitudes of the demographic and epidemiological parameters λ_i, s_i and R_i, but with the rarer genotype enjoying an advantage there is the possibility of a polymorphic equilibrium at an internal point where $W_1 = W_2$.

By substituting the fitness functions of eqs (19) and (20) into eqs (17) and (18), one obtains non-linear 'maps' relating p_{t+1} to p_t:

$$p_{t+1} = F(p_t). \tag{21}$$

These mapping functions $F(p)$ depend explicitly on genetic and epidemiological assumptions about the host–parasite association. Figure 6 displays a typical such map, corresponding to the fitness functions of Fig. 5.

As discussed in detail elsewhere (Levin & Lenski, 1983; Levin et al., 1982; May & Anderson, 1983), the situation depicted in Fig. 6 is typical, in that there exists an 'interior fixed point' or polymorphism, $p_{t+1} = p_t \neq 0$ or 1. The dynamics of this system are, however, not trivial. If non-linearities are not too severe, the map shown in Fig. 6 can give a stable equilibrium or balanced polymorphism. But, with

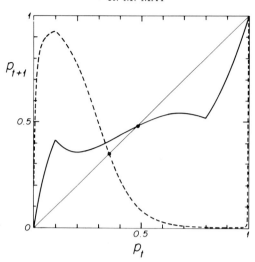

Figure 6. The map relating p_{t+1} to p_t, as given by eq (17), is shown for a haploid host with the fitness functions illustrated in Fig. 5: the solid and dashed curves correspond to the solid and dashed curves in Fig. 5, respectively. The stability of the fixed points where the map $p_{t+1} = F(p_t)$ intersects the 45° line, $p_{t+1} = p_t$, are as discussed as in the text (from May & Anderson, 1983).

sufficient non-linearity, there can easily arise stable cycles in which host gene frequencies alternate high and low in successive generations, or there can even be chaotic fluctuations in gene frequency. This range of possibilities — stable point, cycles, or chaos — is illustrated in Fig. 7. The underlying mathematics is in some ways similar to, but in other ways more complicated than, that found in simple population models (May, 1976: the familiar population models have 'maps with one lump'; the maps in Fig. 6 are messier in possessing 'two humps'). The details

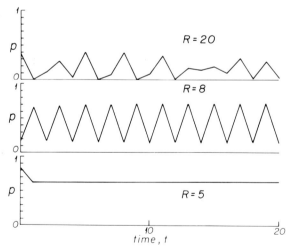

Figure 7. The gene frequency, p, of the A allele in the host population can exhibit a range of dynamical behaviour, as illustrated here. As shown, increasing R values tend to take the system from a stable point, through stable cycles, to apparently chaotic dynamics. The example shown here is for a haploid host system whose fitnesses are given by eqs (19) and (20) with $R_1 = 5, 8, 20$ (as labelled), $R_2 = 0$ (so that host genotype a or 2 is resistant to infection, $I_2 = 0$), $s_1 = 1$, and $\lambda_2 = 0.95\lambda_1$. For a more full discussion, see May & Anderson (1983).

of this array of dynamical behaviour are presented elsewhere (May & Anderson, 1983; May, 1979).

In short, gene-for-gene associations between hosts and pathogens will typically give rise to polymorphism, which may be stable, or may oscillate in stable cycles, or may vary chaotically. Some of the biological consequences, and some possible observational tests of the ideas, have been developed by Hamilton (1980), May & Anderson (1983) and Levin *et al.* (1982).

Evolution of virulence

The models of the second section (p. 245) (involving only epidemiological dynamics) and the models of this section (involving both epidemiology and genetics) have both been used to explore the extent to which 'successful' parasites will evolve towards avirulence (Levin & Pimentel, 1981; Anderson & May, 1982a; May & Anderson, 1983; Bremermann & Pickering, 1983; Levin *et al.*, 1982). On theoretical grounds, it would indeed appear that parasites evolve to be avirulent or 'harmless', provided the transmissibility and duration of infectiousness are entirely independent of virulence. More generally, however, many co-evolutionary endpoints are possible, with the outcome in any one instance depending on the relationships among parasite virulence and transmissibility and the costs of host resistance.

A specific analysis of the Australian rabbit-myxoma virus interaction has found theory in broad agreement with experimental observations, with the system apparently having settled to an equilibrium in which the predominant grade of virus is one of intermediate virulence (May & Anderson, 1983).

DYNAMICS AND GENETICS COMBINED

The preceding section dealt only with frequency-dependent selection, with the parasites affecting the relative proportions of the host genotypes but not the total number of hosts (which was taken to be constant, $N_t = K$). More generally, we may return to eqs (17)–(19), and let the parasites alone be responsible for regulating the density of the host population. In this case, the fitnesses W_i of eq (19) will all depend (via the infected fractions I_i) both on the gene frequency p_t and on the total host density at the start of generation t, N_t: for hosts of genotype i, I_i is given from eq (2) by

$$1 - I_i = \exp[-I_i N_t f_i / N_{T,i}]. \tag{22}$$

Here, as before, $f_1 = p_t$ and $f_2 = 1 - p_t$ for this haploid system. Eq (17) now gives, via eqs (19) and (22), an expression for p_{t+1} in terms of p_t and N_t. It remains to obtain a parallel relation for N_{t+1} in terms of p_t and N_t; such a relation comes from the basic definition of the fitness functions, and is

$$N_{t+1} = \sum_i N_i W_i = N_t \overline{W}_t. \tag{23}$$

This frequency and density dependent system can now be studied, both analytically and numerically (May and Anderson, 1983). As in the purely frequency-dependent case, polymorphism usually exists unless resistance can arise with essentially no cost, or unless parasite virulence can become very low with no loss in transmissibility. Such polymorphisms are more liable to exhibit cyclic or chaotic oscillations than are the corresponding cases with no parasite-induced density dependence. Figure 8 illustrates a typical example, which in some ways is a direct extension (to a genetically polymorphic system) of the interaction studied in the second section (p. 245) between a host with discrete generations and a microparasite.

Thus, the phenomenon noted in the fourth section (p. 255), whereby gene-for-gene associations between hosts and parasites may promote the maintenance of genetic diversity (either stably, or cyclically, or with chaotic dynamics), is also manifested when the parasites are the regulators of host population density. A variety of other complications and suggestions for further work are discussed in May & Anderson (1983).

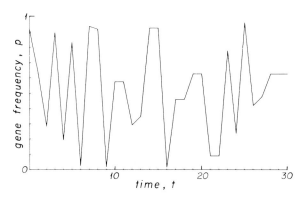

Figure 8. This figures shows the highly chaotic dynamical behaviour in the gene frequency, p, that can arise once the selective forces exerted by the pathogen are both frequency and density dependent. The figure is for a haploid host, where the fitness functions are given by eq (19) in conjunction with the density dependent eq (22): $\lambda_1 = \lambda_2 = e^2$; $s_1 = s_2 = 1$; and $N_{T,1} = N_{T,2} = 2$.

CONCLUSIONS

Both in their population dynamics and in their population genetics, host–parasite associations represent a special class of prey–predator systems. Despite the many complexities of specific interactions, host–parasite associations are, in general, simpler and more amenable to manipulation and quantitative study than are other prey–predator associations. They thus can provide a testing ground for ideas about the ecology and evolution of prey–predator interactions. In particular, we have seen how some of the focal concepts of contemporary population biology are borne out in a simple and natural way in host–parasite associations: bifurcating cascades of stable cycles and apparently chaotic orbits arise in many situations, and indeed the simplest model for a univoltine insect regulated by a pathogen exhibits pure chaos; the aggregative behaviour of predators (macroparasites) in an environment comprising many patches (individual hosts) is the basic mechanism stabilizing many prey–predator (host–macroparasite) interactions.

There is, however, great need for more data directed toward answering particular questions. Thus, although parasites are capable of regulating their host populations, the extent to which they do so in nature is debatable (Holmes, 1982; Hassell *et al.*, 1982). For naturally occurring host–parasite associations, it would be preferable to have more demographic and epidemiological data that were collected with an eye on these questions. Similarly, the extent to which parasites will tend to evolve toward avirulence depends on the degree to which transmissibility is ineluctably linked with harmful effects on host physiology or behaviour; essentially no information is available about these kinds of linkages; yet, without such information, studies of the evolution of virulence are doomed to sterile abstraction.

ACKNOWLEDGEMENTS

I am indebted to Roy M. Anderson and Andrew P. Dobson for many helpful conversations. This work was supported in part by the Rockefeller Foundation and by the U.S. National Science Foundation under grant BSR83-03772.

REFERENCES

ANDERSON, R. M. & MAY, R. M., 1978. Regulation and stability of host–parasite population interactions: I, regulatory processes. *Journal of Animal Ecology, 47:* 219–247.

ANDERSON, R. M. & MAY, R. M., 1979. Population biology of infectious diseases. *Nature, 280:* 361–367 and 455–461.

ANDERSON, R. M. & MAY, R. M., 1981. The population dynamics of microparasites and their invertebrate hosts. *Philosophical Transactions of the Royal Society B, 291:* 451–524.

ANDERSON, R. M. & MAY, R. M., 1982a. Coevolution of hosts and parasites. *Parasitology, 85:* 411–426.

ANDERSON, R. M. & MAY, R. M., 1982b. The population dynamics and control of human helminth infections. *Nature, 297:* 557–563.

ANDERSON, R. M. & MAY, R. M., 1982c. Directly transmitted infectious diseases: control by vaccination. *Science, 215:* 1053–1060.

ANDERSON, R. M. & MAY, R. M., 1983. Vaccination against rubella and measles: quantitative investigations of different policies. *Journal of Hygiene, 90:* 259–325.

ANDERSON, R. M. & MAY, R. M., in press. Age related changes in the rate of disease transmission: implications for the design of vaccination programmes. *Journal of Hygiene.*

ANDERSON, R. M. & MAY, R. M., 1985. Helminth infections of humans: mathematical models, population dynamics and control. *Advances in Parasitology, 24:* 1–101.

ANDERSON, R. M., GRENFELL, B. T. & MAY, R. M., 1984. Oscillatory fluctuations in the incidence of infectious disease and the impact of vaccination: time series analysis. *Journal of Hygiene, 93:* 587–608.

BAILEY, N. J. T., 1975. *The Mathematical Theory of Infectious Diseases* (2nd edition): New York: Macmillan.

BARTLETT, M. S., 1960. *Stochastic Population Models.* London: Methuen and Co.

BECK, K., in press. Coevolution: mathematical analysis of host–parasite interactions. *Journal of Theoretical Biology.*

BRADLEY, D. J. & MAY, R. M., 1978. Consequences of helminth aggregation for the dynamics of schistosomiasis. *Transactions of the Royal Society for Tropical Medicine and Hygiene, 72:* 262–273.

BREMERMANN, H. J. & PICKERING, J., 1983. A game-theoretical model of parasite virulence. *Journal of Theoretical Biology, 100:* 411–426.

CROFTON, H. D., 1971a. A quantitative approach to parasitism. *Parasitology, 63:* 179–193.

CROFTON, H. D., 1971b. A model of host–parasite relationships. *Parasitology, 63:* 343–364.

DIETZ, K., 1975. Transmission and control of arbovirus diseases. In D. Ludwig & K. L. Cooke (Eds), *Epidemiology:* 104–121. Philadelphia: Society for Industrial and Applied Mathematics.

FINE, P. E. M. & CLARKSON, J. A., 1982. Measles in England and Wales, II: The impact of the measles vaccination programme on the distribution of immunity in the population. *International Journal of Epidemiology, 11:* 15–25.

FINE, P. E. M. *et al.*, 1982. Control of infectious diseases (group report). In R. M. Anderson and R. M. May (Eds), *Population Biology of Infectious Diseases:* 121–148. New York: Springer Verlag.

GETZ, W. M. & PICKERING, J., 1983. Epidemic models: thresholds and population regulation. *American Naturalist, 121:* 892–898.

GILLESPIE, J. H., 1975. Natural selection for resistance to epidemics. *Ecology, 56:* 493–495.

HAMILTON, W. D., 1980. Sex versus non-sex versus parasite. *Oikos, 35:* 282–290.

HASSELL, M. P., 1978. *The Dynamics of Arthropod Predator–Prey Associations.* Princeton: Princeton University Press.

HASSELL, M. P. & MAY, R. M., 1984. From individual behavior to population dynamics. In R. Sibly & R. Smith (Eds), *Behavioural Ecology:* 3–32. Oxford: Blackwell.

HASSELL, M. P. *et al.*, 1982. Impact of infectious diseases on host populations (group report). In R. M. Anderson & R. M. May (Eds), *Population Biology of Infectious Diseases*: 15–35. New York: Springer Verlag.

HOLMES, J. C., 1982. Impact of infectious disease agents on the population growth and geographical distribution of animals. In R. M. Anderson & R. M. May (Eds), *Population Biology of Infectious Diseases*: 37–51. New York: Springer Verlag.

KERMACK, W. O. & McKENDRICK, A. G., 1927. A contribution to the mathematical theory of epidemics. *Proceedings of the Royal Society A, 115:* 700–721.

KNOX, E. G., 1980. Strategy for rubella vaccinations. *International Journal of Epidemiology, 9:* 13–23.

LEVIN, B. R., *et al.*, 1982. Evolution of parasites and hosts (group report). In R. M. Anderson & R. M. May (Eds), *Population Biology of Infectious Diseases*: 212–243. New York: Springer Verlag.

LEVIN, B. R. & LENSKI, R. E., 1983. Coevolution in bacteria and their viruses and plasmids. In D. J. Futuyma & M. Slatkin (Eds), *Coevolution*: 99–127. Sunderland, Mass.: Sinauer.

LEVIN, S. A., 1983. Some approaches to the modelling of coevolutionary interactions. In M. Nitecki (Ed.), *Coevolution:* 21–66. Chicago: University of Chicago Press.

LEVIN, S. A. & PIMENTEL, D., 1981. Selection of intermediate rates of increase in parasite–host systems. *American Naturalist, 117:* 308–315.

MACDONALD, G., 1952. The analysis of equilibrium in malaria. *Tropical Disease Bulletin, 49:* 813–829.

MACDONALD, G., 1965. The dynamics of helminth infections, with special reference to schistosomes. *Transactions of Royal Society of Tropical Medical Hygiene, 59:* 489–506.

MACDONALD, G., 1973. (Collected papers, L. J. Bruce-Chwatt & V. J. Glanville (Eds), *Dynamics of Tropical Disease*. Oxford: Oxford University Press.

MAY, R. M., 1976. Simple mathematical models with very complicated dynamics. *Nature, 261:* 459–467.

MAY, R. M., 1977a. Dynamical aspects of host–parasite associations: Crofton's model revisited. *Parasitology, 75:* 259–276.

MAY, R. M., 1977b. Togetherness among schistosomes: its effects on the dynamics of the infection. *Mathematical Biosciences, 35:* 301–343.

MAY, R. M., 1979. Bifurcations and dynamic complexity in ecological systems. *Annals of New York Academy of Sciences, 316:* 517–529.

MAY, R. M., 1983. Parasitic infections as regulators of animal populations. *American Science, 71:* 36–45.

MAY, R. M., 1985. Regulation of populations with non-overlapping generations by microparasites: a purely chaotic system. *American Naturalist, 125:* 573–584.

MAY, R. M. & ANDERSON, R. M., 1978. Regulation and stability of host–parasite population interactions: II, destabilizing processes. *Journal of Animal Ecology, 47:* 249–267.

MAY, R. M. & ANDERSON, R. M., 1983. Epidemiology and genetics in the co-evolution of parasites and hosts. *Proceedings of Royal Society, B219:* 281–313.

MAY, R. M. & ANDERSON, R. M., 1984. Spatial heterogeneity and the design of immunization programs. *Mathematical Bioscience, 72:* 83–111.

MODE, C. J., 1958. A mathematical model for the co-evolution of obligate parasites and their hosts. *Evolution, 12:* 158–165.

NASELL, I. & HIRSCH, W. M., 1973. The transmission dynamics of schistosomiasis. *Comm. Pure and Applied Mathematics, 26:* 395–453.

REGNIERE, J., 1984. Vertical transmission of diseases and population dynamics of insects with discrete generations: a model. *Journal of Theoretical Biology, 107:* 287–308.

SCHENZLE, D., 1984. Control of virus transmission in age-structured populations. In V. Capasso (Ed.), *Mathematics in Biology and Medicine*. New York: Springer Verlag.

SMITH, C. E. G., 1970. Prospects for the control of infectious disease. *Proceedings of the Royal Society of Medicine, 63:* 1181–1190.

WARREN, K. S., 1981. The control of helminths: non-replicating infectious agents of man. *Annual Reviews of Public Health, 2:* 101–115.

WARREN, K. S., *et al.*, 1982. Transmission: Patterns and dynamics of infectious diseases (group report). In R. M. Anderson & R. M. May (Eds), *Population Biology of Infectious Diseases*: 67–85. New York: Springer Verlag.

Subject index